P9-AET-453

Psycho-Analytic Explorations

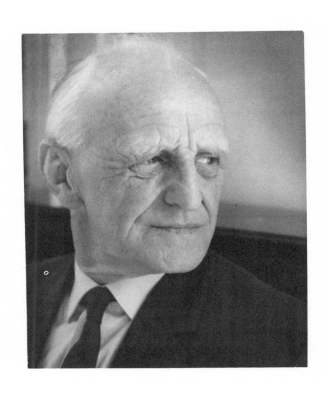

D. W. WINNICOTT

Psycho-Analytic Explorations

EDITED BY

Clare Winnicott

Ray Shepherd

Madeleine Davis

HARVARD UNIVERSITY PRESS

Cambridge, Massachusetts

Copyright © 1989 by The Winnicott Trust
By arrangement with Mark Paterson
All rights reserved
Printed in the United States of America

FOURTH PRINTING, 1994

First Harvard University Press paperback edition, 1992

Library of Congress Cataloging-in-Publication Data

Winnicott, D. W. (Donald Woods), 1896–1971.
  Psycho-analytic explorations / D. W. Winnicott; edited by Clare
Winnicott, Ray Shepherd, Madeleine Davis.
     p.   cm.
  Includes index.
  ISBN 0-674-72090-3 (alk. paper) (cloth)
  ISBN 0-674-72091-1 (paper)
  1. Psychoanalysis. 2. Psychotherapy. 3. Child Analysis.
4. Child psychotherapy.   I. Winnicott, Clare.   II. Shepherd, Ray.
III. Davis, Madeleine.   IV. Title.
RC501.2.W56   1989   88-21465
616.89'17—dc19   CIP

Contents

Preface

When Donald Winnicott died in 1971 he left more than one hundred lectures and articles, both longer and shorter, which had never been published. There were also many papers published in anthologies and journals that were not always easy to obtain. Our aim has been to bring this material together in books under his own name; and, because the nature of the papers varied so much with the different audiences that he addressed, we decided to make our collections as far as possible according to the audiences for whom they were intended.

The papers in this volume are those we consider of greatest interest to psycho-analysts and psychotherapists, for whom, indeed, most of them were written. This was the last collection that we worked on with Clare Winnicott before her death in April 1984; and for us it is therefore a vivid reminder of what she shared with us in order to make this work possible. It is appropriate that her reflections on Donald Winnicott as a person should come at the beginning of this collection. After her death, while her house at 49 Lower Belgrave Street was being cleared, some papers—among them a number of short ones—were found; nearly all of these have been included here.

The editing of the text of the papers has been kept to a minimum. Naturally there were least difficulties where a paper had already been published, but in one or two cases where we found the original manuscript of such a paper we preferred this version to the one that had ended up in print.

Before he died Winnicott himself had intended to make new collections of his work. With this in mind he prepared (probably in 1968 or early 1969) two separate lists of papers, which included amongst much else nearly all the material that made up his posthumously published book *Playing and Reality* (1971). The following papers from these lists are contained in the present work:

"Excitement in the Aetiology of Coronary Thrombosis" (1957)
"Psychoneurosis in Childhood" (1961)
"Psycho-Somatic Illness in Its Positive and Negative Aspects" (1964)

"New Light on Children's Thinking" (1965)

"The Concept of Trauma in Relation to the Development of the Individual within the Family" (1965)

"The Psychology of Madness" (1965)

"The Concept of Clinical Regression as Compared with Defence Organisation" (1967)

"The Use of the Word 'Use'" (1968)

"Physical and Emotional Disturbances in an Adolescent Girl" (1968)

"The Mother-Infant Experience of Mutuality" (1969)

"Physiotherapy and Human Relations" (1969)

As well as his lists, two piles of papers, which he had placed in order, were found after his death. These contained most of the papers on the lists as well as a few others, one of which, "Fear of Breakdown" (1963?), is included here. There were also some papers found marked at the top with the words "Belonging to Book," and it is likely that Winnicott considered using these (though he did not in fact include them) when he was compiling *Playing and Reality*. They include:

"Addendum to 'The Location of Cultural Experience'" (1967)

"Interpretation in Psychoanalysis" (1968)

"Thinking and Symbol-Formation" (1968)

"Roots of Aggression" (1968)

Apart from these papers, some written in 1969 and 1970 and therefore not included in Winnicott's lists fulfill the strictest criteria for inclusion in this book. Among these are:

"Mother's Madness Appearing in the Clinical Material As an Ego-Alien Factor" (1969)

"Basis for Self in Body" (1970)

"Individuation" (1970)

And we should certainly also include in this class of eligibility his account, previously published in an anthology in 1965, of "A Child Psychiatry Case Illustrating Delayed Reaction to Loss."

Aside from these considerations, which are already moving from evidence to speculation, we have no way of telling how much of the material reproduced in this collection Winnicott would have considered for publication or re-publication; or whether he would have left such material in its present form. Sixteen years, however, have now passed since his death, and it seems to us that in this time interest in his work has increased rather than diminished. His major contributions to psycho-analytic thought are no doubt already known, but at

the present time it seems appropriate to reproduce here, even if sometimes in note form, work done around such concepts as "playing,"
"the split-off male and female elements," and "the use of an object."
We also believe that the inclusion of material written on the work of
Melanie Klein and other analysts, often in the form of reviews of their
books, helps to elucidate, among other things, the still vexed subject
of the relationship of Winnicott's formulations to the work of others.
On a rare occasion, in an informal address to some of his colleagues,
Winnicott spoke even more directly about this relationship; a tape
recording of his talk fortunately survived, and we have included a
transcript of it at the end of the book.

Then, too, we thought it important to publish most of Winnicott's
writing expressing his concern—often passionate—over the use of
leucotomy and shock therapy in the treatment of the mentally ill. In
1943 and 1944 especially he spent much time and energy trying to
get people to think and talk about the psychological effects of ECT,
and in the early 1950s he was particularly active in drawing public
attention to the ethical considerations surrounding the use of leucotomy. Most of what he wrote at the time still has relevance today; for
though treatment by leucotomy has become a rare thing, the tendency—so disturbing to him—to blur the distinction between ethical
considerations and those of efficacy does not seem to have diminished.

Much of the remaining material could be called fragmentary, a lot
of it being in the form of what Winnicott called "snippets" from case
histories. Many of these had obviously been used for teaching; others
had possibly been put aside in case the need arose to illustrate a particular point. Each of them has something to say.

The result of all this is a book of papers uneven in length and content, and uneven also in formality of presentation. We believe that
our justification in having so compiled it lies not only in what it will
contribute to the literature but also in what it may reveal of the development of Winnicott's ideas and of his growth through experience.

Ray Shepherd
London, January 1987   Madeleine Davis

Psycho-Analytic Explorations

D.W.W.: A Reflection

by Clare Winnicott

> O hours of childhood, hours when behind the figures there was
> more than the mere past, and when what lay before us was not the
> future! True, we were growing, and sometimes made haste to be
> grown up, half for the sake of those who'd nothing left but their
> grown-upness. Yet, when alone, we entertained ourselves with ev-
> erlastingness: there we would stand, within the gap left between
> world and toy, upon a spot which, from the first beginning, had
> been established for a pure event.
>
> *Rainer Maria Rilke*

A few years ago the editors of a book on transitional objects and
transitional phenomena[1] invited me to write something of a personal
nature about D.W.W. It seems to me that what I wrote about him
then, though I was naturally keeping the subject of the transitional
area in the forefront of my mind, is central to the whole of his
achievement.

I began with two questions: what was it about D.W.W. that made
the exploration of the transitional area inevitable, and made his use
of it clinically productive? It was my attempt to answer these questions that resulted in the contribution that followed, given here with
a very few alterations.

I suggest that the answers have to be looked for not simply in a
study of the development of D.W.W.'s ideas as he went along, but
essentially in the kind of personality that was functioning behind
them. It could seem therefore as if I were saying that these concepts
arose naturally and easily out of his own way of life. In one sense this
is true; but it is only half the story. The rest concerns the periods of
doubt, uncertainty, and confusion, out of which form and meaning
eventually emerged.

1. *Between Reality and Fantasy,* ed. Simon A. Grolnick and Leonard Barkin (New York,
London: Jason Aronson, 1978).

D.W.W. could be excited by other people's ideas, but could use them and build on them only after they had been through the refinery of his own experience. By that time, unfortunately, he had often forgotten the source, and he could, and did, alienate some people by his lack of acknowledgement. While other people's ideas enriched him as a clinician and as a person, it was the working out of ideas based on clinical practice that really absorbed him and that he grappled with to the end of his life. This was a creative process in which he was totally involved. In his clinical work D.W.W. made it his aim to enter into every situation undefended by his knowledge, so that he could be as exposed as possible to the impact of the situation itself. From his point of view this was the only way in which discovery and growth were possible, both for himself and for his patients. This approach was more than a stance; it was an essential discipline, and it added a dimension to his life as vital to him as fresh air.

The question is sometimes asked as to why D.W.W. in his writings seemed mainly concerned with exploring the area of the first two-person relationship. Strictly speaking this is not true: he wrote on a wide range of topics, including adolescence and delinquency and other matters of medical and sociological concern, and the greater part of his psychoanalytic practice was with adults. However, it could be true to say that his main contribution is likely to turn out to be in the study of the earliest relationships, and its application to the aetiology of psychosis and of the psychotic mechanisms in all of us. I suggest that his study took this direction from two sources. In the first place, he brought with him into psycho-analysis all that he had learnt and went on learning from paediatrics, and secondly, at the time he came to psycho-analysis the area of study just then opening up was that concerning the earliest experiences of life. Given his personality, his training and experience, and his urge for discovery, it seems inevitable that he would concentrate his researches on the so far comparatively unexplored area of earliest infancy and childhood. His findings, however, are recognised by many as having implications far beyond the immediate area of study. It is the expressed opinion of some that they throw light on all areas of living.

As I have suggested, the essential clue to D.W.W.'s work on transitional objects and phenomena is to be found in his own personality, in his way of relating and being related to, and in his whole style of life. What I mean is that it was his *capacity to play*, which never deserted him, that led him inevitably into the area of research that he conceptualised in terms of the transitional objects and phenomena. It is not my purpose here to discuss the details of his work, but it seems important to note that in his terms the capacity to play is equated with a *quality of living*. In his own words, "Playing is an experience, always a creative experience, and it is an experience in the space-time continuum, a basic form of living."[2]

This quality of living permeates all levels and aspects of experiencing and relating, up to and including the sophisticated level described in his paper "The Use of an Object" at which, in his own words, "It is the destructive drive that creates the quality of externality"; and again, "this quality of 'always being destroyed' makes the reality of the surviving object felt as such, strengthens the feeling tone, and contributes to object constancy."[3] For him, the destroying of the object in unconscious fantasy is like a cleansing process, which facilitates again and again the discovery of the object anew. It is a process of purification and renewal.

Having said that, I see my contribution as an attempt to throw some light on D.W.W.'s capacity for playing. I expect that readers will be familiar enough with his writings on this subject to know that I am not talking about playing games. I am talking about the capacity for operating in the limitless intermediate area where external and internal reality are compounded into the experience of living. I hope I do not suggest that D.W.W. lived in a state of permanent elation, because that was far from the case. He often found life hard and could be despondent and depressed and very angry, but given time he could come through and encompass these experiences in his own way and free himself from being cluttered up with resentment and prejudices. During the last years of his life the reality of his own death had to be negotiated, and this he did, again gradually and in his own way. I was always urging him to write an autobiography because I felt that his style of writing would lend itself to such a task. He started to do this, but there are only a few pages, and typically he used this exercise to deal with his immediate problem of living, which was that of dying. I know he used it in this way because he kept this notebook to himself and I did not see it until after his death.

The title of the autobiography was to be *Not Less Than Everything,* and the inner flap of the notebook reads as follows:

2. From "Playing: A Theoretical Statement" (1968), in *Playing and Reality* (London: Tavistock; New York: Basic Books, 1971; Penguin, 1974).

3. See *Playing and Reality;* also Chapter 34 of the present book.

T. S. Eliot "Costing not less than everything"
T. S. Eliot "What we call the beginning is often the end
And to make an end is to make a beginning.
The end is where we start from."

Prayer

D.W.W. Oh God! May I be alive when I die.

Following these words he started on the writing, and it begins by imaginatively describing the end of his life. I shall quote his own words:

I died.

It was not very nice, and it took quite a long time as it seemed (but it was only a moment in eternity).

There had been rehearsals (that's a difficult word to spell. I found I had left out the "a." The hearse was cold and unfriendly).

When the time came I knew all about the lung heavy with water that the heart could not negotiate, so that not enough blood circulated in the alveoli, and there was oxygen starvation as well as drowning. But fair enough, I had had a good innings: mustn't grumble as our old gardener used to say . . .

Let me see. What was happening when I died? My prayer had been answered. I was alive when I died. That was all I had asked and I had got it. (This makes me feel awful because so many of my friends and contemporaries died in the first World War, and I have never been free from the feeling that my being alive is a facet of some one thing of which their deaths can be seen as other facets: some huge crystal, a body with integrity and shape intrinsical in it.)

He then goes on to discuss the difficulty that a man has dying without a son to imaginatively kill and to survive him—"to provide the only continuity that men know. Women *are* continuous." This dilemma is discussed in terms of King Lear and his relationship to his daughter who should have been a boy.

I hope that these quotations give some idea of D.W.W.'s capacity to come to terms with internal and external reality in a playful way, which makes reality bearable to the individual, so that denial can be avoided and the experience of living can be as fully realized as possible. In his own words, "playing can be said to reach its own saturation point, which refers to the capacity to contain experience."[4] He

4. From "Playing: A Theoretical Statement."

was avid for experience and would have hated to miss the inner experience of the reality of his own death, and he imaginatively achieved that experience. In conversation he would often refer to his deathday in a lighthearted way, but I knew that he was trying to get me and himself accustomed to the idea that it would come.

Having started at the end of his life, I must now go back to the beginnings and relate something about his earlier years and about the years that he and I spent together. I shall limit what I say to an attempt to illustrate the theme of playing, because that was central to his life and work.

First I must set the scene within which he grew up. It was an essentially English provincial scene in Plymouth, Devon, and it was far from London, not merely in mileage, but in custom and convention. When we drove to Plymouth from London he was always thrilled when we arrived at the place where the soil banked up at the side of the road changed color to the red soil of Devon. The richness of the soil brought back the richness of his early life which he never lost touch with. Of course on the return journey he was always equally pleased to be leaving it behind. But he was proud of being a Devonian, and that there is a village of Winnicott on the map of Devon. We never actually found the village, although we always meant to. It was enough that it was there.

The Winnicott household was a large and lively one with plenty of activity. But there was space for everyone in the large garden and house and there was no shortage of money. There were a vegetable garden, an orchard, a croquet lawn, a tennis court, and a pond, and high trees enclosed the whole garden. There was a special tree, in the branches of which Donald would do his homework in the days before he went to boarding school. Of the three children in the family Donald was the only boy, and his sisters, who still live in the house, were five and six years older than he. There is no doubt that the Winnicott parents were the centre of their children's lives, and that the vitality and stability of the entire household emanated from them. Their mother was vivacious and outgoing and was able to show and express her feelings easily. Sir Frederick Winnicott (as he later became) was slim and tallish and had an old-fashioned quiet dignity and poise about him, and a deep sense of fun. Those who knew him speak of him as a person of high intelligence and sound judgement. Both parents had a sense of humour.

Across the road was another large Winnicott household which contained Uncle Richard Winnicott (Frederick's elder brother) and his wife, and three boy cousins and two girls. The cousins were brought up almost as one family, so there was never a shortage of playmates. One of the sisters said recently that the question "What can I do?" was never asked in their house. There was always something to do— and space to do it in, and someone to do it with if needed. But more important, there was always the vitality and imagination in the children themselves for exploits of all kinds. Donald's family, including his parents, were musical, and one sister later became a gifted painter. The household always included a nanny and a governess, but they do not seem to have hampered the natural energies of the children in any unreasonable way. Perhaps it would be more correct to say that the Winnicott children successfully evaded being hampered. As a small child Donald was certainly devoted to his nanny, and one of the first things I remember doing with him years later in London was to seek her out and ensure that she was all right and living comfortably. We discovered that the most important person in her life then (1950) was her own nephew Donald.

There is no question that from his earliest years Donald Winnicott did not doubt that he was loved, and he experienced a security in the Winnicott home which he could take for granted. In a household of this size there were plenty of chances for many kinds of relationships, and there was scope for the inevitable tensions to be isolated and resolved within the total framework. From this basic position Donald was then free to explore all the available spaces in the house and garden around him and to fill the spaces with bits of himself and so gradually to make his world his own. This capacity *to be at home* served him well throughout his life. There is a pop song which goes "Home is in my heart." That is certainly how Donald experienced it, and this gave him an immense freedom which enabled him to feel at home anywhere. When we were traveling in France and staying in small wayside inns, at each place I would think to myself, "I wonder how long it will be before he's in the kitchen"—the kitchen of course being the centre of the establishment—and sure enough, he would almost always find his way there somehow. Actually, he loved kitchens, and when he was a child his mother complained that he spent more time with the cook in the kitchen than he did in the rest of the house.

Because Donald was so very much the youngest member of the Winnicott household (even the youngest boy cousin living opposite was older than he) and because he was so much loved and was in himself lovable, it seems likely that a deliberate effort was made, particularly on the part of his mother and sisters, not to spoil him. While this did not deprive him of feeling loved, it did I think deprive him of some intimacy and closeness that he needed. But as Donald possessed (as do his sisters still) a natural ability to communicate with children of almost any age, the communication between children and adults in the Winnicott home must have been of a high order. Of course they all possessed an irrepressible sense of humor, and this, together with the happiness and safety of their background, meant that there were no "tragedies" in the Winnicott household—there were only amusing episodes. Not so many years ago, when the tank in the roof leaked, causing considerable flooding and damage, they were more excited and amused than alarmed by this unexpected happening.

At this point I should like to quote another page from Donald's autobiographical notes. Before doing so I should explain that the garden of the Winnicott home is on four levels. On the bottom level was the croquet lawn; then a steep slope (Mount Everest to a small child) leading to the pond level; next another slight slope leading to the lawn which was a tennis court; and, finally a flight of steps leading to the house level.

Now that slope up from the croquet lawn to the flat part where there is a pond and where there was once a huge clump of pampas grass between the weeping ash trees (by the way do you know what exciting noises a pampas grass makes on a hot afternoon, when people are lying out on rugs beside the pond, reading or snoozing?) That slope up is fraught, as people say, fraught with history. It was on that slope that I took my own private croquet mallet (handle about a foot long because I was only three years old) and I bashed flat the nose of the wax doll that belonged to my sisters and that had become a source of irritation in my life because it was over that doll that my father used to tease me. She was called Rosie. Parodying some popular song he used to say (taunting me by the voice he used)
<blockquote>
Rosie said to Donald
I love you
Donald said to Rosie
I don't believe you do.
</blockquote>
(Maybe the verses were the other way round, I forget) so I knew the doll had to be altered for the worse, and much of my life has been founded on the undoubted fact that I actually *did* this deed, not merely wished it and planned it.

I was perhaps somewhat relieved when my father took a series of matches and, warming up the wax nose enough, remoulded it so that the face once more became a face. This early demonstration of the restitutive and reparative act certainly made an impression on me, and perhaps made me able to accept the fact that I myself, dear innocent child, had actually become violent directly with a doll, but indirectly with my good-tempered father who was just then entering my conscious life.

Again, to quote further from the notebook:

Now my sisters were older than I, five and six years; so in a sense I was an only child with multiple mothers and with a father extremely preoccupied in my younger years with town as well as business matters. He was mayor twice and was eventually knighted, and then was made a Freeman of the City (as it has now become) of Plymouth. He was sensitive about his lack of education (he had had learning difficulties) and he always said that because of this he had not aspired to Parliament, but had kept to local politics—lively enough in those days in far away Plymouth.

My father had a simple (religious) faith and once when I asked him a question that could have involved us in a long argument he just said: read the Bible and what you find there will be the true answer for you. So I was left, thank God, to get on with it myself.

But when (at twelve years) I one day came home to midday dinner and said "drat" my father looked pained as only he could look, blamed my mother for not seeing to it that I had decent friends, and from that moment he prepared himself to send me away to boarding school, which he did when I was thirteen.

"Drat" sounds very small as a swear word, but he was right; the boy who was my new friend was no good, and he and I could have got into trouble if left to our own devices.

The friendship was in fact broken up then and there, and this show of strength on the part of his father was a significant factor in Donald's development. In his own words: "So my father was there to kill and be killed, but it is probably true that in the early years he left me too much to all my mothers. Things never quite righted themselves."

And so Donald went away to the Leys School, Cambridge, and was in his element. To his great delight the afternoons were free, and he ran, cycled and swam, played rugger, joined the School Scouts, and made friends and sang in the choir, and each night he read a story aloud to the boys in his dormitory. He read extremely well, and years later I was to benefit from this accomplishment because we were never without a book that he was reading aloud to me. One Christmas Eve sitting on the floor (we never sat on chairs) he read all night because the book was irresistible. He read in a dramatic way, savouring the writing to the full.

Donald described to me his going away to school. The whole family would be there to see him off, and he would wave and be sorry to leave until he was taken from their sight by the train's entering quite a long tunnel just outside Plymouth. All through this tunnel he settled down to the idea of leaving, but then out again the other side he left them behind and looked forward to going on to school. He often blessed that tunnel because he could honestly manage to feel sorry to leave right up to the moment of entering it.

I have in my possession a letter which Donald wrote to his mother from school which shows the kind of interplay that existed between members of the family:

My dearest Mother,
On September 2nd all true Scouts think of their mothers, since that was the birthday of Baden Powell's mother when she was alive.

And so when you get this letter I shall be thinking of you in particular, and I only hope you will get it in the morning.

But to please me very much I must trouble you to do me a little favour. Before turning over the page I want you to go up into my bedroom and in the right-hand cupboard find a small parcel . . . Now, have you opened it? Well I hope you will like it. You can change it at Pophams if you don't. Only if you do so, you must ask to see No. 1 who knows about it.

I have had a ripping holiday, and I cannot thank you enough for all you have done and for your donation to the Scouts.

My home is a beautiful home and I only wish I could live up to it. However I will do my best and work hard and that's all I can do at present.

Give my love to the others: thank Dad for his games of billiards and V and K [his sisters] for being so nice and silly so as to make me laugh. But, it being Mother's day, most love goes to you,
from your loving boy
Donald.

Some who read this abbreviated account of D.W.W.'s early life and family relationships may be inclined to think that it sounds too good to be true. But the truth is that it *was* good, and try as I will I cannot present it in any other light. Essentially he was a deeply happy person whose capacity for enjoyment never failed to triumph over the setbacks and disappointments that came his way. Moreover, there is a sense in which the quality of his early life and his appreciation of it did in itself present him with a major problem, that of freeing himself from the family, and of establishing his own separate life and identity without sacrificing the early richness. It took him a long time to do this.

It was when Donald was in the sick room at school, having broken his collarbone on the sports field, that he consolidated in his own mind the idea of becoming a doctor. Referring to that time he often said: "I could see that for the rest of my life I should have to depend on doctors if I damaged myself or became ill, and the only way out of this position was to become a doctor myself, and from then on the idea as a real proposition was always on my mind, although I know that father expected me to enter his flourishing business and eventually take over from him."

One of Donald's school friends, Stanley Ede (who remained a lifelong friend), had often stayed in the Winnicott household and was well known to all the family. Back at school after a visit to his home Donald, aged sixteen, wrote the following in a letter to the friend who had not yet returned to school:

Dear Stanley,
Thank you so much for the lovely long letter you sent me in the week. It is awfully good of you to take such a lot of trouble and to want to . . .
Father and I have been trying consciously and perhaps unconsciously to find out what the ambition of the other is in regard to my future. From what he had said I was *sure* that he wanted me more than anything else to go into his business. And so, again consciously and not, I have found every argument for the idea and have not thought much about anything else so that I should not be disappointed. And so I have learned to cherish the business life with all my heart, and had intended to enter it and please my father and myself.
When your letter came yesterday you may have expected it to have disappointed me. But—I tell you all I feel—I was so excited that all the stored-up feelings about doctors which I have bottled up for so many years seemed to burst and bubble up at once. Do you know that—in the degree that Algy wanted to go into a monastery—I have for ever so long wanted to be a doctor. But I have always been afraid that my father did not want it, and so I have

never mentioned it and—like Algy—even felt a repulsion at the thought.

This afternoon I went an eight mile walk to the Roman Road with Chandler, and we told each other all we felt, and especially I told him what I have told you now. O, Stanley!

> Your still sober and true—
> although seemingly intoxicated—
> but never-the-less devoted
> friend.
>   Donald

It seems that Stanley, one year older than Donald, had offered to broach the question of Donald's future to his father, and that he did so. There is a postcard to Stanley saying, "Thank you infinitely for having told father when and what you did. I have written Dad a letter which I think pretty nearly convinced him."

Donald recounts that when he summoned up courage to go to the Headmaster at school and tell him that he wanted to be a doctor, the Head grunted and looked at him long and hard before replying slowly: "Boy, not brilliant, but will do." And so he went to Jesus College, Cambridge, and took a degree in biology. His room in College was popular as a meeting place, because he had hired a piano and played it unceasingly and had a good tenor voice for singing.

But the first World War was on, and his first year as a medical student was spent helping in the Cambridge Colleges which had been turned into military hospitals. One of the patients, who became a lifelong friend, remembers Donald in those days: "The first time I saw him was in hospital in Cambridge in 1916 in the first war; he was a medical student who liked to sing a comic song on Saturday evenings in the ward—and sang 'Apple Dumplings' and cheered us all up."

It was a source of deep sorrow and conflict that all his friends went at once into the army, but that as a medical student Donald was exempt. Many close friends were killed early in the war, and his whole life was affected by this, because always he felt that he had a responsibility to live for those who died, as well as for himself.

The kind of relationship with friends that he had at that time in Cambridge is illustrated by a letter from a friend who had already joined up in the army and was on a course for officers in Oxford. It is written from Exeter College Oxford and dated 28 November 1915:

> What are you doing on Saturday for tea? Well, I'll tell you!! *You are going to provide a big Cambridge Tea for yourself, myself and*

Southwell (of Caius) [Caius College Cambridge] whom you've met I think. He's a top-hole chap and has got a commission. If you haven't met him you ought to have, and anyway you've heard me speak of him. Can you manage it? Blow footer etc. etc. or I'll blow you next time I see you. Try and manage it will you? Good man! It's sponging on you I know, but I also know you're a silly idiot and won't mind. Silly ass! Cheer O old son of a gun and get plenty of food.

Feeling as he did Donald could not settle in Cambridge and was not satisfied until he was facing danger for himself, and, coming from Plymouth, he of course wanted to go into the navy. He applied for and was accepted as a surgeon probationer. He was drafted to a destroyer, where he was one of the youngest men on board and the only medical officer in spite of his lack of training; fortunately, there was an experienced medical orderly. He was subject to a great deal of teasing in the Officers' Mess. Most of the officers had been through one or other of the Royal Naval Colleges and came from families with a naval tradition. They were astonished that Donald's father was a *merchant*. This was a novelty, and they made the most of it, and Donald seems to have made the most of their company and of the whole experience. He has often related with amusement the banter that went on at meal times. Although the ship was involved in enemy action and there were casualties, Donald had much free time, which he seems to have spent reading the novels of Henry James.

After the war Donald went straight to St. Bartholomew's Hospital in London to continue his medical training. He soaked himself in medicine and fully committed himself to the whole experience. This included writing for the hospital magazine and joining in the social life: singing sprees, dancing, occasional skiing holidays, and hurrying off at the last minute to hear operas for the first time, where he usually stood in his slippers at the back of the "Gods."

It is difficult to give any dates in relation to Donald's girl friends, but he had quite close attachments to friends of his sisters and later to others he met through his Cambridge friends. He came to the brink of marriage more than once but did not actually marry (for the first time) until the age of twenty-eight.

Donald had some great teachers at the hospital, and he always said that it was Lord Horder who taught him the importance of taking a careful case history, and to listen to what the patient said, rather than simply to ask questions. After qualification he stayed on at Bart's to work as casualty officer for a year. He literally worked almost all day and night, but he would not have missed the experience for the world. It contained the challenge of the unexpected and provided the stimulation that he revelled in.

During his training Donald became ill with what turned out to be an abscess on the lung and was a patient in Bart's for three months. A friend who visited him there remembers it in these words: "It was a gigantic old ward with a high ceiling dwarfing the serried ranks of beds, patients and visitors. He was *intensely* amused and interested at being lost in a crowd and said 'I am convinced that every doctor ought to have been once in his life in a hospital bed as a patient.'"

Donald had always intended to become a general practitioner in a country area, but one day a friend lent him a book by Freud and so he discovered psycho-analysis; deciding that this was for him, he realized that he must therefore stay in London to undergo analysis. During his medical training he had become deeply interested in children's work, and after taking his Membership examination he set up as a consultant in children's medicine (there was no specialty in paediatrics in those days). In 1923 he obtained two hospital appointments, at The Queen's Hospital for Children and at Paddington Green Children's Hospital. The latter appointment he held for forty years. The development of his work at Paddington Green is a story in itself, and many colleagues from all over the world visited him there. Because of his own developing interests and skills over the years, his clinic gradually became a psychiatric clinic, and he used to refer to it as his "Psychiatric Snack Bar" or his clinic for dealing with parents' hypochondria. In 1923 he also acquired a room in the Harley Street area and set up a private consultant practice.

At the beginning he found Harley Street formidable because he had few patients, so in order to impress the very dignified porter who opened the door to patients for all the doctors in the house, he tells how he used to pay the fares of some of his hospital mothers and children so that they could visit him in Harley Street. Of course this procedure was not entirely on behalf of the porter, because he selected cases in which he was particularly interested and to which he wanted to give more time so that he could begin to explore the psychological aspects of illness.

The sheer pressure of the numbers attending his hospital clinics must have been important to him as an incentive to explore as fully as he did how to use the doctor-patient *space* as economically as possible for the therapeutic task. The ways in which he did this have been described in his writing.

However, there is one detail he does not describe, and which I observed both at his Paddington Green Clinic and in his work with evacuee children in Oxfordshire during the last war. He attempted to round off and make significant a child's visit to him by giving the child something to take away which could afterwards be used and/or destroyed or thrown away. He would quickly reach for a piece of paper and fold it into some shape, usually a dart or a fan, which he might play with for a moment and then give to the child as he said goodbye. I never saw this gesture refused by any child. It could be that this simple symbolic act contained the germ of ideas he developed in the "Use of an Object" paper written at the end of his life. There could also be a link here with the transitional object concept.

In attempting to give some idea of D.W.W.'s capacity to play I have somehow slipped into an historical or biographical sequence of writing without intending to do so. This is in no way meant to be a biography. What I have been trying to do is to illustrate how he related to people at different stages of his life and in different situations. But I must now abandon the historical perspective which so far protected me, and bring him briefly into focus for myself and in relation to our life together. From now on "he" becomes "we" and I cannot disentangle us.

Many years ago a visitor staying in our home looked round thoughtfully and said: "You and Donald *play.*" I remember being surprised at this new light that had been thrown on us. We had certainly never *set out* to play; there was nothing self-conscious and deliberate about it. It seems just to have happened that we lived that way, but I could see what our visitor meant. We played with *things*—our possessions—rearranging, acquiring, and discarding according to our mood. We played with ideas, tossing them about at random with the freedom of knowing that we need not agree, and that we were strong enough not to be hurt by each other. In fact the question of hurting each other did not arise because we were operating in the play area where everything is permissible. We each possessed a capacity for enjoyment, and it could take over in the most unlikely places and lead us into exploits we could not have anticipated. After Donald's death an American friend described us as "two crazy people who delighted each other and delighted their friends." Donald would have been pleased with this accolade, so reminiscent of his words: "We are poor indeed if we are only sane." [5]

Early in our relationship I had to settle for the idea that Donald was, and always would be, completely unpredictable in our private life, except for his punctuality at meal times and the fact that he never failed to meet me at the station when I had been away. This unpredictability had its advantages, in that we could never settle back and take each other for granted in day-to-day living. What we could take for granted was something more basic that I can only describe as our recognition and acceptance of each other's separateness. In fact the strength of our unity lay in this recognition, and implicit in it is an acceptance of the unconscious ruthless and destructive drives which were discussed as the final development of his theories in the "Use of an Object" paper. Our separateness left us each free to do our own thing, to think our own thoughts, and possess our own dreams, and in so doing to strengthen the capacity of each of us to experience the joys and sorrows which we shared.

There were some things that were especially important to us, like the Christmas card that Donald drew each year, and which we both painted in hundreds, staying up until 2 A.M., in the days before Christmas. I remember once suggesting to him that the drawing looked better left as it was in black and white. He said, "Yes, I know, but I like painting." There were his endless squiggle drawings which were part of his daily routine. He would play the game with himself and produced some very fearful and some very funny drawings, which often had a powerful integrity of their own. If I was away for a night he would send a drawing through the post for me to receive in the morning, because my part in all this was to enjoy and appreciate his productions, which I certainly did, but sometimes I could wish that there were not quite so many of them.

Donald's knowledge and appreciation of music was a joy to both of us, but it was of particular importance to me because he introduced me to much that was new. He always had a special feeling for the music of Bach, but at the end of his life it was the late Beethoven string quartets that absorbed and fascinated him. It seems as if the refinement and abstraction in the musical idiom of these works

5. From "Primitive Emotional Development" (1945), in *Collected Papers: Through Paediatrics to Psycho-Analysis* (London: Tavistock, 1958; New York: Basic Books, London: Hogarth Press, 1975).

helped him to gather in and realise in himself the rich harvest of a lifetime. On quite another level he also greatly enjoyed the Beatles and bought all their recordings. Donald never had enough time to develop his own piano playing, but he would often dash up to the piano and play for a moment between patients, and invariably he celebrated the end of a day's work by a musical outburst fortissimo. He enjoyed the fact that I knew more about poets than he did, and that I could say a Shakespeare sonnet or some Dylan Thomas or T. S. Eliot to him on demand. He particularly enjoyed Edward Lear's "The Owl and the Pussycat" and couldn't hear it often enough. In the end he memorised it himself.

Our favorite way of celebrating or simply relaxing was to dress up and go out to a long, unhurried dinner in a candle-lit dining room not so far from where we lived. In the early days sometimes we danced. I remember him looking around this room one evening and saying: "Aren't we lucky. We still have things to say to each other."

For years two T.V. programmes that we never missed were "Come Dancing" (a display of all kinds of ballroom dancing) and "Match of the Day," which was the reshowing of the best football or rugger match each Saturday, or in the summer it would be tennis.

I think that the only times when Donald actually showed that he was angry with me were on occasions when I damaged myself or became ill. He hated to have me as a patient, and not as his wife and playmate. He showed this one day when I damaged my foot and it became bruised and swollen. We had no crêpe bandage so he said he would go and buy one and I was to lie down until he returned. He was away for two hours and came back pleased with a gold expanding bracelet he had bought for me—but he had forgotten the bandage.

I was always speculating about Donald's own transitional object. He did not seem to remember one specifically, until suddenly he was able to get into touch with it. He described the experience to me in a letter written early in 1950:

> Last night I got something quite unexpected, through dreaming, out of what you said. Suddenly you joined up with the nearest thing I can get to my transition object: it was something I have always known about but I lost the memory of it, at this moment I became conscious of it. There was a very early doll called Lily belonging to my younger sister and I was fond of it, and very distressed when it fell and broke. After Lily I hated *all* dolls. But I always knew that

before Lily was a quelquechose of my own. I knew retrospectively that it must have been a doll. But it had never occurred to me that it wasn't just like myself, a person, that is to say it was a kind of other me, and a not-me female, and part of me and yet not, and absolutely inseparable from me. I don't know what happened to it. If I love you as I loved this (must I say?) doll, I love you all out. And I believe I do. Of course I love you all sorts of other ways, but this thing came new at me. I felt enriched, and felt once more like going on writing my paper on transition objects (postponed to October). (You don't mind do you—this about you and the T.O.?)

It would not be right to give the impression that Donald and I shared only experiences that lay outside our work. It was our work that brought us together in the first place, and it remained central, and bound us inextricably together. Writing to me in December 1946 he said, "In odd moments I have written quite a lot of the paper for the Psycho-Analytical Society in February, and I spend a lot of time working it out. My work is really quite a lot associated with you. Your effect on me is to make me keen and productive and this is all the more awful—because when I am cut off from you I feel paralyzed for all action and originality."

In fact each of us was essential to the work of the other. During Donald's lifetime we worked in different spheres, and this was an added interest extending the boundaries of our joint existence. We were fortunate that through the years a wide circle of people came to be intimately included in our lives and work, and we in theirs. This was a strong binding force for all concerned because it provided the community of interest which is the prerequisite for creative living. How lucky we were in those who shared our lives; how much we owe to them, and how much we enjoyed their company!

Throughout his life Donald never ceased to be in touch with his dream world and to continue his own analysis. It was the deep undercurrent of his life, the orchestral accompaniment to the main theme. His poem called "Sleep" is relevant here:

> Let down your tap root
> to the centre of your soul
> Suck up the sap
> from the infinite source
> of your unconscious
> And
> Be evergreen.

To conclude, I want to relate a dream about Donald which I had two and a half years after his death.

I dreamt that we were in our favorite shop in London, where there is a circular staircase to all floors. We were running up and down these stairs grabbing things here, there, and everywhere as Christmas presents for our friends. We were really having a spending spree, knowing that as usual we would end up keeping many of the things ourselves. I suddenly realized that Donald was alive after all and I thought with relief, "Now I shan't have to worry about the Christmas card." Then we were sitting in the restaurant having our morning coffee as usual (in fact we always went out to morning coffee on Saturday). We were facing each other, elbows on the table, and I looked at him full in the face and said: "Donald there's something we have to say to each other, some truth that we have to say, what is it?" With his very blue eyes looking unflinchingly into mine he said: "That this is a dream." I replied slowly: "Oh yes, of course, you died, you died a year ago." He reiterated my words: "Yes, I died a year ago."

For me it was through this dream of playing that life and death, his and mine, could be experienced as a reality.

Part One

Psycho-Analysis: Theory and Practice

1
Early Disillusion

Dated 24 October 1939

Our patients, who teach us so much of what we get to know, often make it clear that they met disillusionment very early indeed. They have no doubt of this and can reach deeper and deeper sadness connected with the thought.

The analysis proceeds, and yet a very great amount of work has to be done before the disillusionment can be exactly described in words. Although there is no short-cut to this result it is interesting to record individual results as they come.

The complaint often is that the loved and idealised mother trained the child to be *dishonest*. Honesty seems to be something very nearly fundamental to human nature, and presently I shall say why I think it is not quite fundamental and how I think it can itself be analysed further. But whatever its origin there is no doubt that the little child— I was going to say infant—can get a bad shock from finding it is not good to be honest.

How does it come about that the child is given to understand so early that honesty is not even the best policy, let alone good?

In two words, the baby lies there sucking her thumb and thinking thoughts, and someone comes and takes her thumb out of her mouth. She has to learn to get on with her thoughts *without* the obvious part of the orgastic accompaniment.

No doubt, what makes the parental action effective is the infant's guilt over the destructive elements of the fantasy material. One could say, then, that at one end of the scale is the minimum of guilt and the maximum of parental interference; while at the other end is maximum guilt (because of destructive elements) producing inhibition, with little or no need for parental interference. Roughly speaking it may be said that at the first-mentioned end is a hiding of the *obvious* parts of orgastic functioning with tension from the hidden functioning; whereas at the latter end is a *more* complete inhibition of bodily functioning, a more certain divorce of fantasy material from the body's instinctual life.

In regard to conscious feelings, we get here a wide range extending from a desperate attempt to be honest, one that never succeeds, to the possession of a *secret* fantasy world, to a sense of unreality about fantasy and to a repudiation of fantasy or an inability to accept ownership of whatever fantasy material intrudes itself.

A woman patient is right at the end of her analysis, but cannot finish. One of her difficulties is this: She can at last *say* "thank you." She can at last believe she is grateful, but she cannot feel certain that I (her analyst) can accept her gratitude fully. She can feel the whole thing in quite primary terms. She has been greedy at the breast, has loved it, pulled at it, torn it, scarred it, made it tired and old. Now she wants to give mother something. In herself she feels colour, value, life, but somehow she cannot believe in my acceptance of the perfect motion.

She can get into touch with the destructive parts of her fantasy. In her transference she has experienced hate more acutely than I have known any other patient to do. She can also tell me about her orgastic functions, can show me her thumb-sucking of terrific intensity, her pleasurable wriggling, her erotic excretion functions. Yet one thing is noticeable: in masturbation the *hands are never used* and she insists with great vehemence that there is no lost or forgotten hand-action. "Why should I use my hands when I can get all the bodily parts alive and excited and gratified without using them?" "Why should I rub my genitals when I can get such pleasure (genital included) from sucking my thumb?" and so on.

It has been clear from the start of the analysis that this patient's hands are of great importance. She has had inhibitions of hand function, but has managed to get jobs that essentially involve hand work, and lately there has been a remarkable freeing of her capacity to use the hands (gardening, type-writing etc. etc.).

It is quite clear that this patient cannot let her mother know she masturbates with her hands, that is that her hands, in the fantasy, do steal and kill, and that she enjoys this to a degree. She does know that she enjoys destroying with her hands, and this knowledge goes right back to early childhood. But something is lacking in her ability to be honest and to let her mother know this *through her masturbating.* (She could always let her mother know by tearing up paper compulsively, or by upsetting things and making messes, i.e. defiantly.)

It is likely that in this case the mother really did contribute to the difficulty, not necessarily by taking the child's hands away from her genitals, but more likely by taking her tiny hands from her mouth and smacking them. This pattern remained and perhaps entirely prevented this child from ever using the hands in genital masturbation. I am, of course, not certain of this, and there was certainly a real tussle between the mother and baby over skin-scratching. (In this case I have not finally determined the relative importance of anus-excitement.)

It is now possible to discuss the analysis of honesty.

This young woman wants me to receive a gift from her inside, in return for what I have done. It is a perfect gift and she does not believe I can believe in it. I don't.

The point is, that if I (her mother) cannot stand what in her honesty she tried to show me when she was an infant by her overt orgastic activities, how can I stand the bad things which will certainly be there in the gift from her inside. In fact, a great chunk of good and bad fantasy material has been kept secret from me (mother), and as long as this is so she cannot be happy about her capacity to be grateful.

That is, she knows that she really cannot restore a whole good penis to mother; the penis has been stolen and hurt; but she can do something towards filling the hole in mother's body with some parts of the penis which have been preserved, and even developed lovingly, *if* she can manage the original difficulty about secrecy over the theft.

Extreme honesty has been one of the banes of this person's existence, and she would be very glad of the relief from compulsive honesty which a successful analysis of her original failure to find a mother who could stand her honesty must bring.

2
Knowing and Not Knowing:
A Clinical Example

Undated

The patient, a woman of thirty-five, who has been in analysis for some years, is only just beginning to realise how ill she has been. The nature of her illness was such that she need not know about it, and she has always protested that the analysis started long before she came to analysis, and that it has only helped her to continue a little further than she could have done alone what she had always been able to some extent to do.

In particular she has never acknowledged that she has been unconscious of anything. When the very considerable changes occurred in her as a result of the analysis she always said when she became conscious of material that she was formerly unconscious of "I have always known that," and it is quite certain that she was not just lying as she is by character an extremely reliable person.

An important step in her self-knowledge came as a report of what she had once said to an examiner. She had replied to his question "I know but I have forgotten." In telling me of this, although she was reading it from a script having written it down on paper the day before when it occurred to her, she made a mistake and said that her reply was "I do not know but I have forgotten it." She could not believe that she had made this mistake and hated me for pointing it out to her. And yet it was really the first admission of not knowing. In one sense it was a great advance on what she said to the examiner. To the examiner she in effect said this: "I know this and when I am dispensing medicine I shall be able to use the knowledge, and the fact that when I am talking to you I do not remember it is of no consequence." What she said to me was "I know secretly." In other words in the original way of speaking there was a split personality and by means of split personality she was able to be dishonest and secretive without having to acknowledge it. She knew and she did not know.

In analysis, for instance, she could say to me "I do not dream and, therefore, I am hiding nothing." At the same time she could say "Of course I dream, I dream all night and my life is one dream, but you do not know how to make use of these dreams so I do not tell them to you." In a hundred ways she was able to maintain what was characteristic of her, which was scrupulous honesty by means of this splitting of herself into two or more parts.

The importance of this interpretation in regard to the slip of the tongue was borne out by the fact that she followed it up by saying "last night I pretended to my brother that I had no cigarettes. Well, you see, if I had let him know that I had any he would have taken them all." This was in this patient's case an achievement that she had been able to deceive her brother, and interpretation along these lines produced more confirmation. She said, "This evening I am going with my aunt to a lecture on dreams by Dr Crighton Miller." This was to her a relationship with her aunt which was destructive to me, for she had given me no dreams for two months and when tackled said that this was because I did not know what use to make of them. We were at the point of transition: she first indicated along the old lines that she was not dreaming and this was nearly honest as it would have been in the old days; but soon she had to see that she was dreaming and holding back the dreams and deceiving me. She was, therefore, one person deceiving me instead of two people telling me two sets of truths. From this she went on to say that she had always deceived her father, and I have reason to think that this is the way that her father has really been valuable to her in spite of his many faults or perhaps because of them. It had been impossible on the other hand to deceive her mother, and this seems to connect up with her mother's deception of her. By this I mean her mother's inability to know and acknowledge that she deceived her child. Throughout the analysis there had always been the mother's wig in the foreground as a cover memory for some arch deception. The deception in connection with becoming pregnant and having a son when the patient was three years old we knew to be important, but it is only now that we have understood the importance of the mother's inability to acknowledge that she would deceive a child in certain circumstances. From this it occurred to the patient that it would be wise at times to deceive a child and that I in the analysis might deceive my patient to protect her from external factors which would interfere with the analysis.

3
A Point in Technique

Undated

I have learned recently to adopt the following procedure in analytic practice.

When the fantasy that is represented in the transference material is revealed I ask myself: what and where is the accompanying orgastic bodily functioning? And, *per contra,* when in the analytic situation there is orgastic bodily functioning I ask myself: what fantasy material is the patient telling me about by this functioning?

. . . . .

When I come to expand this statement of a technical procedure I am at a loss to know where to start. I have put dots underneath the statement to represent the months which I hope anyone reading this will take to look into their own clinical behaviour and to see how much they do and do not already act as I have come to do in this special respect.

Assuming that these months have passed, I now attempt to enlarge on this theme, which I must agree is neither original nor revolutionary.

A woman patient has a voice which is characteristic. When she works hard, at analysis for instance, she does a tremendous amount of work with her mouth and with her whole vocal apparatus. She talks loudly, and she has gradually become conscious of the fact that she enjoys the functioning of her speech department almost to a painful degree.

In the course of the analysis fantasy of all kinds has emerged accompanied by feeling of very great intensity.

One day, at a time when ideas of robbing and all sorts of hand actions of love, jealousy, hate and revenge were conscious, I wanted very badly to get her to see me half an hour before the arranged time. This I knew would suit her better and also it made me able to avoid cutting short her hour owing to circumstances outside my control. I therefore risked going to look for her. I knew she would be dining in a certain restaurant, so I went there and attempted to speak to her.

She was eating, eating like a wild animal, and reading the newspaper. It was quite difficult to break through the invisible shell, and to get her to notice me.

The anxiety and rage roused by this action of mine were very great. I had found the hidden orgastic bodily functioning hidden from me in the analysis, but without which the fantasy material, though intensely felt, could never become quite real or personal. Gradually I came to understand that the clue could have been found all along in her voice, which was the part of her that was trying to be honest in spite of her general determination to keep apart (in her relationship to me) the fantasy and the bodily accompaniment.

Analysis along these lines produced material which made clear her thumb-sucking experiences (orgastic pleasure, defiance, guilt feelings, inhibition) and her hand masturbation which had been long inhibited and the idea repudiated.

4

Play in the Analytic Situation

Dated 5 November 1954

I wish to discuss some aspects of play in adult analysis. In child analysis play is nearly always in evidence, but in adult analysis one expects to be able to leave play and to rely on dreams and hallucinations and fantasying.

Occasionally one hears of adult patients who are seen through a sticky patch by being given child-analysis toys which they manipulate over a phase and which enables the analyst to interpret in silent periods. What concerns me at the moment is not the introduction of play material into the analytic hour but the recognition of the importance of play in adult analysis, play being different from fantasy and dream.

An example was given me by a student in a supervision hour. The patient said, "I have just found a short-cut to analysis." In describing the short-cut he said he passed through the children's playground. The student quite rightly made the interpretation that the patient could see the value of play. As this patient has had violent episodes it is very important that in the analysis such things as a sense of humour should not be neglected, because the only hope that this man has of coming through his analysis without periods in which management will become necessary (as indeed it was at one time before the analysis started) is through his being able to play.

After the interpretation given by the student the patient leaned over and rearranged the mat and gave associations to this bit of play. In the circumstances it is understandable that the student neglected to continue on the subject of play and became bogged down in the material of the free associations which indeed were important on their own account.

On one occasion a patient of mine came without having had coffee on the way and was in a dither about wanting coffee and feeling the whole hour would be wasted. I am sure that the management of this situation could be along two or more distinct lines. On this occasion I produced the coffee and we then saw what a tremendous difference there was between the patient's relationship to the coffee, the cup and saucer, the tray and sugar, and her relationship to the idea of wanting coffee from the dream that might have been there of having coffee given her by myself. It became a matter of play and an example of the introduction of play material into adult analysis.

Somewhere about this time another patient, a man, said to me "I have been meaning to let you know that I enjoy coming in and going out because it is playing. There is all the business about a routine and the avoidance of seeing other patients and so on." This was a surprising statement from a man who is unable to play and who comes because of an inability to keep his friendships as he can only talk in a ponderous manner and there is no play available. There was a reason why this man was able to make this observation and that was that in the previous sessions we had been dealing with play and the time had come in his analysis for me to let him see that instead of playing he was masturbating regularly, and the fantasying was locked up in the masturbation. This interpretation coming at the right moment began to free his playing and made him very conscious of his loneliness throughout childhood except when there were organised games. He had been unable to play because sharing the fantasy meant losing so much. A day or two later we came upon a game that he had never known about. We found that he had had an imaginary sister throughout his childhood of whom he was violently jealous, although in fact he was never jealous of either his older sister or his younger sister. This imaginary girl he found had represented his feminine self and had been practically a perfect individual and had had a close relationship with his father which he was unable to have through being a boy. In desperation he had tried dressing up as a girl a great deal during childhood but this had never been satisfactory because of the idealised girl that he always took with him and whom he hated and of course loved in a narcissistic way.

It has certainly been my practice to remember playing in adult analyses and often I have introduced pencil and paper and there have been play aspects, humorous interchanges, and so on, but it is only recently that I have recognised the very important differences between these play episodes and dreams and fantasying. One important thing is the obvious one that in play, although one has to drop a considerable amount which cannot be shared with the other person, there is a great deal to be gained from the overlap of other people's fantasy with one's own, so that there is a shared experience even if over a limited area of the total fantasying.

5
Fragments Concerning Varieties of Clinical Confusion

Dated 13 and 22 February 1956

I

An important feature of obsessional behaviour is the confusion that it implies. Why is it that in health a muddle can be tidied up, and in illness the tidying up that is compulsive is also futile?

The Clue: In obsessional illness the confusion is an organised defence. A degree of confusion is *unconsciously maintained* in order to hide a very simple fact: triumph of bad over good, hate over love, aggression over capacity for preservation, etc.

In this way, the tidying up can never succeed. But there may be found an almost conscious muddling up when tidying seems to succeed.

> O the doing and undoing
> When a lover goes a-wooing!

Clinically we find: confusion as a defence, organised, only altered by analysis of the oral sadism, which in turn alters the balance of forces within, so that there is less of the simple fact of hopelessness which must be hidden by confusion. It can be helpful to the patient, in the process, to be informed of the confusion as a defence. This helps acceptance of the usefulness of the obsessions, which, however, are not "cured" thereby.

There is a relationship between depression and obsession of the following kind: (a) Depressed and obsessed persons are intolerant of each other. (b) One patient moves to and fro from depression to obsession. On the whole the patient feels more real in the depressed state, but the fatuous obsessions can provide temporary relief from mood.

The question arises, what makes one depressed patient able to be obsessional at times, or makes one obsessional patient able to become temporarily depressed; whereas some patients remain in one or other diagnostic category?

This question emphasises the fact that depression as a clinical state is not "the depressive position." The depressive position and the patient's failure to reach it underlie the depression and obsession states equally.

We are concerned with the patient's capacity to tolerate mood. Fear of contra-depressive defences may contribute to adoption of obsessional techniques, for when depression is severe as a mood the opposite is not manic defence but mania. ("Severe as a mood" implies a high degree of repression of aggression or of ruthless love.)

The depressed person despises the obsessional who has fled from feelings. The obsessional cannot stand the depressive's capacity to hold a mood; holding a mood implies hope, and in fact a depressed mood tends to lift spontaneously in time. The depressed person needs, however, to be preserved from suicide at the bottom of the depressed phase.

Depression then implies hope. What sort of hope? I suggest: hope of being held over a period of time, while working through can take place—that is, a sorting out or tidying up within, in the so called inner world. It is only here that sorting out is anything but futile.

There will be an accumulation of "memories" of good mothering at the time of the early achievements in respect of the depressive position. In the case of the obsessional there will be instead an accumulation of "memories" of training, teaching, implantations of morality. Comparison of these two states seems to me to lead us to a contrast between two types of early mothering.

Incidental to this theme is the complication which must be fully acknowledged by the analyst when it is present; namely the organised confusion being a state of the mother, corresponding to the organised defences against depression of which I have written elsewhere.[1]

Confusion as an organised defence must be analysed if the patient is to get to that which is always at the centre of the individual, a primary chaos, out of which samples of individual self-expression organise themselves. In terms of the initial stages of development this is the primary state of unintegration, to which attention is drawn by Glover in his theory of ego nuclei.[2] In our work we find great clinical

1. "The Manic Defence" (1935) and "Reparation in Respect of Mother's Organised Defence against Depression" (1948), in *Collected Papers: Through Paediatrics to Psycho-Analysis* (London: Tavistock, 1958; New York: Basic Books, 1975; Hogarth Press, 1975).
2. E. Glover, *On the Early Development of the Mind* (London: Imago, 1956).

relief when the clearing away of organised defence confusion enables a patient to reach this primary chaos at the centre. This can only be reached of course in an environment that is of the special type that I have called primary maternal preoccupation, when the mother (analyst) who holds is identified to a high degree with the infant held. At this point in an analysis *some* patients do seem to need to be actually held, in some token form, with a modicum of physical contact. Environmental failure at this point means that the unintegrated self falls forever, and the affect belonging to this is anxiety of psychotic intensity. It is here more than anywhere else in an analysis that the patient must take a risk in order to progress to integration.

In making this note I have deliberately gone from one extreme to the other describing the organised confusion of a sophisticated kind and contrasting it with the primary unintegrated state. The intermediate confusions have their own importance. An example is the confusion which can occur at any stage if a demand is made on mental activity which is just beyond the scope of the individual at the moment either because of multiple problems presenting at the same time or because the task is beyond that which fits the state of ego development and organisation.

II

I have long been interested in the relationship between the concept of the depressive position and the mood depression and the emotions called grief, sadness, sense of loss.

A patient brought me up against this problem. The clinical picture is as follows: this patient is not at the moment at the depressive position although near, that is to say there is not an integrative experience of a whole person related to a part object and a whole object, these two being recognized as related.

The analysis had just reached a point at which the patient had found the original confusion state belonging to unintegration, this implying considerable confidence in the environmental factor, namely the analyst in the transference. The analysis was interrupted at this point by my wife's illness. At first the patient came forward in a false way and dealt with the situation with sympathy. After two days this broke down and the patient became confused; this time the confusion was disintegrated or even an organised confusional state and not the primary confusion of unintegration. On returning after four days' interval the patient was at first unable to get back to analysis and was very much concerned with the reality situation. At the end of the hour she had arrived at the stage at which analysis could have continued along the old lines. The next day there was a gradual return to confidence and this led to a piece of acting out which surprised the patient, in which certain things happened that showed me that she had a body memory of suddenly being put down. She had anxiety of the most acute kind and after it was all over we recognised this as a delayed reaction to my abandoning her four days previously, a reaction which had been quite impossible for her to have on her own. The next day confidence had returned in a full way and there was a repetition of the acting out in the session.

It will be noted that in the previous day's acting out there was no rigidity, which is the most primitive reaction; instead there was un-integration changing over into disintegration. On this second occasion there was a much more mature reaction. The patient under the influence of unconscious processes showed quite clearly that she was a tiny infant in great distress holding out her hands and experiencing a sense of loss. It was not quite felt as grief although nearly. Sense of loss certainly was felt in a very acute way and this instead of anxiety. After recovery the patient returned to the confident relationship to myself which had made this bit of acting out possible. Here the patient had gone forward with her discovery and the reaction to my withdrawal. The important thing was that here was a moment of my withdrawing myself to which she could react with a sense of loss, and that this compared with her mother's withdrawn state which gave no moment for such a reaction. In the relationship to the mother there had been simply a withdrawn state more or less evenly distributed. With me, however, she had now experienced my withdrawing at a certain moment and had reacted with acute sense of loss.

Here, then, was nearly grief. At the same time I remember that this patient is not in a state of ego development which makes possible the full experience of the depressive position. No doubt to some extent the experience of grief depends not only on my behaviour but also on the patient's build-up within herself of the idea of a good object. This is closely related to her ability to hold the idea of the mother for a moment when she had withdrawn, thus enabling the sense of loss to be a reality.

6

Excitement in the Aetiology of
Coronary Thrombosis

*Notes for a lecture given to the Society for Psycho-
Somatic Research, University College, London,
5 December 1957*

A. Survey of psycho-somatic disorder
   Coronary thrombosis is a good example of a psycho-somatic disorder.
   1. It can be a purely physical illness.
   2. It becomes a physical illness
      i. arterial changes
      ii. thrombosis
   3. It is not a disease of the working class but of the professional
      class.
   4. It is related to emotional stress.
   5. It is not especially related to a psychiatric diagnostic group
      (though perhaps depression-linked).
   6. It is part of the living of a personal life in an environment, that
      is to say, part of a relationship experience.
   7. Its not being immediately fatal makes it possible for the pa-
      tients to use the tendency as a spur to altering an impossible
      mode of life which had become a habit.
But this is not all. There remains the essential problem of physiology.

B. Literature of coronary thrombosis
   In the literature of coronary thrombosis the psychology of the
   subject is mostly confined to the following three aspects:
   1. The effect of the illness on the patient, who must adjust to a
      lowered ceiling of physical power, and who knows now how
      he will probably die.
   2. The predisposing factors in terms of a description of the envi-
      ronment and the patient's place in it, note being taken of the

stress factors. It is generally recognised that the individual is to some extent responsible for his environment and for continuing to live in it if it is difficult.

3. The beginnings of an understanding of emotional conflict as opposed to emotional strain.

C. Approaches from psychology

Three modes of attack come from psychology:

1. The statistic approach—as applied to gastric ulcer or hypertension. This involves preconceived notions which can be stated and proved to be significant or non-significant.

2. The approach with therapy in it—such as Hambling's observations on hypertension.[1]

3. (At the other extreme) the psychoanalyst who talks in terms of the whole analysis of the patient, in the course of which psycho-somatic disorders come and go; such disorders can not infrequently be seen to be related to unconscious fantasy, to defences against anxiety, to massive introjections of traumatic situations, to the strains and stresses of reality adaptations of all kinds, etc. etc., and also to secondary gain through illness.

D. Appeal to physiology

At this point it ought to be possible to take down a text book of physiology from the shelf, and to look up the changes that belong to excitement, for coronary thrombosis is a disorder of the apparatus of excitement.

It would seem to me that for this one must ask for a new physiological orientation, one which links with the new work of ethologists and also of some neuro-physiologists and endocrinologists.

The physiology I learned was cold, that is to say, it could be checked up by careful examination of a pithed frog or a heart-lung preparation. Every effort was made to eliminate variables such as emotions, and animals as well as human beings seemed to me to be treated as if they were always in a neutral condition in regard to instinctual life. One can see the civilising process which brings a dog into a constant state of frustration. Consider the strain that we impose on a dog that *does not even secrete urine into the bladder* until

1. John Hambling, "Emotions and Symptoms in Essential Hypertension" and "Psychosomatic Aspects of Arterial Hypertension," *British Journal of Medical Psychology* 24 (1951) and 25 (1952).

some indication is given that there will be opportunity for bladder discharge. How much more important it must be that we shall allow physiology to become complicated by emotion and emotional conflict when we study the way the human body works.

A study of the problem of coronary thrombosis as a psycho-somatic disorder requires of us a knowledge of the physiology of excitement. This indeed must be complex but it is not enough. We further need to know what happens in the body when excitement "goes cold," that is to say, does not reach a climax.

In the literature I think there may be a failure to examine coronary thrombosis under the high power of the microscope, largely because of lack of opportunity. In consequence, the psychopathology remains obscure. It will be observed that adverse external factors, however real, become internal strains when one patient comes under scrutiny.

E. Physiology of excitement

    Local .... Preparation (forepleasure)
    General .... Climax
                             Relaxation

(This implies a purely personal experience: i.e. not a relationship.)

To this must be added the relationship factor, all that goes with the attempt to link instinctual experience with other kinds of love and with affectionate regard.

At this point we need some sort of chart which can be modified to cover the degree of excitement that needs to be lost.

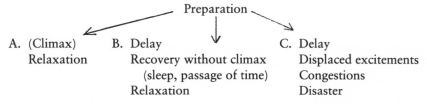

A. (Climax)   B. Delay   C. Delay
   Relaxation   Recovery without climax   Displaced excitements
                  (sleep, passage of time)   Congestions
                  Relaxation   Disaster

It is necessary to take into account the age of the subject, for a young person of 20–30 can hold the tension better than one of 40–50. A young person can even suffer tremendous mental and bodily distress caused by a failure to reach climax without the added insult of a physical accident with irreversible change such as thrombosis of an arteriole.

In the first degree of failure (B) the local excitement dies down, or in a general way the climax is represented by sleep, or a game of golf, or a row with the cook.

The further degree (C) produces a highly complex state of affairs, first with alternative congestions and displaced excitements, and then with any of the mental states that we call abnormal according to the makeup of the individual.

Disaster ......
(hysteria)
depression
depersonalisation
disintegration
sense of unreality
    or a mixture
general tension (chaotic defences)

Only the passage of time cures this phase in which there is impotence or frigidity, and probably there is an incapacity to masturbate, or masturbation is only possible by the dragging in of pervert and regression mechanisms.

F. Elaboration of the theme of excitement
   It will be clear that I am not referring to
   1. Elation, a mental state, a matter of the mind or
   2. Manic defence against depression, the depressed mood being potential but denied (hypomania) or
   3. Manic swing in manic-depressive psychosis.

Excitement is the pre-condition for instinctual experience. There are many zones at which excitement occurs locally, but for the integrated personality local excitements are part of the build-up for a general state of excitement, and purely local satisfaction of a major instinctual locality is a frustration to the whole person who expected more result—in fact, a whole experience on the basis of the experience of the past.

In references to masturbation in adolescence how often this matter of total participation is ignored, so that it is not known whether the local discharge of instinct tension was good or bad for the whole body (this apart altogether from the presence or absence of anxiety or sense of guilt).

When local excitement builds up to become part of a whole body excitement, and of a whole person excitement, we still want to know whether this phenomenon is or is not a part of a relationship, and if it is, whether the other object is a thing or another total human being.

At one extreme, there is no hindrance from outside, no external reason why excitement should not build up into a climax, followed by relaxation. At the other extreme, there is every reason why it is difficult for one individual to get a satisfactory and well-timed personal climax since this climax has to be fitted in with someone else's similar need for a well-timed climax. Except when two romantic persons are in love with each other the conditions for two satisfactions at the same time but seldom obtain.

All this is very obvious, but I am not sure how much attention has been paid to the physiology of impotence and frigidity—more easily do we find the statement that instinctual satisfaction is good, in a physiological sense, producing a state of general release from tension—or a state that is called normal.

The common state of affairs in men and women who like to link their instinctual experiences with the enrichment of relationships is that many excitements must remain unrequited, and must find a way of dying down. Here we come near to the physiology of such a psycho-somatic disorder as coronary thrombosis.

7

Hallucination and Dehallucination

Written for a seminar on 3 October 1957

A woman had the following dream; this is her account:

> I woke up screaming (I suppose soundlessly) from a dream. I was in
> a room when an old-fashioned little boy about six years came run-
> ning towards me as for help. I recognised this at once as an halluci-
> nation and it simply terrified me and I started screaming at the top
> of my voice. As he retreated I threw a cushion after him, then some-
> one like Nannie appeared at the door as if to see what was the mat-
> ter. I wondered whether she too would see the little boy, but it was
> rather blurred in that part of the room. I rather thought she picked
> him up. I hoped W. would hear my screams and come but by now I
> realised that I was actually making no noise. This increased my fears
> and it was in this state that I woke up, still quite disorientated. I did
> not know where or when, even though I heard the clock ticking. I
> remained in a state of fright for some time. Eventually I recovered
> enough to get out and pass water.

There were associations to the dream and the patient felt that it had
to do with an interpretation in relation to dehallucination. The patient described this dream to me as by far the most terrifying of all
her many nightmares.

The associations to the dream and its place in the analysis made
much of its function clear. The point to which I wish to refer concerns
this matter of the relationship of hallucination to dehallucination. I
wish to put forward an idea about this for you to discuss.

It often strikes me as a difficulty which we have not met that sometimes we say a patient is hallucinating and take that as evidence of
psychosis and at other times we refer to patients and especially to
children as hallucinating without thinking of them as being even ill.
They may perhaps be tired and therefore aware of hallucinations
which when they are more alert they hide or confine to the sort of
objects that in fact they can perceive in their environment. Most children hallucinate freely, and I would certainly not diagnose abnormal-

ity when a mother tells me that in her flat there is a cow in the passage and that her four-year-old son has great difficulty in dealing with this obstruction. The same boy has a whole series of imaginary objects which have to be treated with the respect due to them—someone, for instance, called Fluflu, who lives most of the time under a chair and who is in a vague way mixed up with the idea of Jesus. There is no need for me to give examples because anyone in touch with small children knows that the children who hallucinate freely are not necessarily ill.

May we ask a question: Is there some difference between the hallucinating which denotes illness and that which has no such significance? Probably the answer to this question is that there are several ways in which we can distinguish between normal and pathological hallucinating. I wish to refer to one possible difference and in doing so I wish to acknowledge help derived directly from Dr Margaret Little. I do in fact think that the sort of discussion that I am promoting here is related to the discussion of her paper on delusional transference.[1]

In suggesting an answer to this question I am making use of what seems to me to be a valuable piece of new understanding about dehallucination. I have been looking for years for the clue to the special use that children and adults make sometimes of blackness. The dark may be liked and blackness may be for some people the best colour, but black also denotes something evil, terrifying, traumatic. At a Medical Section meeting when I was chairman I organised a discussion round the word "black" and the answer that I wanted was not forthcoming although nearly produced by Dr Robert Moody, a Jungian analyst. I am referring to well-known phenomena such as, for instance, the blacking out of pictures after they have been painted. I know of a patient in a mental hospital at the moment who paints really well but he always blacks out his work of art; sometimes one can be rescued and he does not then object to its being framed and put on the wall, but I think by that time he does not know that it is his.

A schizophrenic boy patient of mine did nothing for a long time but black over the whole of every sheet of paper. Gradually it became clear that there was a picture from his point of view under the black.

---

1. Margaret I. Little, "On Delusional Transference (Transference Psychosis)," *International Journal of Psycho-Analysis* 39 (1958); rpt. in Little, *Transference Neurosis and Transference Psychosis* (New York, London: Jason Aronson, 1981).

Sometimes he would lift the veil and paint or draw and allow me to see what there was to be dehallucinated, but for him it was traumatic if a drawing was snatched from him and displayed, so traumatic that in fact no-one would ever have done anything so awful as to force the issue.

My suggestion is that in some cases we notice that hallucinating is pathological because of a compulsive element in it which can be explained in the following way. Something has been dehallucinated and in a secondary way the patient hallucinates in denial of the dehallucination. It is complex because first of all there was something seen, then something dehallucinated, and then a long series of hallucinations so to speak filling the hole produced by the scotomisation.

The dream that I have given illustrates this point very well. The case is simplified by the fact that the patient is not psychotic but she has had to become psychotic in the transference in order to arrive at a memory of a very distressing kind belonging to the time when she was about two years old. This analysis has gone a very long way and in order to reach the strength to deal with this trauma the patient needed to make a very deep regression. In other words she had to become able to deal with her early difficulties in relation to her mother in order to be able to go on to use the father as a father and then to tolerate the terrific trauma of his exposing himself to her. In the actual setting the father had been so to speak giving the infant child psychotherapy, offering her a nice unexcited penis for play which was compensating for the mother's very early withdrawal of the breast. Suddenly and quite unexpectedly the patient came upon the father sexually excited and the result was absolutely disastrous. I can leave out the whole of the rest of the case description and simply say that when the patient now comes to this traumatic moment (which in fact gathers together multiple traumata) she comes to a dehallucination of the excited genital. In the dream the child coming forward is hallucinated in a compulsive way and in a final attempt to deny the space left in front of the patient at the moment of her dehallucinating the excited genital.

There is a dream of many years ago in which all this was foreshadowed but the feeling belonging to this succession of events—perceiving, scotomisation, compulsive hallucinating—was not attainable until recently. When the patient first came to me, instead of the little boy there was a bright light, and this very nearly started off the patient on a false trail of spiritualism, the trail which indeed has been followed by the other members of the family who are all dealing, as is the patient, with various aspects of the father's abnormal state, which was in turn derived from a seduction which took place during his own early childhood, possibly when he was about two.

My thesis then is that we sometimes notice a special type of hallucinating which is compulsive and which is frightening in spite of the fact that what is hallucinated does not in itself constitute a threat. The clue, I suggest, is that it must be maintained in order to deny the scotomisation or the dehallucination. There must be a very important stage according to whether the emotional trauma was something real or a dream.

8
Ideas and Definitions

Probably early 1950s[1]

The false self. The true self

These terms are used in description of a defensive organisation in which there is a premature taking over of the nursing functions of the mother, so that the infant or child adapts to the environment while at the same time protecting and hiding the true self, or the source of personal impulses. This is similar to the function of the Ego, in early Freud, turned towards the world, between the Id and external reality.

In typical cases the imprisoned true self is unable to function, and by being protected its opportunity for living experience is limited. Life is lived through the compliant false self, and the result clinically is a sense of unreality. Other writers have used the following term to describe similar states: Observing Ego.

Spontaneity and real impulse can only come from the true self, and for this to happen someone needs to take over the defensive functions of the false self.

Transitional object. Transitional phenomena

The term "transitional object" was intended to give significance to the first signs in the developing infant of an acceptance of a symbol. This precursor of a symbol is at one and the same time part of the infant and a part of the mother. Often this symbol precursor is in fact an object, and the infant's addiction to this actual object is recognised and allowed for by the parents. Often there is no materialisation, however, and then certain phenomena may be found later to have the same significance; for instance, watching, thinking, distinguishing between colours, exploitation of body movements and sensations, etc. etc.

The mother herself may become a transitional object, sometimes the thumb. Degenerate forms are represented by rocking, head-bang-

---

1. This paper was found in a file marked "Ideas."—EDS.

ing, highly compulsive thumb-sucking, etc., and later pseudologia fantastica and stealing.

In favourable conditions this object gradually gives place to an ever-widening range of objects, and to the whole cultural life.

Regression (to dependence)

The term "regression" is applied ordinarily in psycho-analytic writings to instinct positions. Regression is from genital to pregenital erotic experience or fantasy, or it is to fixation points belonging to the life of infancy in which pregenital fantasy is naturally dominant.

Regression is also a convenient term for use in description of an adult's or a child's state in the transference (or in any other dependent relationship) when a forward position is given up and an infantile dependence is re-established. Typically, regression of this kind is from independence to dependence. In this use of the term the environment is indirectly brought in since dependence implies an environment that meets dependence. By contrast, in the other use of the term "regression" there is no implied reference to an environment. The term "regression" is also used to describe the *process* that can be observed in a treatment, a gradual shedding of the false or caretaker self, and the approach to a new relationship in which the caretaker self is handed over to the therapist.

Good-enough mother

This term is used in description of the dependence that belongs to earliest infancy. The implication is that mental health has to be founded in every case by the mother who, in health, has it in her to meet the minute-to-minute needs of her infant. What is needed and absolutely needed by the infant is not some kind of perfection of mothering, but a good enough adaptation, that which is part of a living partnership in which the mother temporarily identifies herself with her infant. To be able to identify herself with her infant to the necessary degree the mother needs to be protected from external reality so that she may enjoy a period of preoccupation, the baby being the object of her preoccupation. To be able to lose this high degree of identification at the rate of the infant's journey from dependence to independence the mother needs to be healthy in the sense of not being liable to morbid preoccupation.

9

Psychogenesis of a Beating Fantasy
Dated 11 March 1958

Freud's paper "A Child is Being Beaten" brought the subject of the beating fantasy into focus. The extreme complexity of the organisation behind these fantasies is clearly brought out: also the difference between these fantasies in boys and in girls. The idea that a fantasy of this kind is overdetermined is part of the thesis, and also it is taken for granted that cruelty that is organised in this way is certain to be associated with a fixation at the anal phase. In my experience, these fantasies, which are extremely common and which take innumerable forms, must always be examined afresh in each case, because although there are common denominators there can never be a rule of thumb which can be applied to all cases.

In this brief note I would like to describe the history of a beating fantasy which persisted throughout a long analysis and the elucidation of which only arrived at the end. So many trends were gathered together in this important detail and each trend had its own importance. From the beginning the patient made it quite clear that her analysis would not be successful unless it cleared up this particular pervert idea which was so important to her and which had recurred all her life as a sexual outlet, and yet which had never been acted out. It was indeed an important detail as it turned out that in the fantasy itself there was no suffering.

There had been an early childhood development which resulted in this set piece. From the beginning of the analysis it was known that at a certain stage in the development belonging to the time when the patient was about five years old the thrashing was done by a Mrs Stickland, and it was obvious that the stick in the woman's possession was important. This was not just an idea, it was felt by the patient to be of fundamental importance. In one of the developments of the theme the patient's mother fetches a stick out of her wardrobe, but there were innumerable variations on the theme. At one time it was thought that there had been an episode in which the father of this patient had thrashed her in a moment of sexual excitement. This, however, turned out to be a mistake, and it was a cover fantasy behind which lay a sexual episode in which the father was discovered by the child at an awkward moment. In the end the patient and I have agreed that there is no evidence whatever of there having been any actual beating, even in childhood play.

This patient had had a long analysis before coming to me and also a short one, and in the course of a ten-year analysis with myself she had undergone a very deep regression. In the regression the patient was unmistakably infantile and at the bottom of the regression was in a state of almost total regression, with very little healthy ego that was in touch with external reality. At that stage, as I have described elsewhere, I was visiting the patient and indeed managing her affairs and buying her food. During the phase of deepest regression a Home Help was preparing food and coping with the housework. Eventually the patient came out of her regressed state, making a forward development which had many unexpected interruptions, each one of which was extremely painful to both the patient and to myself, because of the strain that this treatment was putting on both of us.

It was interesting that in the course of this deep regression and the forward movement following it, the beating fantasy was the one thing which remained constant in spite of its belonging to a forward stage of development. Whenever the patient developed sexual tension the relief was obtained alongside the fantasy which I am describing. It was perhaps the only reliable sexual outlet, for quite early in the treatment sexual contact with men had become meaningless. It has to be noted in passing that this patient, for certain reasons which became fairly clear eventually, had had no manifest homosexuality experiences although she had attracted the sort of people who might have formed this kind of a relationship with her. The absence of homosexual experience was part of her extreme hopelessness in relationship to her mother, the same that appears also in the beating fantasy.

Right at the end of the treatment the patient brings forward for analysis this same unaltered constellation, both she and I knowing that the analysis could not end without its resolution. Eventually the way was paved for a better understanding of it by material which required the interpretation that the idea of the beating was supplanting an extreme hopelessness about communicating with the mother at an anal level. All her life the patient had manipulated her flatus and had indeed evolved a specialist's technique in this respect, but it was all wasted and there was a period of deep depression associated with a full recognition of the absolute hopelessness that she had as an infant in regard to any communication with the mother in this way. This followed of course a deeper hopelessness about communicating at the oral level, but the failure here went so deep and involved such primitive processes that the patient's ego was not sufficiently organised for her to experience grief or hopelessness. Here she could only feel that her mouth and appetite had gone off with the mother who weaned her and abandoned her to a nurse at the age of two months.

The patient felt that the beating fantasy was related to a fixation.

If can be said that nothing would have altered the patient's feeling about the beating fantasy until it was possible to make the interpretation from the material in the hour that the fixation was in the mother. It was the mother's repressed sadism which was the unalterable factor. In life the mother's masochism was evident and had always been a very important element affecting indeed her husband and all the children. It could be said that she married and had children as a masochistic experience, sometimes going over into a more evident self-punishing position with a suicidal element in it. The underlying sadism did indeed emerge in her old age and was particularly evident in her treatment of a woman who was devoted to her and who was rather obviously a homosexual in type.

Following this interpretation and the hour which made sense of this interpretation there was a sense of there having been a change made in the patient's lifelong association with the beating fantasy. It is perhaps possible to link the detail that there was never any sensation of being hurt with the fact that it was the mother's masochism and the mother's fixation which was operative.

It may be mentioned that all along throughout the analysis the patient's relationship to the mother's repressed unconscious has been important and also the patient's relationship to the mother as an organisation of defences against anxiety. The hopelessness in the patient's relationship to the mother was simply another expression of the fact that the mother as a person was not available, although she became available when the patient was older and indeed became a good friend of a sad and suffering kind.

There is one further point and that is that the patient's own anal fixation was also important but it needs to be noted that clinically no shift could be made until in this case the mother's fixation at this level was brought in as significant. In reviewing the material I cannot believe that a knowledge of this would have made it possible for the analyst to have shortened the analysis by making this sort of interpretation at an earlier date. I think in fact that the interpretation of the mother's anal fixation and repressed sadism could not have been made until the end of the patient's analysis, and I base this view on the fact that it was only then that the material was given in the analysis for this interpretation.

10

Nothing at the Centre

Dated 19 June 1959

The patient, a woman of thirty who is an actress, came to analysis in a rather friendly state. She talked about many things that were going on in her life. She has an attractive personality and there was much that she could say which indicated that people actively like her. I am able to tell that this is an example of this patient's major defence.

The previous hour had been extremely unsatisfactory. The patient had not been able to find any particular thing to react to. She is between jobs but there is no new job pending and there is a gap of several weeks in which perhaps nothing will come her way. One could see that she was agitated, frightened of the state of affairs produced by there being nothing to which she could react. As she said, she might go home and find an invitation to dinner or a message from her agent, and she would be quite all right again, happy and lively and well orientated. In this previous hour she had reached a state of doldrums and was intensely irritated with me for seeming to be in favour of it. What she meant was that I was not adopting the attitude, which she adopts herself and which her parents and friends adopt, "for heaven's sake get a job, do something, pull your socks up," and so on.

This girl has worked very hard from the age of ten, when she started acting. She had a period at the beginning of the treatment in a mental hospital where she was allowed to be depressed and this was of immense value to her, but again she was not floundering because she was all the time dealing with a depression. She felt she knew where she was going. Now that she is nearly recovered she finds herself, however, in this very frightened state with lack of orientation.

In this patient's analysis the really difficult thing was to get at eating and the fantasy of eating, i.e. the oral erotism and sadism that complicate other kinds of relationships to objects. The patient had been so irritated with me the hour before that when I coughed she could not stand it and in any case she knew that she was irritated with me for unknown reasons. She was able to report that she had had the idea of a baby somewhere in her mind, indicating that analysis was no good because it had not produced in her a pregnancy. This was only one aspect, however, of the whole frustration of the analysis which in fact has been steadily successful and productive.

On the occasion of this particular hour that I am referring to the patient was in her usual state of manic defence in which all goes well and everyone likes her, but both she and I knew that this was precarious and that just behind it all was something else.

The striking thing was what happened when I made a certain interpretation. It was she who pointed out that her happiness was due to the fact that some things had been happening to her but that she was the same underneath. I interpreted that if nothing was happening for her to react to then she came to the centre of herself where she knows that there is nothing. I said this nothingness at the centre is her tremendous hunger. The hole in the middle which is herself is a hunger for everything and belongs to the whole of her life and includes the emptiness before impregnation as well as sexual and oral desire. As soon as the trend of my interpretation became clear to her, and the interpretation was not altogether new, she fell dead asleep and stayed asleep for about twenty minutes. When she began to waken and to become impatient with having been to sleep and missed the hour, I began again on the interpretation, whereupon she went suddenly into a new sleep and stayed like it until the end of the hour. When she wakened she said: "I have been glued to the couch." She tore herself off the couch in order to sit up and put on her shoes because in spite of having slept she knew when it was time to go and so she went. By the time she had reached the front door she had regained her usual attractive liveliness.

This patient often goes to sleep but then she is usually in an exhausted state from overworking physically and from staying up late in the way that belongs to the actress life. This time the sleep had a new quality to it, I thought, one which she described as being glued to the couch. I assumed that the sleep represented a particular kind of resistance to the interpretation. The essence of the interpretation was that there is a dissociated self which is nothing; it is nothing but a void; it is only emptiness and when this emptiness comes alive she is nothing but one huge hunger. This is the first time that she and I in the course of four years' analysis have found together a satisfactory statement of her true self and at the same time of her appetite.

At the same time in my practice I have a patient, a man who is a doctor. He too has had to discover in himself a central nothingness. For a long time this has turned up in the analysis as a state of floundering which was very alarming to him. We have had to deal with it in various layers. In one layer when we gradually eliminated all the impingements so that he had nothing to react to he became a thing in space, unaware of time and unaware of position. In three successive hours this week the patient arrived at a different statement of this which is to him part of his search for a self that would feel real. With great difficulty he eliminates all the tremendous number of things in his life to which he reacts and which he copes with successfully. This includes his relationship to his family and to a wife who undoubtedly does present him with great difficulties because of her own ability to fit in exactly with the pattern of his mother. He had chosen her on this account, as he now knows only too well. In this particular patient it was vitally important that I must recognize that at the centre there is nothing. He has had to discard even his potency because it was reactive. He not only has no belief that there is anything there which could be called he; rather he knows that at the centre there is nothing and it is only this that he can tolerate. If I were to provide any hope that there is something there he would have to destroy me. It was interesting how this patient began to turn up in a positive way when he had sufficiently established himself as a nothing. What he reported at the end of these three hours in which this theme had been thoroughly worked through and in which he had been able to maintain a state of nothingness was expressed in the following way. He said he felt tightly wrapped round between the legs and he went on to describe the effect of this on his genitals and his capacity to pee. I had a very great deal of material available which enabled me to make the following interpretation. He was telling me in physical terms how his mother conveyed to him when he was a tiny infant that he was from her point of view a girl and not a boy. There is substance in this as he was the second boy and the attitude of the parents all the way along betrayed the fact that they would have liked to have had a girl for the second child. I was able to say that the mother did up his napkin in a way that would be appropriate for a girl baby, perhaps like a sanitary towel. The result of this was that he had no freedom to pee and when I pointed out to him that as a native child living in a hut in the wilds it would have been different he suddenly got the meaning of my interpretation and through this he arrived at the idea of a boy peeing freely. This is the first time that he can remember that his penis has felt to be his own. It looks as if this is the beginning of his potency which he has never had although in fact he has a family. Here in a different way as compared with the first case was a man having to reach to the central nothingness. In his case what emerged was not hunger but peeing. The two cases can perhaps be compared for the purposes of discussion.

11

The Fate of the Transitional Object

*Preparation for a talk given to the Association
for Child Psychology and Psychiatry, Glasgow,
5 December 1959*

Although many of you are very familiar with what I have said about transitional objects I would like first of all to re-state my view of them, and then pass on to my main subject which is the question of their fate. Here is a statement then of the way in which transitional objects seem to me to have significance. They seem to me to be in several lines of transition. One of these has to do with object relationships; the infant has a fist in the mouth, then a thumb, then there is an admixture of the use of the thumb or fingers, and some object which is chosen by the infant for handling. Gradually there is a use of objects which are not part of the infant nor are they part of the mother.

Another kind of transition has to do with the changeover from an object which is subjective for the infant to one which is objectively perceived or external. At first whatever object gains a relationship with the infant is created by the infant, or at least that is the theory of it to which I adhere. It is like an hallucination. Some cheating takes place and an object that is ready to hand overlaps with an hallucination. Obviously the way the mother or her substitute behaves is of paramount importance here. One mother is good and another bad at letting a real object be just where the infant is hallucinating an object so that in fact the infant gains the illusion that the world can be created and that what is created is the world.

At this point you will think of Mme Sechehaye's term "symbolic realisation,"[1] the making real of the symbol, only from our point of view dealing with earliest infancy, we are thinking of the making real of the hallucination. This does in fact initiate the infant's capacity for using symbols, and where growth is straightforward the transitional

1. M. A. Sechehaye, *Symbolic Realization* (New York: International Universities Press, 1951).

object is the first symbol. Here the symbol is at the same time both the hallucination and an objectively perceived part of external reality.

From all this it will be seen that we are describing the life of an infant which means also the relationship of the environment through the mother or her substitute to the infant. We are talking about a "nursing couple," to use Merrill Middlemore's term.[2] We are referring to the fact that there is no such thing as an infant because when we see an infant at this early stage we know that we will find infant-care with the infant as part of that infant-care.

This way of stating the meaning of the transitional object makes it necessary for us to use the word "illusion." The mother is enabling the infant to have the illusion that objects in external reality can be real to the infant, that is to say they can be hallucinations since it is only hallucinations that feel real. If an external object is to seem real then the relationship to it must be that of the relationship to an hallucination. As you will readily agree, this goes bang into an ancient philosophical conundrum, and you will be thinking of the two limericks, one of them by Ronald Knox:

> Do the stone and the tree
> Continue to be
> When there's no-one about in the quad?

and the reply:

> The stone and the tree
> Do continue to be
> As observed by yours faithfully, . . .

The fact is that an external object has no being for you or me except in so far as you or I hallucinate it, but being sane we take care not to hallucinate except where we know what to see. Of course when we are tired or it is twilight we may make a few mistakes. The infant with a transitional object is in my opinion all the time in this state in which we allow him or her to be and although it is mad we do not call it mad. If the infant could speak the claim would be: "This object is part of external reality and I created it." If you or I said that we would be locked up or perhaps leucotomised. This gives us a meaning for the word "omnipotence" which we really need because when we talk about the omnipotence of early infancy we do not only mean omnipotence of thought; we intend to indicate that the infant believes

2. M. P. Middlemore, *The Nursing Couple* (London: Hamish Hamilton, 1941).

in an omnipotence which extends to certain objects and perhaps extends to cover the mother and some of the others in the immediate environment. One transition is from omnipotent control of external objects to the relinquishment of control and eventually to the acknowledgement that there are phenomena outside one's personal control. The transitional object that is both part of the infant and part of the mother acquires the new status called "possession."

There are other transitions which I think are in process during the period of time in which the infant uses transitional objects. For instance, there is that which belongs to the developing powers of the infant, developing co-ordination, and a gradual enrichment of sensibility. The sense of smell is at its highest and probably will never be so high again, except perhaps during psychotic episodes. Texture means as much as it can ever mean, and dryness and dampness and also what feels cold and what feels warm; these things have tremendous meaning.

Alongside this one has to mention the extreme sensitivity of the infantile lips and no doubt of the sense of taste. The word "disgusting" has not come to mean anything yet for the infant and at the beginning the infant has not even become concerned with excretions. The dribbling and drooling that characterises early infancy covers the object and reminds one of the lion in the cage at the zoo, who almost seems to soften up the bone with saliva before eventually bringing its existence to an end by biting it up and eating it. How easy to imagine the lion with very tender caressing feelings towards the bone which is just going to be destroyed. So in transitional phenomena we see the initiation of the capacity for affectionate feelings, with the instinctual direct relationship sinking into primary repression.

In this way we can see that the infant's use of an object can be in one way or another joined up with body functioning, and indeed one cannot imagine that an object can have meaning for an infant unless it is so joined. This is another way of stating that the ego is based on a body ego.

I have given some examples just to remind you of all sorts of possibilities which exist and which are illustrated in the case of your own children as well as the children who are your clients. Sometimes we find the mother used as if she herself were a transitional object, and this may persist and give rise to great trouble; for instance, a patient that I have had to deal with recently used the lobe of his mother's ear. You will guess that in these cases where the mother is used, there is almost certainly something in the mother—an unconscious need of her child—into the pattern of which the child is fitting himself or herself.

Then there is the use of the thumb or fingers which may persist and there may or may not be an affectionate caressing of some part of the face or some part of the mother or of an object going on at the same time. In some cases the caressing continues and the thumb- or finger-sucking is lost sight of. Then it often happens that an infant who did not use the hand or thumb for autoerotic gratification nevertheless may use an object of some kind or other. Where an object is employed one usually finds an extension of interest so that soon other objects become important. For some reason or other girls tend to persist with soft objects until they use dolls, and boys tend to go more quickly over to an adoption of hard objects. One could perhaps better say that the boy in children goes over to hard objects and the girl in children of both sexes tends to retain the interest in softness and in texture, and this may join eventually on to the maternal identification. Often where there is a clear-cut transitional object dating from early times this persists although in fact the child is employed more in using the next and less important objects; perhaps at times of great distress, sadness or deprivation there is a return to the original or to the thumb or a loss altogether of the capacity to use symbols and substitutes at all.

I want to leave it at that. There is an infinite variety in the clinical picture, and all we can talk about usefully is the theoretical implications.

The Passing of the Transitional Object

There are two approaches to this subject:

A. Old soldiers never die, they simply fade away. The transitional object tends to be relegated to the limbo of half-forgotten things at the bottom of the chest of drawers, or at the back of the toy cupboard. It is usual, however, for the child to know. For example, a boy who has forgotten his transitional object has a regression phase following a deprivation. He goes back to his transitional object. There is then a gradual return to the other later-acquired possessions. So the transitional object may be

   i. supplanted but kept

   ii. worn out

iii. given away (not satisfactory)
iv. kept by mother—relic of a precious time in her life (identification)
v. etc.

This refers to the fate of the object itself.

B. I come now to the main point that I want to put forward for discussion. This is not a new idea although I believe it was new when I described it in my original paper. (I fear now that I come to it that you will feel it is too obvious, unless of course you disagree.)

If it is true that the transitional object and the transitional phenomena are at the very basis of symbolism, then I think we may fairly claim that these phenomena mark the origin in the life of the infant and child of a sort of third area of existing, a third area which I think has been difficult to fit into psycho-analytic theory which has had to build up gradually according to the stone-by-stone method of a science.

This third area might turn out to be the cultural life of the individual.

What are the three areas? One, the fundamental one, is the individual psychic or inner reality, the unconscious if you like (not the repressed unconscious which comes very soon but definitely later). The personal psychic reality is that from which the individual "hallucinates" or "creates" or "thinks up" or "conceives of." From it dreams are made, though they are clothed in the materials gathered in from external reality.

The second area is external reality, the world that is gradually recognised as NOT-ME by the healthy developing infant who has established a self, with a limiting membrane and an inside and an outside. The expanding universe which man contracts out of, so to speak.

Now infants and children and adults take external reality in, as clothing for their dreams, and they project themselves into external objects and people and enrich external reality by their imaginative perceptions.

But I think we really do find a third area, an area of living which corresponds to the infant's transitional phenomena and which actually derives from them. In so far as the infant has not achieved transitional phenomena I think the acceptance of symbols is deficient, and the cultural life is poverty-stricken.

No doubt you easily see what I mean. Put rather crudely: we go to a concert and I hear a late Beethoven string quartet (you see I'm highbrow). This quartet is not just an external fact produced by Beethoven and played by the musicians; and it is not my dream, which as a matter of fact would not have been so good. The experience, coupled with my preparation of myself for it, enables me to create a glorious fact. I enjoy it because I say I created it, I hallucinated it, and it is real and would have been there even if I had been neither conceived of nor conceived.

This is mad. But in our cultural life we accept the madness, exactly as we accept the madness of the infant who claims (though in unuttered mutterings) "I hallucinated that and it is part of mother who was there before I came along."

From this you will see why I think the transitional object is essentially different from the internal object of Melanie Klein's terminology. The internal object is a matter of the inner reality, which becomes more and more complex with every moment of the infant's life. The transitional object is for us a bit of the blanket but for the infant a representative both of the mother's breast, say, and of the internalised mother's breast.

Watch the sequence when the mother is absent. The infant clings to the transitional object. After a length of time the internalised mother fades, and then the transitional object ceases to mean anything. In other words the transitional object is symbolical of the internal object which is kept alive by the alive mother's presence.

In the same way, perhaps, an adult may mourn someone, and in the course of mourning cease to enjoy cultural pursuits; recovery from mourning is accompanied by a return of all the intermediate interests (including the religious experiences) which enrich the individual's life in health.

In this way I feel that transitional phenomena do not pass, at least not in health. They may become a lost art, but this is part of an illness in the patient, a depression, and something equivalent to the reaction to deprivation in infancy, when the transitional object and transitional phenomena are temporarily (or sometimes permanently) meaningless or non-existent.

I would very much like to hear your reactions to this idea of a third area of experiencing, its relation to the cultural life, and its suggested derivation from the transitional phenomena of infancy.

12
Notes on Play

Undated[1]

I

The characteristic of play is pleasure
Observations of animal young including human young

II

Satisfaction in play depends on the use of symbols, although, at base, the drive comes from instinct.
Symbols: This stands for that.
            If *that* is loved *this* can be used and enjoyed.
            If *that* is hated *this* can be knocked over, hurt, killed etc.,
            and restored, and hurt again.
That is: the capacity to play is an *achievement* in the emotional development of every human child.

III

Play as an achievement in individual emotional growth
   A. The tendency that is inherited that propels the child onwards and (owing to the extreme dependence of the human infant)
   B. The provision in the environment for conditions that meet the infant's and small child's needs, so that development is not interrupted by reactions to impingement (cold, heat, bad holding, faulty handling, starvation, etc.),
      and
   C. Play starts as a symbol of the infant's and the small child's trust in the mother (or substitute mother).

1. These handwritten notes were found in D.W.W.'s "Ideas" file. It is likely that they date from before the late 1960s, when it became his custom to use the verbal noun "playing" rather than (as mostly here) "play."—EDS.

IV

Play is an *imaginative elaboration* around bodily functions, relating to objects, and anxiety.

Gradually as the child becomes more complex as a personality, with a personal or inner reality, play becomes an expression in terms of external materials of inner relationships and anxieties. This leads on to the idea of play as an expression of identifications with persons, animals and objects of the inanimate environment.

V

Play is primarily a *creative activity* (as in dream) performed
    1. in terms of the actual (own body and objects at hand)
    2. under conditions in which the child is confident in someone, or has become confident generally through adequate experience of good care.

By contrast, inadequate care, producing lack of trust, makes the capacity to play diminish.

VI

Products of play

Besides the essential element which is pleasure, play gives the child practice in
    a. manipulation of objects
    b. management of power of co-ordination, skills, judgements etc.
    c. control over a limited area. While the child finds limited power to control he or she at the same time discovers the unlimited scope of the imagination.

Through play the child deals with external reality creatively. In the end this produces creative living, and leads to the capacity to feel real and to feel life can be used and enriched. Without play the child is unable to see the world creatively, and in consequence is thrown back on compliance and a sense of futility, or on the exploitation of direct instinctual satisfactions.

Especially in the management of aggression and destructiveness has play a vital function when a child has the capacity to enjoy manipulation of symbols. In play an object can be

destroyed and restored
hurt and mended
dirtied and cleaned
killed and brought alive
with the added achievement of ambivalence in place of splitting the object (and self) into good and bad.

VII

Developments of the capacity for playing (socialisation)
From playing comes
a. playing along with others with gains in the exercise of
b. playing according to rules: child's own, other's rules, shared regulations
c. playing games with rules and regulations pre-arranged
d. allowing for complexities in terms of leader and led.

VIII

Psychopathology of play
A. The *loss of the capacity* associated with lack of trust, anxiety associated with insecurity
B. *Stereotypy* in play patterns (anxiety re free fantasy)
C. Flight into *daydreaming* (a manipulated state halfway between true dream and play)
D. *Sensualisation*—instinct appearing in crude form along with failure of symbolisation
E. *Domination*—one child only able to play his own game but involving other children who must comply
F. *Failure to play a game* (restless, deprived children) unless dominated by strict rules and a games-officer
G. Flight to *physical exercise* from calisthenics right up to a need to be drilled, if to avoid inertia

IX

Relation to masturbation in adolescence
At this age phase there can be a thin line between physical masturbation with fantasy unconscious and the compulsive acting out of

masturbation fantasy as part of an attempt (largely unconscious) to cope with conflict or guilt over actual masturbation.

x

Towards adolescence

Play helps during this phase of indeterminate sex because in acting and dressing up there is infinite scope for cross-identifications—legitimate transvestism.

Also—expressed in character types

tomboy (girl)	pash
maternal type or hero-worship (boy)	homosexual involvement

XI

Adolescence (early)

Instinctual tensions become intense, so that play capacity may be lost, and compulsive masturbation (especially in boys) be substituted.

In this phase especially is there a liability for the compulsive acting out of masturbation fantasy to displace play.

In public school culture games are typically exploited to distract boys from the conflicts arising out of sexual tensions and masturbation compulsion. With girls this ruse is not so successful as it works only with girls who are male-identified. Woman-identified girls are relatively uncatered for in social provision, and they go through periods of intense depression (say at fourteen) perhaps unsuccessfully competing against the career girls who seem to be generally accepted and successful.

In the case of boys who are maternal in the quality of their typical identifications, there is considerable suffering to be expected where the local culture expects games and exploits to do instead of a personal life. Those who protest are clinical failures at this age and they have a struggle to gain social recognition; to compensate they band together in groups that isolate them from society.

XII

Adolescence

Characteristic of play in adolescence is the fact that the "toys" are world affairs.

1. They "play" with world politics, and feel intensely, and shame the adults by really minding   or

2. they "play" at fathers and mothers in the sense of having love affairs and perhaps marrying and having children   or

3. they "play" at imaginative construction, by becoming or learning to become artists, musicians, philosophers, architects, religious enthusiasts, etc.   or

4. they "play" at games by becoming professionals or competing for world championships   or

5. they "play" at war by going and fighting, or doing things that involve them in real risk. If delinquent they "play" at robbers by being robbers   or

6. they fail to play having lost the capacity and so get thrown back on

    i. paralysis (introversion or schizoid non-living) including bed, drugs, outbursts of mania or suicidal impulses

    ii. the exploitation of instinct and fantasy-free activity (at best this is the extrovert life).

13

Psycho-Neurosis in Childhood

*A paper given to the Scandinavian Orthopsychiatric
Congress, Helsinki, 8 September 1961*

Originally the title of my talk was given out as "The Neurotic Child."
We thought, however, that these words, at any rate in the English
language, are popular rather than diagnostic terminology. In fact, so-
called neurotic children are often, in an analytic treatment, found to
be in part psychotic. A psychotic element is hidden in the neurotic
child, and it can be this psychotic element that must be reached and
treated if the clinical state of the child is to be mended.

To make my task a little easier we decided to alter the title to "Psycho-Neurosis in Childhood." In this way I am to try to give you a
statement of something that is different from psychosis. There remains one difficulty, however, in that there are two possible ways of
dealing with even this simplified title. Shall I talk about the origins of
psycho-neurosis, origins which are always to be found in the childhood of the individual under study, or shall I talk about the clinical
state of children who are themselves, at the time, during childhood,
psycho-neurotic? I think I shall not try to be too careful about this
dilemma.

I am therefore describing psycho-neurosis and distinguishing it
from other psychiatric states. Of course, in psychiatry there are no
clear borderlines between clinical states, but in order to get anywhere
at all we need to pretend that borderlines exist. The main alternative
to psycho-neurosis is psychosis. Let us say that in psychosis there is a
disorder involving the structure of the personality. The patient can be
shown to be disintegrated, or unreal, or out of touch with his or her
own body, or with what we as observers call external reality. The
psychotic's troubles are of this order. By contrast, in psycho-neurosis
the patient exists as a person, is a whole person, recognising objects
as whole; the patient is well lodged in his or her own body, and the
capacity for object relationships is well established. From this vantage
point the patient is in difficulties, and these difficulties arise from the
conflicts that result from the experience of object relationships. Nat-

urally, the most severe conflicts arise in connection with the instinctual life, that is, the various excitements with bodily accompaniment that have as their source the body's capacity for getting excited—generally and locally.

Here then we have two sets of children, those whose earliest stages of development have been satisfactory, and who have troubles that we call psycho-neurotic, and those whose earliest stages of development are incomplete and the incompleteness dominates the clinical picture. So the thing about psycho-neurosis is that it is a disorder of those children who are healthy enough not to be psychotic.

Of course, this division of clinical states into two is much too simple. There are three complications which I must mention if you are to be satisfied with what I say.

1. Somewhere between psychosis and psycho-neurosis comes depression. In depression the personality structure is relatively well established. We can deal with this complication by saying that there are depressions that are rather psychotic, with such things as depersonalisation states as part of the picture, and there are depressions that are practically psycho-neuroses. In either case the patient is in difficulties over the destructive impulses and ideas that go with the experience of object relationships; I mean the experience of object relationships that have excitements to them, that is to say, that are more vital and intense than feelings that can be described by words like affectionate, and that include climax or orgasm.

2. The second complication comes from the fact that in some patients there is a persecutory expectation, and this may date from even very early infancy.

3. The third complication has to do with the state that is sometimes referred to by the word "psychopathy." I mean, children with an antisocial tendency deserve a classification all to themselves, because they may be essentially normal or psycho-neurotic or depressive or psychotic. The fact is that their symptomatology is to be thought of in terms of nuisance value. The antisocial tendency represents the S.O.S. or *cri de coeur* of the child who has been at some stage or other deprived, deprived of the environmental provision which was appropriate at the age at which it failed. The deprivation altered the child's life; it caused intolerable distress, and the child is right in crying out for recognition of the fact that "things were all right, and then they weren't all right," and this was an external factor outside the child's control.

Such a child is engaged in trying to get back through the deprivation, and back through the intolerable distress to the state that existed before the deprivation, when things weren't too bad. We cannot classify this state, that may lead on to delinquency or to recidivism, along with the other states that we label with the words psychosis, depression and psycho-neurosis.

You will, I hope, agree that first I had to lay out the psychiatric map in this way so that I might pursue my thesis that psycho-neurosis is a state of children (or adults) who in their emotional development have reached a state of relative mental health. Having been brought through the earliest stages that belong to extreme dependence, and having come through the rather later stages in which deprivation traumatises, these individuals are now in a position to have *their very own difficulties*. These difficulties belong essentially to life and to interpersonal relationships, and on the whole people do not resent these difficulties because they are their own, that is, are not the result of environmental failures or of neglect.

Looked at in this way psycho-neurosis takes on a form, and can be described with considerable clarity. I would say that Anna Freud's *The Ego and the Mechanisms of Defence*[1] gives a good picture, and probably you all know this book.

You might be wondering what ages I am thinking about when I speak of the origins of psychosis and of psycho-neurosis. In regard to psychosis I think of earliest infancy as the stage of extreme dependence, when it scarcely makes sense in psychology to speak of an infant, because the mother's presence and attitude are so vital a part of what could be called the infant potential in process of becoming infant.

I think of later infancy, while dependence is becoming less severe, when I refer to the origins of depressive anxieties. I think of the period (roughly 10 months to 2–3 years) when I refer to the age at which deprivation leads to the setting up of an antisocial tendency, and here I am agreeing with John Bowlby whose work you all know. Then, when I come to the place where psycho-neurosis appears I refer to the toddler age, to the time when the little child in the family is working up to the full blast of the Oedipus complex. That is, if he or she is healthy enough to get there.

But I don't want you to pin me down too precisely to these ages. We are talking of stages rather than of ages. The stages of infancy and dependence reappear and so do all the later stages, so that there is no

1. London: Hogarth Press, 1937.

age corresponding exactly to a stage, and at puberty much has to be re-enacted, if the boy or girl is to carry forward the early development into adult life.

Here we are then at the age of 3–4–5 years. The boy or girl has developed well, and in play and in dream is capable of identification with either parent, and along with the play or the dream there is the instinctual life and the bodily excitements. We take for granted a satisfactory development of the use of symbols. Much of the child's life remains unconscious, but as the child becomes more and more self-conscious so the distinction between what is conscious and what is unconscious becomes more distinct. The unconscious life, or the child's psychic reality, appears mainly through symbolic representation.

We now have to make a general statement about children of toddler age, and we will refer to children living at home in good homes.

You see, this is the age at which, in health, psycho-neurosis is becoming established, and is forming its pattern. If we analyse patients of any age we find the origins of psycho-neurosis at this the 2–3–4–5 period. What happens, though, if we look directly at the toddler himself or herself?

We must say clearly that the healthy toddler has every possible kind of psycho-neurotic symptom. (Let's take a boy, so that I don't have to keep on saying he or she.) He is vital and physically active, and also he goes white and limp, so that his mother thinks the life has gone out of him. He is kind and sweet and also cruel to the cat, and to insects he may be like the worst of the world's torturers. He is affectionate and also he hurts, he kicks his mother's belly if it seems to be getting big, he tells his father to go away, or perhaps he joins up with father and despises women. He has temper tantrums, which can be awkward in the middle of the High Street; he has nightmares, and when his mother comes to console him he says: "go away you witch, I want my mother." He is afraid of this and that, although very brave or too brave. He is highly suspicious of food that has a hair in it, or that is the wrong colour, or that is not cooked by his mother—or perhaps he refuses food at home, and eats voraciously with his aunt or grandmother.

It is quite likely that there are all sorts of imaginary people or animals in the corridor of the flat, or there are imaginary children that have to be laid for at dinner table. It's easier to accept these delusions than to reach out for sanity.

Every now and again the child tells you he loves you, or makes a spontaneous gesture that indicates as much. A mixture of everything.

At this stage of development the child is in process of working out a relationship between the dream potential or the total imaginative life with the available environmental reliability. For instance, if father will be there at breakfast (I refer to England) then it is safe to dream that father got run over, or to have a dream in which in symbolic form the burglar shoots the rich lady's husband in order to get at her jewel box. If father is not present such a dream is too frightening, and leads to a guilt feeling or a depressed mood. And so on.

I must now try to state what is happening.

Even in the most satisfactory environment possible the child has impulses, ideas and dreams in which there is intolerable conflict: conflict between love and hate, between the wish to preserve and the wish to destroy; and in a more sophisticated way, between the heterosexual and the homosexual positions in parent-identification. Such anxieties are to be expected; they are part of the story and imply that the child is alive.

However, the child finds certain aspects of the anxieties intolerable, and so begins to set up defences. These defences organise and we then speak of psycho-neurosis. Psycho-neurosis is the organisation of defences against anxiety of the kind I am describing.

Of course the child may regress to infantile dependence and to infantile patterns, may lose the phallic and genital qualities that have become a feature in the fantasy and play going with excitement, and may go back to oral or to alimentary tract existence, or even to a loss of the early attainments of integration, and of having a capacity for object relationships; or may even lose some of the close contact that has developed between his psyche and his body. We would not then speak here of psycho-neurosis.

Keeping strictly to our subject we say that in psycho-neurosis the child loses none of the early integrative development, but defends against anxiety by one of several ways, ways that Miss Freud describes with clarity in the book to which I have referred.

First there is repression—a special kind of unconscious develops, the repressed unconscious. Much of the life of the toddler age goes under repression, and becomes unconscious. The repressed unconscious is of course a nuisance because repression is expensive in terms of energy, and also what is repressed is always liable to turn up in some form or other, in a dream, or perhaps projected on to outside phenomena. Nevertheless the gain is to be measured in terms of the child's lessened liability to clinical or manifest anxiety. A special aspect of repression is inhibition of the impulse, a loss of some of the instinctual drive in the relating to objects. This amounts to serious impoverishment of the child's living experience.

Secondly, repressed fantasy may appear and give trouble in the form of psycho-somatic disorder, so-called conversion symptoms, whose fantasy content is lost; or in hypochondriacal anxieties about parts of the body, or of the soul; and there is no solution to such symptomatology except by recovery of the lost fantasy content.[2]

Thirdly, there become organised certain phobias. For instance, fear of wolves, or of rats if these are nearer home. Such a phobia may do very well to safeguard a child against sibling rivalry, for instance, and the fear of the hated siblings.

Fourthly, an obsessional tendency may be organised to deal with confusion and to prevent the dangerous return of the destructive impulse. In perfectionism a hate of the world that would turn it upside down is dealt with in advance. This is a poor substitute for the sequence of health—(1) destructive impulse and idea, (2) sense of guilt, (3) reparation or constructive activity—but for the neurotic it has to serve.

You may be able to add to this list several more types of psycho-neurotic pattern-formation. In each case the pattern of the defences is against anxiety at the Oedipus complex level, and is determined to some extent by the character of the environment, but the drive to psycho-neurotic symptom formation comes from the essential conflicts in the individual between love and hate, conflicts that indicate healthy emotional development in the sense of ego structuring and ego strength, and that also indicate a failure of the ego to tolerate the consequences of id or instinct tensions.

And the main defence is repression. This is the reason why psycho-analysis in its classical form is a treatment dealing with patients who are ego-healthy to the extent that they have dealt with ambivalence by means of repression and without a break-up of ego structure; and the main work of the analysis of the patient with psycho-neurotic

---

2. It occurs to me that I may be using the word "fantasy" in a way that is not familiar to some of you. I am not talking about fantasying, or about contrived fantasy. I am thinking of the whole of the child's personal or psychic reality, some of it conscious, but mostly unconscious, and including that which is not verbalised or pictured or heard in a structural way because it is primitive and near the almost physiological roots from which it springs.— D.W.W.

symptoms consists in the bringing of the repressed unconscious into consciousness. This is done through the day-by-day interpretation of the relationship of the patient to the analyst, as this relationship gradually evolves, and in evolving reveals the pattern of the patient's own history at the level of the Oedipus complex, and at the 2–3–4 age.

What part is played in these matters by the environment? I have indicated the vital part played at the beginning at the stage of very great dependence, I have referred to the special period during which the small child can easily be turned into a deprived child, and in several ways I have shown, I hope, that at the stage of the Oedipus complex it is *immensely valuable* if the child can be going on living in a settled home environment so that it is safe to play and to dream, and so that the impulse to be loving can be made into an effective gesture at the appropriate moment.

The environment is something that we take for granted. A child in an institution has a different task at this the stage of the first triangular relationships from that which the child has who is living in his or her own home with his or her own parents and siblings. Also the good home absorbs much difficulty which becomes only too apparent when the home breaks or when the home is disturbed by illness, especially psychiatric abnormalities in the parents. Nevertheless, if I keep strictly to my point, which is the study of psycho-neurosis, it is necessary for me to emphasise that it is just here and exactly here that we are dealing with the *internal* strains and stresses, the conflicts, chiefly unconscious and belonging to the realms of the individual's personal psychic reality.

The patient who is suffering from psycho-neurosis wants personal help of the kind that makes possible the lessening of the forces of repression, and the freeing of personal energy for unpremeditated impulse.

Psycho-neurotic illness can be measured according to the rigidity of the defences, defences against anxiety belonging to the real and imaginary experience of triangular relationships, as between whole persons.

You will see that the environment comes into the picture of psycho-neurosis in partly determining the nature of the defence pattern. Psycho-neurosis does not find its aetiology, however, in the environmental condition, but in the personal conflicts that belong specifically to the individual. By contrast, the antisocial child is quite clearly antisocial as a result of a deprivation. Also, to our surprise, we find that in the aetiology of the most severe psychiatric disorder, schizophrenia, a failure of care in the earliest phase of absolute dependence of infancy is even more important than the hereditary factor.

In practice this view of psycho-neurosis is made obscure by the fact that we do not commonly find patients who are, so to speak, "pure" psycho-neurosis cases. Moreover, as Melanie Klein showed us,[3] the origin of the child's failure to avoid psycho-neurotic defence organisations lies in developmental failures at earlier stages. But this must not muddle us up. We have to talk as if illnesses were either psycho-neuroses, affective disorders, or psychoses, or the anti-social tendency, in order to sort ourselves out.

The question arises, what is normality? Well—we can say that in health the individual has been able to organise his or her defences against the intolerable conflicts of the personal psychic reality—but in contrast to the person ill with psycho-neurosis the healthy person is relatively free from massive repression and inhibition of instinct. Also in health the individual can employ all manner of defences, and can shift round from one kind to another, and in fact he or she does not display that rigidity of defence organisation which characterises the ill person.

Having said all this I want to suggest that *clinically* the really healthy individual is nearer to depression and to madness than to psycho-neurosis. Psycho-neurosis is boring. It is a relief when an individual is able to be mad and to be serious and to enjoy the relief afforded by a sense of humour, and to be able, so to speak, to flirt with the psychoses. Through modern art we experience the undoing of the processes that constitute sanity and psycho-neurotic defence organisations, and the safety-first principle.

Let me add a word about the vast subject of adolescence. In the period of adolescence, puberty threatens and then develops and dominates the scene. A description of the adolescent would be rather like a description of the child of 2–3–4–5—a collection of self-contradicting tendencies. Because of the gradual maturing of the instincts the adolescent is for a few years in a state of *not accepting false solutions*. This brings about our difficulty in dealing with adolescents, the fact

3. "The Oedipus Complex in the Light of Early Anxieties" (1945), in Melanie Klein, *Contributions to Psycho-Analysis, 1921–1945* (London: Hogarth Press, 1948).

that we have to tolerate their refusal to find a way out of doubt and dilemma. The only solution to adolescence is the maturation that time will bring so that adolescence turns into adulthood.

So psycho-neurosis comes into the picture of adolescence as a threat of false solutions, false solutions coming from within the individual, inhibitions, obsessional rituals, phobias and conversion symptoms, defences against anxiety associated with the instinctual life that now threatens in a new way. It is part of the worldwide adolescence problem at the present time that we have to watch each child stoutly defending his or her right *not to find a false solution,* either in psycho-neurosis or through acceptance of the various kinds of help that we helplessly offer.

Psycho-neurosis persisting in adult life is clearly seen and felt as a nuisance and as an abnormality, and the only thing I need say here about adult psycho-neurosis is that its aetiology belongs to the individual's 2–5-year period of childhood, to the period of the first establishment of interpersonal relationships, and to the development of a capacity in the child for making an identification with the parents in their instinctual lives.

14
Further Remarks on the Theory of the Parent-Infant Relationship

Part of a discussion of papers by Phyllis Greenacre and Winnicott which took place at the Twenty-Second International Psycho-Analytic Congress, Edinburgh, 1961[1]

I have looked forward with excitement to the discussion of these two papers and of the vast subject that they introduce.

It is, of course, important to me that there is a measure of agreement between Dr Greenacre and myself. For instance, we both assume the innate maturational processes of the infant, and we see these in a setting of dependence. I shall not go further, at the moment, into Dr Greenacre's contribution. She has developed in a most interesting way the theme of the maturational processes, and I have chosen out of this huge subject to deal with the subject of dependence.

In regard to my own contribution it interests me that this subject is not psycho-analysis—it is: "psycho-analysts discussing something which is very important to them." When we are seeing mothers and babies in an infant welfare clinic some of the babies that we see are already ill in the sense that when they grow up they will not be accepted for treatment by a classical psycho-analysis. They may be, of course, physically quite healthy. Perhaps the problem, as I am putting it in my limited way, is: Is an infant a phenomenon that can be isolated, at least hypothetically, for observation and conceptualisation? And I am suggesting that the answer is no. When we look back through our analyses of children and adults we tend to see mecha-

---

1. The two papers discussed at the conference are to be found in the *International Journal of Psycho-Analysis* 41 (1960). Winnicott's paper also appears under the title "The Theory of the Parent-Infant Relationship" in *The Maturational Processes and the Facilitating Environment* (London: Hogarth Press; New York: International Universities Press, 1965). The discussion from which these remarks are extracted contains comments by Greenacre and many other analysts, and ends with a reply by Winnicott not published here; it can be found in the *International Journal of Psycho-Analysis* 43 (1962).

nisms rather than infants. But if we look at an infant we see an infant in care. The processes of integration, and of separating out, of getting to live in the body and of relating to objects, these are all matters of maturation and achievement. Conversely, the state of not being separated, of not being integrated, of not being related to body functions, of not being related to objects, this state is very real; we must believe in these states that belong to immaturity. The problem is: How does the infant survive such conditions?

In preparing this paper I find I reached a deeper understanding than I had before of the parental function in terms of this problem, of the way infants survive immaturity. I have seen more clearly than I did that in introducing the world to the child in small doses, that is to say in her adaptation to the ego-needs of her infant, the mother gives time for the development of the extensions to the infant's powers that come with maturation. In a discussion like this one, in which the state of dependence of the infant must be given an important place, we do indeed need to come to terms with the paradoxical. For instance, the baby knows only how to allow, or to disallow, the parental union that produced his own conception. The baby does not at first know how to let parental intercourse precede his existence. But the infant's body-scheme eventually comes to include everything. In a good enough environment the infant gradually begins to find ways of including not-me objects and not-me phenomena in his own body-scheme and therefore to avoid narcissistic wounds. If steady growth is facilitated, then omnipotence and omniscience are retained, *along with* an intellectual acceptance of the reality-principle. In a psycho-analytic statement of theory we say that defences are formed in relation to anxiety. Watching a living infant we say that the infant experiences intolerable anxiety with recovery through the organisation of defences. From this it follows that the successful outcome of an analysis depends, not on the patient's understanding of the meaning of the defences, but on the patient's ability, through the analysis, and in the transference, *to re-experience this intolerable anxiety* on account of which defences were organised.

In a so-called borderline case there has to be discovered not only intolerable anxiety but also the actual clinical breakdown of infancy, the overstretch of omnipotence, the annihilation that constituted the narcissistic wound. All this gives, for me, a vivid colouring to our picture of the parent-infant relationship, and to our view of the actual care of an infant. The word "love" is not sufficiently specific. And the word "separation" is crude for our use. All along, according to the age and the maturational stage of the infant, the parent is engaged in preventing clinical breakdown from which recovery occurs only through organisation and reorganisation of defences. It is by minute-to-minute care that the parent is laying down the basis of the future mental health of the infant. And this is the tremendous parental task. Its size is reflected in the length of a psycho-analytic treatment, and in the duration of mental illness, even when the patient is given the best possible mental nursing. And on the whole, parents have always tended to succeed in this, their essential, tremendous task, the reason being that for this purpose what they need to be is themselves, and to be and do exactly what they like being and doing; and by doing just this they save their children from jerky reorganisations of defences, and from the clinical distress that lies behind each of these reorganisations.

In the psycho-analysis of the case well chosen for classical analysis the clinical distress comes in the form of anxiety, associated with memories and dreams and phantasies. But as analysts we get involved in the treatment of patients whose *actual clinical breakdowns of infancy* must be remembered by being re-lived in the transference. In all cases relief comes only through a reviving of the original intolerable anxiety or the original mental breakdown. The breakdown is associated with an environmental factor that could not at the time be gathered into the area of the infant's omnipotence, as I put it. The infant knows no external factor, good or bad, and suffers a threat of annihilation. In a successful treatment the patient becomes able to stage the trauma or environmental failure and to experience it within the area of personal omnipotence, and so with a diminished narcissistic wound. Thus it is that as analysts we repeatedly become involved in the role of failure, and it is not easy for us to accept this role unless we see its positive value. We get made into parents who fail, and only so do we succeed as therapists. This is just one more example of the multiple paradox of the parent-infant relationship.

I like to remind myself that when their children are ill, and when things are not going well, we can tell them how to behave as therapists. But, by contrast, we cannot tell parents how to behave as parents if all goes well. If all goes well it just happens. What we can do then is to study what is happening, and properly to evaluate this parental function, and so to recognise and support it, and to see that it is not interfered with when it exists.

I thought I would not make a summary of my paper, but make this comment, and leave it at that.

15

A Note on a Case Involving Envy

Dated January 1963

This patient has had about three years' analysis with me after three previous treatments with other therapists, the whole lasting about twenty-five years. The end of the treatment is in sight although a date has not been arranged.

The patient lay on the couch as usual and said: "Well here's a day in which I don't know what is going to happen." Yesterday's hour was important because it was an hour without feelings. The patient then went on to describe with considerable feeling the behaviour of a colleague who often comes into the material presented. This colleague I will call Dr X. He happens to be a paediatrician who hates psychology. The patient described, accurately as far as I know, how Dr X is arrogant, self-satisfied, vain, self-confident, authoritative, etc. He said: "I envy him" and he was rather surprised about this because he himself is, as he said, lacking in confidence in himself and self-effacing and sensitive.

After he had spent some minutes expressing his feelings about this man, I interpreted that he was using Dr X in order to express feelings about me. In spite of having very considerable insight at this stage in his analysis, the patient had been unaware of this and yet he felt that I was making the right interpretation. He spent several minutes telling me how pleased he was that he was no longer doing his own analysis, that he could leave it to me. This had only recently become possible. He reminded me of the fact that he had only recently reached the position of being glad to find that I am more than a projection of his own capacities.

I further interpreted his hate of me for being the person to whom he lent all his own self-assurance and understanding. In the course of reacting to my interpretation in which he reiterated his feeling of relief in being able to leave the analysis to me, he went on to deal with his hate of me but interrupting this was the following episode. He said at this point: "My nose has got stuffy and I have got a pain in my belly and I am fighting the idea of going over to my coat to get the ephedrine bottle." In the coat he also has tablets for indigestion and other things. It is necessary in order to make this intelligible to report that in yesterday's session these things had been referred to as part of his hypochondria which is very much associated with his strongly developed maternal identification. This in turn has had to be freed from his far-reaching delusion which he has always had that he is truly female. The playing at being a woman of the female identification which is much more flexible had now come into the analysis and I had made the interpretation that his hypochondria was the precursor of the fantasy of impregnation.

Today I had to make use of the interruption in which he referred to these matters which took us back to the previous session. My interpretation was that in talking he was reaching towards his destruction of me as a male but on the way he found his hypochondria which was to do with the possibility of his being in love with me as a male. There is a great deal of history behind all this. Also in the early part of the hour the patient had described his own management of his daughter in which he was adopting a maternal role.

I continued with the interpretation that in his woman-identification and his search for a male which in his case had never taken him to open homosexual practice but had led him very near it, he had evidently been in search of the man that he wanted to castrate.

He was interested in this interpretation but was unable to feel it in great depth. We talked about the time factor in the reaction to interpretation which has to go along with that other thing which is the sifting of interpretations which can be wrong as well as right. I risked repeating the interpretation in terms of his father. I said that if he were now to find that his father had been strong and useful he would be so pleased to find this that he would not like the discovery that this is the father that he wishes to castrate because he is the potent father in the Oedipus triangle. For a time the patient felt this was rather good intellectual stuff but not acceptable deep down. He then said that the thing about Dr X is that he is arrogant and conceited and self-satisfied and that really the patient admires this, although it is exactly what he does not like in people. We then worked out together that it was necessary to state that Dr X had been brought in to boost the idea of the analyst's potency. Dr X was a young man and gave the impression of being potent and the patient feared that I was old and rather tired and feeble in potency so that I needed this boost. In order to get to his envy of me he had to make his analyst into a Dr X analyst. It was now evident that he admired the Dr X analyst and here was the basis for the maternal identification and the homosexual position and the hypochondria which was a potential pregnancy fantasy.

I now discovered that my earlier interpretation had produced in this patient a whole lot of secondary ideas to which he was reacting. These included the notion that he would have to go through a homosexual phase in relation to me, that is to say a new one ignoring the earlier examples of this in the analysis, and he was thoroughly bored at the prospect. I discovered this when I made the interpretation that he found it painful to feel love and the urge to castrate the Dr X analyst, the ambivalence here being crude. This made the patient report his idea that he would have to have a phase of homosexuality in the transference. He was now nearly able to accept the fact that he is looking for a potent Dr X analyst in order to find a father figure for castration, and that in flight from the conflict of this he would be liable to organise a homosexual phase. This threw considerable light on his behaviour pattern in adolescence and in early manhood and much of the material of his subsequent life in which he struggled to become heterosexual in order to get away from homosexuality. (Hopelessness about all this had led to the fullest possible exploitation of his fundamental delusion of being female which appears to have had a very early root in his emotional development.) In this way the patient's envy of me had many features. It belonged to the extreme pleasure which he has derived from at last handing over the analysis to someone who is not himself and getting the interpretations that he needs without having to tell the analyst what to say. Also the envy belongs to his having achieved in recent months a recognition of my existence as a separate person that he can use for the projection of his own analytic capacity, and his own maternal and paternal functioning, and his own intellectual powers. In relation to all this he hates me for being necessary and for being in his personal opinion the only person that he could have made use of in this way, at last coming to the surrender of all responsibility to me as his analyst.

To bring his envy to full pitch he had to give me the Dr X boost and then there was the trap into which he would have fallen without appropriate interpretations of avoiding the castration or hate by exploiting an intermediate area in which he was pleased to find the potent analyst and fall in love with him.

16
Perversions and Pregenital Fantasy

Unfinished paper written in 1963

The main aim of this paper is to point out the link that seems to exist between pregenital impregnation fantasy and the perversions.

A student once said to me, "Such-and-such a lecturer makes even the perversions dull." This struck me as very funny. The joke, such as it is, may serve to introduce a topic which is in some ways irksome, in that it brings us to discussion of everyday matters that do in fact involve everyone, and that are best left alone except where a scientific interest can be served.

The postulate is that whereas in genital maturity there is a direct relation between potency and impregnation, in immaturity there are innumerable fantasies that eventually become an idea of impregnation; moreover it is these pregenital fantasies that in health provide the imaginative fringe around the stark fact of the baby in the womb.

Out of this postulate arises the idea that in the immature individual there can be a persistence of pregenital impregnation fantasies, these having a symptomatic quality, and being exaggerated by a relative block in the developmental process; these are then to some extent substitutes for the real thing. Further, in male homosexuality these pregenital fixations become exploited because they are the nearest the male can get to pregnancy.

To some extent this is an idea that has been well stated in the literature, but it would seem that there is room for a further development of the theme. For instance, Klein pointed out that for full potency in the male—boy or man—there must be included the anxiety drive that is clearly described in what she called "the depressive position in emotional development."

On the female side, in so far as hypochondriacal anxieties dominate the picture, the interior of the body as opposed to the interior of the uterus is the place where the baby is expected to grow. The womb baby is a miracle and reassures the parents who expect a product of the inner world of contending objects and forces, or an anal baby that has to be cleaned up and taught to be human and to behave, or a lump of dead clay that has to be licked into shape and brought to life and kept alive. In this way we pass from normality to depression in our description of the parents.

17
Two Notes on the Use of Silence

Written in 1963

I

In this case I am not taking notes although I realise that my patient will one day wish that I had done so. I did make an attempt to keep notes in the early stages but I found that this interfered with my analysis of her by keeping the details over-emphasised in the conscious mind. In this way the unconscious or less conscious reaction became distorted.

Looking at the past two weeks I feel that a description might be valuable for reference at a later date and that the sort of things that happened illustrate the pattern of this analysis. Also the patient's reactions are less violent than they were at an earlier stage so that I can now even make mistakes or "blobs" as they are called in this treatment without a big risk that the patient will have a really serious reaction or seek another analyst.

The basis of the treatment at the present time is my silence. Last week I was absolutely silent the whole week except for a remark at the very beginning. This feels to the patient like something that she has achieved, getting me to be silent. There are many languages for describing this and one of them is that an interpretation is a male penis bursting across the field, the field being the breast with the infant unable to cope with the idea of a penis. The breast here is a field rather than an object for sucking or eating, and in the patient's associations it would be represented by a cushion rather than a source of food or of instinct gratification.

Last week was perhaps the most "successful" week in this respect of all weeks, and the patient was very appreciative of my playing this role, which she balances by a very close study that she is making of Henry James. In Henry James she finds a male analyst who deals in words and who has a very particular and comprehensive understanding but who is celibate.

This almost perfect week ended strangely. I had no idea of any trouble but on Monday the patient reported to me that what I had done at the end of the hour on Friday was very disturbing. In consequence all her old defences had returned in moderate degree over the weekend. It appears that as she got up to go there was a sound as if paper were bring crinkled. On Monday she was able to talk about this and her reaction to it but not until she had found ways of complaining about me which were less delusional. From my point of view it is quite clear that my perfect behaviour during the week is something that she cannot believe in and that at the end she had a delusion of some kind which indicated that I am extremely impatient in this role of not speaking. She says that by making me not speak she is turning me into a woman, castrating me, making me impotent, etc. etc., and she quite understands that I cannot stand this, and eventually she came to the idea that I am jealous of her when I give her what she needs because I never had it myself.

At another layer this noise meant to her that I had been masturbating, which was another evidence of my inability to stand doing nothing. The only reality basis for this delusion that I can discover would be that at the end of the hour I sometimes put my handkerchief in my pocket if I have had it in my hand. I am not sure, however, that anything at all took place which would form a reality basis for this delusion on this occasion.

On Monday I did say two things, and I said them not because I found it difficult to be silent but because I thought they ought to be said. She asked me to let her know what I was doing in the summer and next Christmas because of arrangements that had to be made, and she said that she thought she really wanted a reply. I meant to say: "I am not in a position to give you the answer that you require." What I said, however, was: "You want an answer here which I am not in a position to give." As I put it this way round she took it that I had rebuked her, telling her that she ought not to ask this sort of thing. Then again I made an interpretation when she said that she thought she might be able to stand just a little bit of an interpretation from me. I referred to a dream of the previous week and pointed out that a big solid object in amongst material which had to do with delicate tracery of one kind and another represented fact or external reality bursting in on fantasy. This is another version of the penis across the breast and of several other similar figures of speech. The trouble with this interpretation was that I was only repeating an interpretation that she had made herself. The patient now had two blobs which she could use and on the Tuesday she felt that she was in the same position that she had been in near the beginning of the analysis when she did not come back. She had studied my Ordinary Devoted Mother papers again and had underlined the relevant passages and she knew that I really do understand what she needs. "The only explanation can be," she said, "that you cannot do what you know is needed and that the whole thing is phony. The reason must be (she continued) that you can't stand being womanised or whatever silence means to you." And she had already stated that at the present time Henry James has all the male functioning and what she needs in the analysis is absolutely pure mothering. To meet this she is in the analytic session extremely regressed and dependent although able to function well most of the time in her work. Her private life at this stage is almost confined to very great activity in her own room and this includes reading and studying Henry James and his biography voraciously.

First of all I had to accept my position as someone who does not say anything. This was extremely difficult on Tuesday morning, not because I mind being silent but because I could see what was happening and there is nothing more difficult for an analyst to bear than the patient's delusional transference. The effect of this on me was that I got a tickling in the throat which, however, I was able to hide, and I recognised that if I had been able to speak three words the tickle would have gone. Not being able to talk has a curious effect in that it demands a listening which is different from my ordinary way of listening. To some extent I always listen with my throat, and my larynx follows the sounds that I hear in the world and particularly a voice of someone talking to me. This has always been characteristic of me and at one time was a serious symptom. After half an hour the patient said: "Now I feel quite different having said all that and I can stand your saying something; in fact I think I need it." The relief of this was great and I was quite clear that this was not because of my being silent; in fact I rather like it. The reason it was a relief to me was that I could then begin to do something about the patient's delusion, but of course I would not be able to do very much. In this sort of analysis it is essential to accept certain ideas about oneself which are untrue.

This permission to talk gave me a chance to interpret that the trouble was what happened at the end of Friday's session. This had very little basis in fact and it was easier for her to take the two blobs on Monday and talk about these as destroying the otherwise good analysis in which I am silent. I took a risk and said that the way I had put my information about the holiday did in fact make it look as if I was reproving her. Also there is not much point in making an interpretation which has already been made by the patient. These two things therefore had a reality basis as compared with which what happened at the end of Friday was tenuous and almost entirely dependent on her expectations. By the technique of silence I could have given conditions in which the patient herself would have solved the Friday problem. All she needed was time and opportunity without the "penis coming across the breast field." By this time the patient had almost returned to being able to believe in my silence as something that I could give because of her need. It has to be emphasised, however, that the patient retained a strong delusional idea that in fact I cannot stand being silent. Eventually she turned up with an interpretation of my inability to be silent in order to help me. This was that if I do something good for the patient I am jealous of the patient because nobody did that for me ever.

In the course of all this fortnight a very great deal has happened and I am quite confident about the technique of silence which I am very willing to employ except in so far as the patient cannot believe in it.

I do happen to know with a fair degree of certainty an interpretation which would be applicable to this whole phase. It is necessary, however, for me to wait for the patient to make this interpretation herself. As she has said: "With my history of an excitable father constantly breaking into whatever there was of mother-infant experience it is necessary for me to be able to reach the interpretations myself." It is of course compatible with this that there are moments when an interpretation is needed because of the fact that the patient needs something more than she has it in her to see. Nevertheless in this phase the patient is perfectly capable of reaching to the understanding which is needed and in fact has nearly reached this during the last week. I will make an attempt to state this interpretation:

The patient is at a very delicate point of transition from eating and being eaten, the latter being a talion reaction, and eating and being eaten in which this duality is simply an expression of the identification of infant and mother each with the other, or the lack of differentiation from the infant. The stage is represented in my writings which the patient has read in which a twelve-week infant feeds the mother with his finger while breast-feeding, and the patient has said that she feels like bringing me something to feed me with. I do, however, feel that she is trying to reach to the idea of being eaten by the mother and she feels that her own mother failed her in this area of experience. She did of course experience the fear of being eaten talionwise but the basis for this was lacking which is being eaten simply because whatever the infant feels the mother is also feeling.

II

Several problems are outstanding in a general way. Behind everything else is the problem that arises out of not speaking. I seldom make an interpretation and the analysis proceeds best on the basis of my saying nothing at all. This does, however, produce complications, because it becomes more and more evident that one of the purposes of interpreting is to establish the limits of the analyst's understanding. The basis for not interpreting and in fact not making any sound at all is the theoretical assumption that the analyst really does know what is going on. Probably up to the present I am able to say that I do know what is going on in this analysis and for this reason I continue with the policy of not speaking which is certainly what the patient asks of me. Within this framework there are two themes. More on the surface is the whole matter of triangular relationships as between whole people; the Oedipus complex, Electra, Cressida, etc. This theme started with "blond hair" etc. and it has included the idea of my being jealous of the patient's sexual relationship with men and also the idea of my wife being jealous of the patient in her relationship to me (umbrellas in stand; my wife might take her umbrella by mistake, etc). There is a very great deal of material around this theme and there has been acting out which is very much part of the analysis. All this is altered by the fact of the other theme which could be called the theme of doom or fate. In this way everything of Oedipus nature is either inside or outside the doom area. The main statement about doom happened before the Easter holiday when the whole interpersonal problem was stated in terms of Greek mythology, so much so that I studied Bowra's *Sophoclean Tragedy* to be prepared for it. The operative phrase was "not a pawn of fate but an agent of fate." After the Easter holiday the same theme turned up in another language. "I have always been a part object." "For the first time I can say I am a very neurotic person; the accent is on the word person." Here the interpretation if it had been made would have been that a part object cannot experience omnipotence. The patient is not, however, prepared for being a whole person experiencing omnipotence and has not sufficient confidence in the facilitating environment to borrow strength from the maternal ego. Here comes the very well behaved analyst who nevertheless cannot be trusted to be well behaved except negatively, i.e. not behaving badly.

The main interpretation which cannot be made because of the circumstances is that the infantile omnipotence which evidently the patient does not experience in her relationship with her mother has been projected wholesale on Greek mythology and now since the holiday onto ancient Irish history, Druids, the roots of Christianity in Ireland, the Irish cross which is in a circle. Re-stating this: for this patient with an insufficient experience of omnipotent living, the Oedipus complex and all triangular relationships and in fact all relationships are outside the projected omnipotence (part objects inter-related) or else they are doomed, caught up in fate, i.e. with the patient's infantile omnipotence projected wholesale.

18
Fear of Breakdown
Written in 1963? [1]

Preliminary Statement

My clinical experiences have brought me recently to a new understanding, as I believe, of the meaning of a fear of breakdown.

It is my purpose here to state as simply as possible this which is new for me and which perhaps is new for others who work in psychotherapy. Naturally, if what I say has truth in it, this will already have been dealt with by the world's poets, but the flashes of insight that come in poetry cannot absolve us from our painful task of getting step by step away from ignorance towards our goal. It is my opinion that a study of this limited area leads to a restatement of several other problems that puzzle us as we fail to do as well clinically as we would wish to do, and I shall indicate at the end what extensions of the theory I propose for discussion.

Individual Variations

Fear of breakdown is a feature of significance in some of our patients, but not in others. From this observation, if it be a correct one, the conclusion can be drawn that fear of breakdown is related to the individual's past experience, and to environmental vagaries. At the same time there must be expected a common denominator of the

1. This paper was published in the *International Review of Psycho-Analysis* (1974). The date of its composition is uncertain. There is some evidence that it was written as a lecture to be given at the Davidson Clinic in Edinburgh in 1963, but that another paper was given instead; it was around this time that Winnicott used the same material in the postscript to his paper "Classification" (1964), in *The Maturational Processes and the Facilitating Environment* (London: Hogarth Press; New York: International Universities Press, 1965). In the paper "The Psychology of Madness" (1965), Chapter 21 in this volume, Winnicott further addresses a difficulty that he encountered in the idea behind "Fear of Breakdown": namely, whether or not it is possible for a complete breakdown of defences *to be experienced.*—EDS.

same fear, indicating the existence of universal phenomena; these indeed make it possible for everyone to know empathetically what it feels like when one of our patients shows this fear in a big way. (The same can be said, indeed, of every detail of the insane person's insanity. We all know about it, although this particular detail may not be bothering us.)

Emergence of the Symptom

Not all our patients who have this fear complain of it at the outset of a treatment. Some do; but others have their defences so well organised that it is only after a treatment has made considerable progress that the fear of breakdown comes to the fore as a dominating factor.

For instance, a patient may have various phobias and a complex organisation for dealing with these phobias, so that dependence does not come quickly into the transference. At length dependence becomes a main feature, and then the analyst's mistakes and failures become direct causes of localised phobias and so of the outbreak of fear of breakdown.

Meaning of "Breakdown"

I have purposely used the term "breakdown" because it is rather vague and because it could mean various things. On the whole the word can be taken in this context to mean a failure of a defence organisation. But immediately we ask: a defence against what? And this leads us to the deeper meaning of the term, since we need to use the word "breakdown" to describe the unthinkable state of affairs that underlies the defence organisation.

It will be noted that whereas there is value in thinking that in the area of psycho-neurosis it is castration anxiety that lies behind the defences, in the more psychotic phenomena that we are examining it is a breakdown of the establishment of the unit self that is indicated. The ego organises defences against breakdown of the ego-organisation, and it is the ego-organisation that is threatened. But the ego cannot organise against environmental failure in so far as dependence is a living fact.

In other words, we are examining a reversal of the individual's maturational process. This makes it necessary for me briefly to reformulate the early stages of emotional growth.

Emotional Growth, Early Stages

The individual inherits a maturational process. This carries the individual along in so far as there exists a facilitating environment, and only in so far as this exists. The facilitating environment is itself a complex phenomenon and needs special study in its own right; the essential feature is that it has a kind of growth of its own, being adapted to the changing needs of the growing individual.

The individual proceeds from absolute dependence to relative dependence and towards independence. In health the development takes place at a pace that does not outstrip the development of complexity in the mental mechanisms, this being linked to neuro-physiological development.

The facilitating environment can be described as *holding,* developing into *handling,* to which is added *object-presenting.*

In such a facilitating environment the individual undergoes development which can be classified as *integrating,* to which is added *indwelling* (or *psycho-somatic collusion*) and then *object-relating.*

This is a gross over-simplification but it must suffice in this context.

It will be observed that in such a description forward movement in development corresponds closely with the threat of retrograde movement (and defences against this threat) in schizophrenic illness.

Absolute Dependence

At the time of absolute dependence, with the mother supplying an auxiliary ego-function, it has to be remembered that the infant has not yet separated out the "not-me" from the "me"—this cannot happen apart from the establishment of "me."

Primitive Agonies

From this chart it is possible to make a list of primitive agonies (anxiety is not a strong enough word here).

Here are a few:

1. A return to an unintegrated state. (Defence: disintegration.)

2. Falling for ever. (Defence: self-holding.)

3. Loss of psycho-somatic collusion, failure of indwelling. (Defence: depersonalisation.)

4. Loss of sense of real. (Defence: exploitation of primary narcissism, etc.)

5. Loss of capacity to relate to objects. (Defence: autistic states, relating only to self-phenomena.)

And so on.

Psychotic Illness as a Defence

It is my intention to show here that what we see clinically is always a defence organisation, even in the autism of childhood schizophrenia. The underlying agony is unthinkable.

It is wrong to think of psychotic illness as a breakdown, it is a defence organisation relative to a primitive agony, and it is usually successful (except when the facilitating environment has been not deficient but tantalising, perhaps the worst thing that can happen to a human baby).

Statement of Main Theme

I can now state my main contention, and it turns out to be very simple. I contend that clinical fear of breakdown is *the fear of a breakdown that has already been experienced*. It is a fear of the original agony which caused the defence organisation which the patient displays as an illness syndrome.

This idea may or may not prove immediately useful to the clinician. We cannot hurry up our patients. Nevertheless we can hold up their progress because of genuinely not knowing; any little piece of our understanding may help us to keep up with a patient's needs.

There are moments, according to my experience, when a patient needs to be told that the breakdown, a fear of which destroys his or her life, *has already been*. It is a fact that is carried round hidden away in the unconscious. The unconscious here is not exactly the repressed unconscious of psycho-neurosis, nor is it the unconscious of Freud's formulation of the part of the psyche that is very close to neurophysiological functioning. Nor is it the unconscious of Jung's which I would call: all those things that go on in underground caves, or (in other words) the world's mythology, in which there is collusion between the individual and the maternal inner psychic realities. In this special context the unconscious means that the ego integration is not able to encompass something. The ego is too immature to gather all the phenomena into the area of personal omnipotence.

It must be asked here: why does the patient go on being worried by this that belongs to the past? The answer must be that the original experience of primitive agony cannot get into the past tense unless the ego can first gather it into its own present time experience and into omnipotent control now (assuming the auxiliary ego-supporting function of the mother [analyst]).

In other words the patient must go on looking for the past detail which is *not yet experienced*. This search takes the form of a looking for this detail in the future.

Unless the therapist can work successfully on the basis that this detail is already a fact, the patient must go on fearing to find what is being compulsively looked for in the future.

On the other hand, if the patient is ready for some kind of acceptance of this queer kind of truth, that what is not yet experienced did nevertheless happen in the past, then the way is open for the agony to be experienced in the transference, in reaction to the analyst's failures and mistakes. These latter can be dealt with by the patient in doses that are not excessive, and the patient can account for each technical failure of the analyst as countertransference. In other words, gradually the patient gathers the original failure of the facilitating environment into the area of his or her omnipotence and the experience of omnipotence which belongs to the state of dependence (transference fact).

All this is very difficult, time-consuming and painful, but it at any rate is not futile. What is futile is the alternative, and it is this that must now be examined.

Futility in Analysis

I must take for granted an understanding and acceptance of the analysis of psycho-neurosis. On the basis of this assumption I say that in cases I am discussing the analysis starts off well, the analysis goes with a swing; what is happening, however, is that the analyst and the patient are having a good time colluding in a psycho-neurotic analysis, when in fact the illness is psychotic.

Over and over again the analysing couple are pleased with what they have done together. It was valid, it was clever, it was cosy because of the collusion. But each so-called advance ends in destruction.

The patient breaks it up and says: So what? In fact the advance was not an advance; it was a new example of the analyst's playing the patient's game of postponing the main issue. And who can blame either the patient or the analyst? (Unless of course there can be an analyst who plays the psychotic fish on a very long psycho-neurotic line, and hopes thereby to avoid the final catch by some trick of fate, such as the death of one or other of the couple, or a failure of financial backing.)

We must assume that both patient and analyst really do wish to end the analysis, but alas, there is no end unless the bottom of the trough has been reached, unless *the thing feared has been experienced*. And indeed one way out is for the patient to have a breakdown (physical or mental) and this can work very well. However, the solution is not good enough if it does not include analytic understanding and insight on the part of the patient, and indeed, many of the patients I am referring to are valuable people who cannot afford to break down in the sense of going to a mental hospital.

The purpose of this paper is to draw attention to the possibility that the breakdown has already happened, near the beginning of the individual's life. The patient needs to "remember" this but it is not possible to remember something that has not yet happened, and this thing of the past has not happened yet because the patient was not there for it to happen to. The only way to "remember" in this case is for the patient to experience this past thing for the first time in the present, that is to say, in the transference. This past and future thing then becomes a matter of the here and now, and becomes experienced by the patient for the first time. This is the equivalent of remembering, and this outcome is the equivalent of the lifting of repression that occurs in the analysis of the psycho-neurotic patient (classical Freudian analysis).

Further Applications of This Theory

Fear of Death

Little alteration is needed to transfer the general thesis of fear of breakdown to a specific fear of death. This is perhaps a more common fear, and one that is absorbed in the religious teachings about an after-life, as if to deny the fact of death.

When fear of death is a significant symptom the promise of an after-life fails to give relief, and the reason is that the patient has a compulsion to look for death. Again, it is the death that happened but was not experienced that is sought.

When Keats was "half in love with easeful death" he was, according to my idea that I am putting forward here, longing for the ease that would come if he could "remember" having died; but to remember he must experience death now.

Most of my ideas are inspired by patients, to whom I acknowledge debt. It is to one of these that I owe the phrase "phenomenal death." What happened in the past was death as a phenomenon, but not as the sort of fact that we observe. Many men and woman spend their lives wondering whether to find a solution by suicide, that is, sending the body to death which has already happened to the psyche. Suicide is no answer, however, but is a despair gesture. I now understand for the first time what my schizophrenic patient (who did kill herself) meant when she said: "All I ask you to do is to help me to commit suicide for the right reason instead of for the wrong reason." I did not succeed, and she killed herself in despair of finding the solution. Her aim (as I now see) was to get it stated by me that she died in early infancy. On this basis I think she and I could have enabled her to put off body death till old age took its toll.

Death, looked at in this way as something that happened to the patient but which the patient was not mature enough to experience, has the meaning of annihilation. It is like this, that a pattern developed in which the continuity of being was interrupted by the patient's infantile reactions to impingement, these being environmental factors that were allowed to impinge by failures of the facilitating environment. (In the case of this patient troubles started very early, for there was a premature awareness awakened before birth because of a maternal panic, and added to this the birth was complicated by undiagnosed placenta praevia.)

Emptiness

Again my patients show me that the concept of emptiness can be looked at through these same spectacles.

In some patients emptiness needs to be experienced, and this emptiness belongs to the past, to the time before the degree of maturity had made it possible for emptiness to be experienced.

To understand this it is necessary to think not of trauma but of nothing happening when something might profitably have happened.

It is easier for a patient to remember trauma than to remember nothing happening when it might have happened. At the time the patient did not know what might have happened, and so could not experience anything except to note that something might have been.

Example

A phase in a patient's treatment illustrates this. This young woman lay uselessly on the couch, and all she could do was to say: "Nothing is happening in this analysis!"

At the stage that I am describing the patient had supplied material of an indirect kind so that I could know that she was probably feeling something. I was able to say that she had been feeling feelings, and she had been experiencing these gradually fading, according to her pattern, a pattern which made her despair. The feelings were sexual and female. They did not show clinically.

Here in the transference was myself (nearly) being the cause now of her female sexuality fizzling out; when this was properly stated we had an example in the present of what had happened to her innumerable times. In her case (to simplify for the sake of description) there was a father who at first was scarcely ever present, and then when he came to her home when she was a little girl he did not want his daughter's female self, and had nothing to give by way of male stimulus.

Now, emptiness is a prerequisite for eagerness to gather in. Primary emptiness simply means: before starting to fill up. A considerable maturity is needed for this state to be meaningful.

Emptiness occurring in a treatment is a state that the patient is trying to experience, a past state that cannot be remembered except by being experienced for the first time now.

In practice the difficulty is that the patient fears the awfulness of emptiness, and in defence will organise a controlled emptiness by not eating or not learning, or else will ruthlessly fill up by a greediness which is compulsive and which feels mad. When the patient can reach to emptiness itself and tolerate this state because of dependence on the auxiliary ego of the analyst, then, taking in can start up as a pleasurable function; here can begin eating that is not a function dissociated (or split off) as part of the personality; also it is in this way that some of our patients who cannot learn can begin to learn pleasurably.

The basis of all learning (as well as of eating) is emptiness. But if emptiness was not experienced as such at the beginning, then it turns up as a state that is feared, yet compulsively sought after.

Non-Existence

The search for personal non-existence can be examined in the same way. It will be found that non-existence here is part of a defence. Personal existence is represented by the projection elements, and the person is making an attempt to project everything that could be personal. This can be a relatively sophisticated defence, and the aim is to avoid responsibility (at the depressive position) or to avoid persecution (at what I would call the stage of self-assertion [i.e. the stage of I AM with the inherent implication I REPUDIATE EVERYTHING THAT IS NOT ME]. It is convenient here to use in illustration the childhood game of "I'm the king of the castle—you're the dirty rascal").

In the religions this idea can appear in the concept of one-ness with God or with the Universe. It is possible to see this defence being negatived in existentialist writings and teachings, in which existing is made into a cult, in an attempt to counter the personal tendency towards a non-existence that is part of an organised defence.

There can be a positive element in all this, that is, an element that is not a defence. It can be said that *only out of non-existence can existence start*. It is surprising how early (even before birth, certainly during the birth process) awareness or a premature ego can be mobilised. But the individual cannot develop from an ego root if this is divorced from psycho-somatic experience and from primary narcissism. It is just here that begins the intellectualisation of the ego-functions. It can be noted here that all this is a long distance in time prior to the establishment of anything that could usefully be called the self.

Summary

I have attempted to show that fear of breakdown can be a fear of a past event that has not yet been experienced. The need to experience it is equivalent to a need to remember in terms of the analysis of psycho-neurotics.

This idea can be applied to other allied fears, and I have mentioned the fear of death and the search for emptiness.

19

The Importance of the Setting in
Meeting Regression in Psycho-Analysis

*Written for a seminar given to third-year students at
the Institute of Psycho-Analysis, 9 July 1964*

I have given my three official seminars in which I attempted to talk
about psycho-analysis without allowing my own personal ideas to
encroach too much. The wish has been expressed, however, that I
should talk about my personal views in this unofficial seminar. In
particular I have been asked to talk about regression.

Naturally this opens up very wide territory. I must adapt myself to
giving essentials and attempting to state something which can be
understood and discussed.

Perhaps my main aim will be to counteract some of the misconcep-
tions which so easily cluster round the idea of meeting a regression.
The most important mistake that is made is that regression is some
easy way out in analytic work.

I want to make it quite clear that it is fortunate when the question
of meeting a regression does not arise in a big way in an analysis.

It will be understood that the basic principles of analysis are accepted by myself and that what I try to do is to follow the principles
laid down by Freud which seem to me to be fundamental to all our
work. In a certain setting Freud dealt with the material produced by
the patient and a great deal of his work was concerned with the immense problem of how to deal with this material.

In some cases, however, it turns out in the end or even at the beginning that the setting and the maintenance of the setting are as important as the way one deals with the material. In some patients with a
certain type of diagnosis the provision and maintenance of the setting
are more important than the interpretative work. When this is true
one may feel challenged and it is quite possible that the right thing to
do is to end the treatment on the grounds that one is not able to meet
the demands of the patient.

In the ordinary case one is cashing in on the work done by the parents, and particularly by the mother, in the early childhood and infancy of the patient. It was not too difficult for the mother to adapt to the needs of her infant because she only needed to do this over a relatively short period of time, a few months, and usually this is what she likes to do. She knows that she will recover her own independence in the course of time.

As soon as we have to deal with a patient who did not receive this early good-enough treatment, it is not certain that we can correct what has been faulty. The demands made on us are severe indeed. It is not as if we know immediately what demands are to be made on us. At first we can easily meet them. It is as if the patient gradually seduces us into collusion, collusion with the infant in the patient who in some way or other received inadequate attention at the earliest stages.

The reason why the onset of all this is insidious is that the patient only gradually begins to get hope that these demands will be met. It is because of the development in the patient that there is this gradual increase of the need for a specialised environmental provision. In the kind of case I am talking about it is never a question of giving satisfactions in the ordinary manner of succumbing to a seduction. It is always that if one provides certain conditions work can be done and if one does not provide these conditions work cannot be done and one might as well not try. The patient is not there to work with us except when we provide the conditions which are necessary.

Let me take a very crude example. A patient of mine went to an analyst and very quickly she got confidence in him and therefore she began to cover herself over with a rug and lie curled up on the couch with nothing happening. This analyst said to her: "Sit up! Look at me! Talk! You are not to lie like that doing nothing; nothing will happen!" The patient felt that this was a good thing for the analyst to do. He acknowledged straight off that he could not meet her basic needs. She sat up and talked and she got on very well with the analyst on the basis of a mutual interest in modern art. They looked at books together and they talked about very deep things. It was a matter of how to get away from this analyst, and she hung on to him until she could find another who would not tell her to pull her socks up. She had no resentment about this failed treatment because the analyst never pretended that he could do what he was unable to do. He could not possibly have met her needs which, once they had started, would become very exacting.

Of course the patient was not aware of all this; her insight was limited but she had some insight, enough to make her know how to choose an analyst who would adopt a different attitude and at least make an attempt to meet her basic needs.

I would be quite content if my talking about this subject were to lead analysts into consciously acting as this analyst did, letting the patient know as soon as possible that what the patient needs cannot be given.

By contrast I would quote another case. Before doing so, however, I want to say that gradually if one attempts to meet the patient's needs of the kind I am describing, the demands made on the analyst become very great and there comes a moment when the patient says to the analyst something like this: "The time has now come for you to decide whether to go the whole hog or whether to withdraw. I don't mind if you say now that you can't do it, but if you go further then I am handing over to you something of myself and I am becoming dangerously dependent and your mistakes will matter seriously."

Often at this point it is a matter of life and death and the wise analyst stops the analysis knowing and acknowledging openly that he is unable to do the next part which is what the patient wanted. He will not be blamed for this by the patient.

In illustration I will give a detail in the analysis of a patient who has a tremendous area of healthy personality and yet her analysis inevitably leads to this very deep dependence which is so dangerous. She is past the point of no return.

This patient comes into my room on a Friday, Friday being a day for cashing in on the work of the week. In this patient the pattern of the week is clearly set and Friday on this occasion was to be characterised by calm after storm with some kind of preparation for the weekend contained in it.

In regard to this patient there are certain things that have to be the same always. The curtains are drawn; the door is on the latch so that the patient can come straight in; all the arrangements in the room must be constant and also there are some objects which are variable but which belong to the transference relationship. At the time that I am describing the constant object is placed in a certain position on the desk and there are certain papers which have accumulated which I put beside me waiting for the moment when the patient will want them back.

This Friday in spite of careful inspection of my arrangements of the room I leave the papers on top of the other object instead of putting them beside me. The patient comes into the room and sees these alterations, and when I arrive on the scene I find that this is a complete disaster. I see at the moment of entering the room what has happened and I know that I shall be very lucky if we recover from this disaster in a matter of weeks.

Perhaps this illustrates the way in which the patient becomes sensitised to the setting and its details. In another analysis there are alterations all the time. They may be noticed; they may be important; but they are not disastrous. This patient could not do anything about her reactions except to let them happen. After her initial reaction, which was unreasonable in the extreme, she began to become reasonable and eventually came round to asking what it was in herself that made people behave badly. Eventually she asked me to talk about this, what had she done that made me make this mistake?—a mistake which completely broke up the process of the analysis and of her development, and ruined the whole work of the week?

Before the end of the hour in this case I was able to talk about the whole thing in the way that she asked me to do, which is rather different from giving an interpretation. This is a favourable outcome, which one must not always expect. It could easily have happened that a patient highly sensitised in this way could have a suicidal episode in the weekend or could leave the analysis or could do a piece of acting out from which it would be very difficult ever to recover, like marrying the wrong person. I have had all these things happen in my practice and that is why I am trying to convey how difficult it is to do this work well. On this particular day with this patient I was able to say that as far as I could see this disastrous mistake that I had made had unconscious motivation. I could guess at some of my reasons for making the mistake but in my own opinion, I said, the mistake lies within me and is not a reaction to something in the patient.

I went on, because of the material I had at hand, to show that the patient would much prefer to find that what I had done disastrously was a reaction to something in herself, because this would bring the whole thing into her control and give her some hope for bringing about a change in me because of a change in herself.

From this the patient took the matter back to certain things about her father which she had always tried hard to explain as reactions to something in herself, whereas she had to admit that they were characteristics of her father dating from the time before she was born and indeed explicable in terms of his own family history.

In the end I was able to say: "The thing is, this is what I am like, and if you continue with me you will find I shall do similar things with unconscious motivation again because that is what I am like."

I give this example because although it was a narrow shave I did come out of it without having to deceive anyone and with no more than a statement of my own imperfections. It can easily be seen that one simply cannot afford to make these mistakes with patients who are more ill. By more ill I mean patients who have less healthy personality alongside their ill bit. The ill bit is just as ill in one as it is in another, and one cannot in any way lessen the adaptation to the patient's needs by knowing that the patient has a considerable amount of healthy personality. It is the ill bit that one is dealing with and it is as ill as possible.

The astounding thing is that if one has a patient going through one of these phases one can adapt in a very detailed way to the patient's needs over a period of time; that is to say, in the hour that is set aside for this patient one can have a professional reliability which is very much unlike one's own unreliable personality. In time, however, one's own unreliability begins to seep through, and one of the dangers is that as soon as the patient begins to get better in the sense of being able to allow one to lessen vigilance, one is liable to take a holiday, so to speak, and to rush forward with a show of one's own impulse. One cannot be blamed for being like this but it may lose a case that is going well.

Everything then points to the fact that this work is not only difficult but it absorbs a great deal of one's capacity for cathexis, and it may easily be that one can carry two or perhaps even three cases but not four at the same time. On the whole it is possible to have only one patient at a time who is maximally ill in this way.

Principles

The theory of this work depends on certain principles. These have already been formulated, and once formulated it can be seen that they are to a large extent obvious.

The basic statement is that emotional development is a process of maturation to which is added growth based on the accumulation of experiences.

The maturational process is that which is inherited.

It does not become actual except in a facilitating environment.

The facilitating environment needs to be studied in relation to the details of the maturational process.

The maturational process includes integration in its various forms, as follows:

1. The indwelling of the psyche in the soma.
2. Object-relating.
3. The interaction of the intellectual processes with psychosomatic experience.

Corresponding to these and other details of the maturational process are the three following aspects of the facilitating environment:

a. Holding
b. Handling
c. Realising

The operation of the facilitating environment starts with near 100 percent adaptation, rapidly diminishing according to the growing needs of the baby. These needs include opportunity for object-relating through aggression.

Prior to this comes erotic satisfaction through successful realising. In the emotional growth of the baby the journey is from absolute dependence to dependence and towards independence. In the early stages the baby is unaware of dependence and is related to subjective objects.

An important aspect of growth is the change from relating to subjective objects to a recognition of objects that are outside the area of omnipotence, that is to say that are objectively perceived but not explained on the basis of projection. In this area of change there is the maximum opportunity for the individual to make sense of the aggressive components. Making sense of the aggressive components leads to the baby's experience of anger (related to the Klein concept of envy of the good breast) and leads on in the favourable case to fusion of aggressive and erotic components eventuating in eating. In health by the time eating has become established as part of the relationship to objects there has become organised a fantasy existence which is parallel to actual living and which carries its own sense of real.

It is not possible to give a direct answer to the question: has the baby an ego from the beginning? The reason for this is that at the start the baby's ego is both feeble and powerful. It is feeble in the extreme if there is no satisfactory facilitating environment. In nearly every case, however, the mother or mother-figure supplies the ego support, and if she does this well enough the infant's ego is very strong and has its own organisation. The mother is able to give this ego support through her ability and willingness to identify temporarily with her infant.

It is important to distinguish between a mother's capacity to identify with her infant, retaining of course her own autonomy, and the infant's state of not yet having emerged from absolute dependence. Only gradually does the infant separate out the not-me from the me, and it is an important stage of emotional development when the infant becomes able to recognise the fact of dependence and be able to have a self which is only relatively dependent instead of absolutely dependent on the mother's temporary state in which she colludes with the infant so that the infant has, because of her collusion, an ego and an ego-organisation and a degree of ego strength and resilience.

20
Psycho-Somatic Disorder

I. Psycho-Somatic Illness in Its Positive and Negative Aspects

Originally a lecture given to the Society for Psycho-Somatic Research, 21 May 1964[1]

Preview

1. The word "psycho-somatic" is needed because no simple word exists which is appropriate in description of certain clinical states.

2. The hyphen both joins and separates the two aspects of medical practice which are constantly under review in any discussion of this theme.

3. The word accurately describes something that is inherent in this work.

4. The psycho-somatist prides himself on his capacity to ride two horses, one foot on each of the two saddles, with both reins in his deft hands.

5. Some agent has to be found that tends to separate the two aspects of psycho-somatic disorder, to give the hyphen a place.

6. This agent is, in fact, a dissociation in the patient.

7. The illness in psycho-somatic disorder is not the clinical state expressed in terms of somatic pathology or pathological functioning (colitis, asthma, chronic eczema). It is the persistence of a split in the patient's ego-organisation, or of multiple dissociations, that constitutes the true illness.

8. This illness state in the patient is itself a defence organisation with very powerful determinants, and for this reason it is very common for well-meaning and well-informed and even exceptionally well-equipped doctors to fail in their efforts to cure patients with psycho-somatic disorder.

1. Published in its present form in the *International Journal of Psycho-Analysis* (1966). Copyright © Institute of Psycho-Analysis.

9. If the reasons for this tendency to fail are not understood, medical practitioners lose heart. Then the subject of psycho-somatics becomes a subject for non-clinical or *theoretical* survey, and this is relatively easy because the theoretician is detached, and is not cluttered up by responsibility for actual patients. The theoretician is the very one who is apt to lose touch with the dissociation, and he is able to see from both sides only too easily.

I have a desire to make it plain that *the forces at work in the patient are tremendously strong.* The dilemma of the practising psychosomatist is indeed a reality.

One or two complications should be mentioned at this stage in the argument:

a. Some practising doctors are not really able to ride the two horses. They sit in one saddle and lead the other horse by the bridle or lose touch with it. After all, why should doctors be more healthy in a psychiatric sense than their patients? They have not been selected on a psychiatric basis. The doctor's own dissociations need to be considered along with the dissociations in the personalities of the patients.

b. Patients can have more than one illness. A man with a coronary spasm tendency, secondary to emotional confusion, may also have calcified arteries, or a woman with fibroids and menorrhagia may also have a sexual immaturity. And so on. On the whole it is the hypochondriacs who fail to get examined when they have cancer of the breast or a hypernephroma, and it is the patients who are physically ill who put themselves forward as needing psycho-analysis or hypnotism. And patients who are always pestering a succession of doctors to examine them very seldom have anything to be discovered by physical test. In this way doctors get led astray, and amazing stories of neglect are told, some of which one must believe.

c. Many patients do not split their medical care into two; the split is into many fragments, and as doctors we find ourselves acting in the role of one of these fragments. I have (1958) used the term "scatter of responsible agents"[2] to describe this tendency. Such patients provide the examples quoted in social casework surveys in which twenty or thirty or more agencies have been found to have been involved in relief of one family's distress. Patients with multiple dissociations also exploit the natural splits in the medical profession such as:

---

2. See Winnicott's review of Michael Balint's *The Doctor, His Patient and the Illness* (1958), in Chapter 52 of this volume.

$$
\left\{
\begin{array}{l}
\left\{
\begin{array}{l}
\text{medical} \\
\text{surgical}
\end{array}
\right. \\
\left\{
\begin{array}{l}
\text{psychiatric} \\
\text{psycho-analytic} \\
\text{psychotherapeutic}
\end{array}
\right.
\end{array}
\right.
$$

$$
\left\{
\begin{array}{l}
\text{homeopathic} \\
\text{osteopathic} \\
\text{faith-healing}
\end{array}
\right.
$$

various ancillary services

Psycho-Somatics as a Subject

Psycho-somatics is in many ways a curious subject, for if one ascends into the sphere of intellectualisation and loses contact with the actual patient, one soon finds that the term psycho-somatics loses its integrative function. One soon asks oneself, why is there this speciality? Does it not concern every aspect of human growth, except perhaps that of behaviour? I find myself involved in the same considerations that I tried to clarify for my own benefit in "Mind and Its Relation to the Psyche-Soma" (1949),[3] because it was in the writing of that paper that I became aware of the confusion that exists through the use of the term "mental disorder," a term that somehow fails to cover the case of a child with a bilious attack, or the case of a person with a fatal physical disease who does not become devoid of hope.

I suggest that any intellectualised attempt to make psycho-somatics easy keeps clear of the very clinical clutter-up which bogs us down in our actual work. We find ourselves involved in attempts to build a *theory* where the word should be *theories* (in the plural). My aim is not to state a final truth, but to make my point, and so to provide material for consideration.

The element that gives our work on psycho-somatics cohesion, as I have stated, seems to me to be the patient's pathological splitting of the environmental provision. The split is certainly one that separates off physical care from intellectual understanding; more important, it separates psyche-care from soma-care.

If I take a case in my practice now and try to describe the dilemma, I run the risk of ruining my treatment, because however carefully I word what I have to report I cannot satisfy my patient, who might

---

3. In *Collected Papers: Through Paediatrics to Psycho-Analysis* (London: Tavistock, 1958; New York: Basic Books, 1975; London: Hogarth Press, 1975).

read what is reported. The solution in the case of any one patient is not to be sought in a more and more careful reporting; the solution can only come through the success of the treatment which, if time be allowed, may result in the patient's becoming able to need no longer the split which creates the medical dilemma which I am describing. As I am in practice I need to be very careful in presenting my illustrative material.

Let us pretend that I have a patient among the readers, a patient with a variety of this disorder that we label psycho-somatic. The patient will probably not mind being quoted, that is not the trouble here. The trouble is that *it would not be possible for me to give an acceptable account of something that has not yet become acceptable in that patient's internal economy.* Only the continuation of the treatment is of use in the actual case, and in the course of time the patient whose existence I am postulating may come to relieve me of the dilemma that his illness places me in, the dilemma that is the subject of my paper. And one thing I would hate to do would be to seduce the patient to an agreed statement which would involve an abandonment of the psyche-soma and a flight into intellectual collusion.

Am I beginning to convey my meaning that *in practice* there does exist a real and insuperable difficulty, the dissociation in the patient which, as an organised defence, keeps separate the somatic dysfunction and the conflict in the psyche? Given time and favourable circumstances the patient will tend to recover from the dissociation. Integrative forces in the patient tend to make the patient abandon the defence. I must try to make a statement that avoids the dilemma.

It will be evident that I am making a distinction between the true psycho-somatic case and the almost universal clinical problem of functional involvement in emotional processes and mental conflicts. I do not necessarily call my patient whose dysmenorrhoea is related to anal components in the genital organisation a psycho-somatic case, nor the man who must micturate urgently in certain circumstances. This is just life, and living. But my patient who claims that his slipped disc is due to a draught might claim to be labelled psycho-somatic, and so qualify for our attention in this paper.

Illustrative Material

When I reach for clinical examples, I am of course overwhelmed by a mass of material. There must be a hundred ways of proceeding from this place in my exposition of my point of view.

Case of Anorexia Nervosa

There are certain common features in anorexia cases, though in one case the child may be almost normal and in another she (sometimes he) may be very ill. One child may nearly die of starvation in a phase-disturbance, and yet recover spontaneously, and in another less dangerous example the child may remain a psychiatric casualty.

I describe briefly a girl of ten years who is in analysis. She is physically well because she is taking food as a medicine. She eats nothing at all as food. You can imagine that this girl is very suspicious of talk between her physical doctors and her analyst. At the same time she absolutely and consciously relies on a close co-operation between the analyst and the doctors and the nursing staff. There are multiple splits; nurses and doctors are classified by the patient into those who understand and those who could never understand. Every effort is made by all concerned to avoid the moment when logic appears on the scene and makes plain the existence of the dissociation in the patient. The worst possible thing would be to force this issue. One doctor said to her: "You are wasting your time, you must do school lessons." This produced a threat of anxiety of extreme intensity, and the situation was only saved by the fact that the analytic session came soon after this dangerous event. The patient knew she could rely on the analyst to forbid teaching. But I did not need to do anything because she soon found one of the other doctors, "the one who understands," and he of course proscribed teaching and put the whole matter straight. One of the ward nurses, however, and one of the ward charwomen, could be relied on to say something tactless, that is to say, something that ignored the dissociation in the patient. I do believe that by now no-one within ten miles of this girl would actually tell her to *eat,* so well has her very great need to be left alone in this respect become known and reluctantly accepted.

Here is another way of describing this aspect of this case. For many months in this analysis the patient's sensations and agonies and dreams appeared in the form of urgent material related to the belly. There was a whole world of objects in and falling out of her front. In a dream there were filing cabinets and even steel doors with sharp edges that gave her acute belly pain. These could not be altered by interpretations relative to internal objects. One day (after years) she reported a *headache.* Here at last was a shift from the dissociated state since headache could be accepted as associated with a confusion of ideas and of responsibilities. I now interpreted that she was telling me about an illness of her *mind,* and I therefore slipped over from being part of a psycho-somatic team into the role of psychotherapist. This has persisted, and for many months now there has been hardly any report to me in terms of belly stuff. Now, as a mental patient, she is able to give me material that I can interpret in inner object terminology, if I feel so disposed, and I can work with the patient on the nature of her fantasy of her inside, and what is there to be found, and how it got there, and what to do with it. In the previous phase, by contrast, there was a flight to delusional belly-symptoms, and a denial of mind content.

If this patient were here now, reading this paper, she would find herself ill at ease, because she would realise that the doctors who look after her are her analyst's friends. Psycho-somatic patients are always complaining that the various doctors do not co-operate, but they become anxious when in fact they do meet to discuss the case. Mercifully, my paediatric colleagues are not wholly committed to this point of view of the dynamic psychologist or of the psycho-analyst, and so there is some split actually present in the medical environment; this makes the child feel she has allies whichever side she happens to be on in her internal conflict arising out of the dissociation.[4]

In the practice of psycho-somatics what the psychotherapist needs is the co-operation of a *not too scientific* physical doctor. This sounds very bad, and I expect opposition when I make this claim. Yet I must state what I feel. When doing the analysis of a psycho-somatic case I would like my opposite number to be *a scientist on holiday from science.* What is needed is science-fiction rather than a rigid and compulsive application of medical theory on the basis of perception of objective reality.

An Adult Patient

A psycho-analytic patient of mine, a woman in mid-life, has depended on many beside her analyst in the course of her treatment. Let me list a few:

The family G.P. and a group of gynaecologists and pathologists.
Her osteopath.

---

4. 1965–66. Since this was written in 1964 the nature of this patient's illness has altered. She is now not a psycho-somatic case. She has a severe disturbance of emotional development and she is using the analysis for the relief of mental conflict and agony, without employing the psycho-somatic defence. (Later note: this patient has done well.)—D.W.W.

Her dermatologist.

Her former analysts.

Her masseuse.

Her hairdresser, especially the *other* one who cures her occasional alopoecia without charge.

A spiritualist with clairvoyance.

The special parson.

The nannie of her children, very carefully chosen to be good enough in the care of infants and therefore capable of turning into a mental nurse for herself.

The very special garage for her car.

Etc.

Here is a "scatter of responsible agents" secondary to an active disintegration in the economy of the patient's personality. Integration in her analysis has been a gradual undoing of the organised scatter of therapeutic agents and the multiple dissociation of her personality by which she defended herself against loss of identity in a merging in with her mother. Is it clear that initially the patient used all these helpers in a dissociated way? There was a flitting from one to every other, and as there was an essential multiple dissociation the patient was never all at once in one place and in touch with each and every aspect of the care that she organised.

But in the course of the treatment a very big change occurred. I have watched all these agents gradually settle down to being *aspects of the transference*. When the patient was near to this achievement she was able for the first time to love someone, her husband. The personality splitting was related to a need the patient had to rescue a personal identity and to avoid merging in with the mother. It was a red-letter day for me when the patient rang me up by mistake when intending to ring her butcher.[5]

A Case of Colitis

In a third case, a less happy outcome can be reported to balance this. A child was having analysis by me because of colitis, certainly a good example of the type of disorder that appears along with the split that I am trying to describe. Unfortunately I was unable to see early

5. In case this patient should read these words I would wish to state that this description is not only inadequate in every way, it is not even accurate. But I am using it to illustrate an idea. (Later note: this patient has done well.)—D.W.W.

enough that the ill person in this case was the mother. It was the mother who had the essential split, and the child who had the colitis. But it was the child who was brought to me for treatment.

I was doing very well with the child and I thought I had the mother's co-operation. I certainly had her friendliness. When the girl was eight years old I said she could go to school, as she wished to do so, and this produced a change in the mother's unconscious attitude. The child got to school but soon became very ill indeed.

I now found that it was at eight years that the mother had herself been a school-refusal case, and certainly this in turn had to do with her own mother's psychopathology. The mother, though unconscious of the fact, could not allow her daughter, who was living her life for her again, to go outside the pattern.

After the unexpected breakdown of my treatment I found that the child was under several general practitioners, and also in the care of a paediatrician, and also, at one time towards the end of my ministration, was attending a hypnotist and another psychotherapist. It was not long before she had her colon removed by a surgeon, and I dropped out of the case, my going being scarcely noticed. I was not even dismissed. Yet three months earlier I had the whole case in my hands, as it seemed, and I thought I had the full confidence of the family, and I certainly had the confidence of the child in so far as she was an autonomous human being. Unfortunately, this was precisely what she was not.

I do not know the outcome and I have not the heart to enquire. My error was to treat the child when the illness was in the mother, and the illness included the essential psycho-somatic dissociation that is the subject of this paper. Not that I neglected the mother's psychopathology, which the child knew about, and which was all the time an important element in the work done between the child and myself. But I had forgotten the tremendously powerful unconscious need that exists in such a mother to scatter the responsible agents and to maintain the *status quo* of which, here, the child's somatic illness was an integral part. The mother could have a healthy body while the illness was in the child.

Recapitulation

A multiplication of clinical examples would not further the argument. There is no area of personality development that escapes being involved in a study of psycho-somatic disorder. A severe disintegration threat can be hidden in a cricked neck; an insignificant skin rash may hide a depersonalisation; blushing may be all that shows of an infantile failure to establish a human relationship through the passing of water, perhaps because no-one would look and admire in the phase of micturition potency. Moreover suicide may be gathered into a hard patch on the inner maleolus, produced and maintained by constant kicking; delusions of persecution may be confined clinically to the wearing of dark glasses or a screwing up of the eyes; an antisocial tendency belonging to a serious deprivation may show as simple bedwetting; indifference to crippling or painful disease may be a relief from a sado-masochistic sexual organisation; chronic hypertension may be the clinical equivalent of a psycho-neurotic anxiety state or of a long-continued traumatic factor, such as a parent who is loved but who is a psychiatric casualty. And so one might go on, but all this is familiar ground.

My contention is that *these things do not of themselves constitute psycho-somatic disorder,* nor do they justify the use of a special term or the organisation of a *Psycho-Somatic Group* within the general medical and surgical profession. What makes sense of this grouping is the need that some patients have to keep the doctors on two or more sides of a fence, because of an inner need; also that this inner need is part of a highly organised and powerfully maintained defensive system, the defences being against the dangers that arise out of integration and out of the achievement of a unified personality. These patients need us to be split up (yet essentially united in the far background that they cannot allow themselves to know about).

For a long time I have been puzzled by our failures to classify psycho-somatic disorders and our inability to state a theory, a unified theory of this illness group. When I found a way of saying to myself what psycho-somatic disorder really is I found myself with a ready-made classification which I will give (for what it is worth). But first let me re-state my main thesis, linking it with the theory of maturation in individual growth.

The Positive Element in the Psycho-Somatic Defence

Psycho-somatic illness is the negative of a positive; the positive being the tendency towards integration in several of its meanings and including what I have referred to (1963)[6] as personalisation. The positive is the inherited tendency of each individual to achieve a unity of the psyche and the soma, an experiential identity of the spirit or psyche and the totality of physical functioning. A tendency takes the infant and child towards a functioning body on which and out of which there develops a functioning personality, complete with defences against anxiety of all degrees and kinds. In other words, as Freud said many decades ago, the ego is based on a body ego. Freud might have gone on to say that *in health* the self retains this seeming identity with the body and its functioning. (The whole complex theory of introjection and projection, as well as conceptualisation around the term "internal object," is a development of this theme.)

This stage in the integrating process is one that might be called the "I AM" stage (Winnicott, 1965).[7] I like this name because it reminds me of the evolution of the idea of monotheism and of the designation of God as the "Great I AM." In terms of childhood play this stage is celebrated (though at a later age than I have in mind now) by the game "I'm the king of the castle—you're the dirty rascal." It is the meaning of "I" and "I am" that is altered by the psycho-somatic dissociation.

The splitting of the psyche from the soma is a retrogressive phenomenon employing archaic residues in the setting up of a defence organisation. By contrast the tendency towards psycho-somatic integration is a part of forward movement in the developmental process. "Splitting" is here the representative of "repression" that is the appropriate term in a more sophisticated organisation.

Classification

If this be true then it should be possible to classify psycho-somatic illness according to the theory of the maturational processes, including two main ideas:

1. A primary unintegrated state, with a tendency towards integration. Result dependent on
   Mother's ego reinforcement, based on her adapting capacity, giving the infant's ego a reality in dependence.

6. "The Mentally Ill in Your Caseload," in *The Maturational Processes and the Facilitating Environment* (London: Hogarth Press, 1965).

7. Various chapters in *The Maturational Processes and the Facilitating Environment* and *The Family and Individual Development* (London: Tavistock, 1965).

Maternal failure which leaves the infant without the essentials for the operation of the maturational processes.

2. Psycho-somatic integration or the achievement of the "indwelling" of the psyche in the soma, and this to be followed by the enjoyment of a psycho-somatic unity in experience.

In the process of integration the infant (in healthy development) gains a foothold in the "I AM" or the "king of the castle" position in emotional development, and then not only does the enjoyment of body functioning reinforce ego development, but also ego development reinforces body functioning (influences muscle tone, coordination, adaptation to temperature change, etc., etc.). Developmental failure in these respects results in uncertainty of "indwelling," or leads to depersonalisation in so far as indwelling has become a feature that can be lost. The term indwelling is used here to describe the dwelling of the psyche in the personal soma, or *vice versa*.

At the "I AM," or "king of the castle" position the individual may or may not for internal or for external reasons (and the infant is still highly dependent) be able to cope with the rivalry that this engenders ("you're the dirty[8] rascal"). In health rivalry becomes an added stimulus to growth and to the zest for living.

Hence, psycho-somatic disorder relates to

Weak ego (dependent largely on not good-enough mothering) with a feeble establishment of indwelling in personal development;

and/or

Retreat from I AM and from the world made hostile by the individual's repudiation of the NOT-ME, to a special form of splitting which is in the mind but which is along psycho-somatic lines.

(Here an actual persecuting environmental detail may determine the individual's retreat to some form of splitting.)

In this way, psycho-somatic illness implies a split in the individual's personality, with weakness of the linkage between psyche and soma, or a split organised in the mind in defence against generalised persecution from the repudiated world. There remains in the individual ill person, however, a tendency *not* altogether to lose the psycho-somatic linkage.

Here, then, is *the positive value of somatic involvement.* The indi-

---

8. This word here implies: "You are not (as I am) a womb-baby capable of integration and autonomy, but you are an excretory product of your mother, without form or maturational process."—D.W.W.

vidual values the potential psycho-somatic linkage. To understand this one must remember that defence is organised not only in terms of splitting, which protects against annihilation, but also in terms of protection of the psyche-soma from a flight into an intellectualised or a spiritual existence, or into compulsive sexual exploits which would ignore the claims of a psyche that is built and maintained on a basis of somatic functioning.

One more complication. Naturally, when the personality is dissociated, dissociations in the environment are exploited by the individual. An example would be the use made of a tendency in the mother towards disintegration or depersonalisation, of parental discord, or of the break-up of the family unit, or of antagonism (especially unconscious antagonism) between family and school. In the same way, use is made of the splits (to which I have referred) in the matter of medical provision.

Here there can be a return to my main idea, which is that the existence of a "psycho-somatic" or (psycho somatic) group of doctors depends on the patients' need for us to split up for practical purposes, but to remain theoretically united by a common discipline and profession.

Our difficult job is to take a unified view of the patient and of the illness *without seeming to do so in a way that goes ahead of the patient's ability to achieve integration to a unit.* Often, very often, we must be contented to let the patient have it, and to manipulate the symptomatology, in a box-and-cox relation to our opposite numbers, without attempting to cure the real illness, the real illness being the patient's personality split which is organised out of ego weakness and maintained as a defence against the threat of annihilation at the moment of integration.

Psycho-somatic illness, like the antisocial tendency, has this hopeful aspect, that the patient is in touch with the possibility of psycho-somatic unity (or personalisation), and dependence, even though his or her clinical condition actively illustrates the opposite of this through splitting, through various dissociations, through a persistent attempt to split the medical provision, and through omnipotent self care-taking.

II. Additional Note on Psycho-Somatic Disorder

Dated 16 September 1969

It has been pointed out that the chronic skin diseases are related in an obscure way to psychotic disorder of the mind. Obviously some chronic diseases are physically determined. Roughly the statement is that the chronic skin irritation or discomfort emphasises the limiting membrane of the body and therefore of the personality and behind this is the threat of depersonalisation and a loss of body boundaries and of the unthinkable almost physical anxiety which belongs to the reverse process of that which is called integration.

One example of this unthinkable anxiety is the state in which there is no frame to the picture; nothing to contain the interweaving of forces in the inner psychic reality, and in practical terms no-one to hold the baby.

A patient, a woman of middle age, has come to a very full recognition of this state of affairs in herself, and she was able to add to the clinical picture certain details which had value for me as an observer. Along with various forms of chronic pruritis, some turning up spontaneously and some produced or exaggerated by scratching, the patient recognised other ways that she had of keeping in her body. It could be said that she has not till recently become aware of the threat of depersonalisation. What she has known about is her skin and her interest in a chronic skin disease of a friend, but also she has a technique for resting which means that she never rests. In bed she is never still. She never lies down because of difficult breathing which she maintains by over-smoking. She always lies in some kind of exaggerated position so that she is conscious of herself in physical terms. She always arranges it that all her muscles are strained. She said: "I can't stop it. I can get as far as trying to think why I do these things and even understanding what it is all about, but it has to go on all the time."

This material was given by this patient on a day when she described the way that she felt cut off from her family because she had not been able to bring herself to enjoy a family ceremony. She felt that she had been unable to take part in the religious rite that had to do with a new baby because it was all connected with the moment of separation of a baby from the mother. She associated this with a sudden thought that she had had (while engaged in a futile obsessional practice) that she would give up her analysis because it can get nowhere. She recognised fairly easily at this stage that she does not want it to get anywhere and that in order to make this gesture she had to forget what she had told me on the previous occasion which is that she has certainly recently made a great step forward and has been able to have a period of time in which she actually lived in the present. In other words her main symptoms had been in abeyance for a period of weeks. Because of the essential dissociation in her nature she knows that she is very ill when she is very ill, and she knows she is well when she feels well, but these two states do not link together, and in order to get a link she has to think of my knowing about her two states. She related this to failure at the stage at which the mother sits happily occupied but available while the child plays. At the extreme of the experience of failure in the infant-mother relationship and the memories of the failure there comes the scream which this patient is always not experiencing. It is always true to say when reviewing one of this patient's sessions that if she could scream she would be well. The great non-event of every session is screaming. It is of course of no use whatever encouraging this patient to scream, and it would not be valuable to introduce something frightening or hurtful to provoke crying. The patient usually knows that not screaming is the subject matter behind all the material that she produces, but how can she alter this state of affairs? She feels trapped, as she said on this occasion, and she remembered her biggest cry when she came back after her mother's funeral and there was a letter from her landlady about some triviality. This letter had been sufficiently persecutory, coming at the exact moment it did, to produce something near a scream, and it is a relief to get towards the scream even with a wrong basis. She is too sane to be able to organise, as some patients do, a paranoid situation and then scream in fear of some threat. With this patient a different approach is necessary.

If we take the situation in which she is a child playing while her mother is occupied with some activity such as sewing, this is the good pattern in which growth is taking place. At any moment the child may make a gesture and the mother will transfer her interest from her sewing to the child. If the mother is preoccupied and does not at first notice the child's need, the child has only to begin to cry and the mother is available. In the bad pattern which is at the root of this patient's illness, the child cried and the mother did not appear. In other words the scream that she is looking for is *the last scream just before hope was abandoned*. Since then screaming has been of no use because it fails in its purpose. The best that the analyst can do is to give understanding at this point as this begins to alter the bad pattern which stopped emotional growth and points towards the good pattern in which crying was taking place. Profound understanding on the part of the analyst on the basis of the material presented by this patient leads of course towards screaming, that is to say towards screaming again, this time with hope.

The relevance of this to the earlier part of this statement which had to do with psycho-somatic interplay is this, that the non-event or the not screaming is in itself a negation or a blotting out of one of the very important things which link the psyche and the soma; that is to say crying, screaming, yelling, angry protest. It is possible already to predict that this patient on becoming able to scream will have an immense strengthening of the psycho-somatic interrelationship and a lessening of the need to employ the somewhat artificial experience of psycho-somatic interplay as described above.

The question naturally arises, does this patient really need to scream in the analytic session? The answer might be yes, but already this patient has had a *dream* in which screaming took place. Alongside this dream came clinical relief in the waking state; that is to say before reporting the dream she reported that she had been able to sing in a community situation, something that she had not been able to do for years, and also at the same time in her behaviour in the transference situation she had been able to make a noise and shout and protest (in a civilised way as it happened) when I was late for the session and she feared that I was ill or that I had forgotten her. The key to the situation therefore is the dream. But the dream only becomes possible as a result of the analysis, in which hope about screaming returns and is recaptured from the time before she became ill when the good pattern changed into the bad pattern either at a certain moment of her babyhood or spread over a period of time.

Clinically there appears along with these changes towards psycho-somatic interplay an enhanced interest on the part of the patient in the shape of her body and in the texture of her clothes. It will be direct evidence of success in this area of the analysis if the patient becomes able to relax in bed and in her waking life to exist in the here and now instead of in a gap between the past and the future.

In this hour the patient referred to the previous hour in which I had given as an interpretation: "It is this non-scream that is in the way, that is to say the fear of not being heard or the hopelessness about screaming producing an effect." She said: "When you told me that I felt it was cruel. What is the use to say such a terrible thing to me?" I had joined it up with my failure in the transference, especially at the point of being unavailable when she arrived for the previous session. She now said: "It was really rather clever. It is not just a physical response to the scream that matters, you know, it is understanding. What you said felt awful. The fact was that *you* knew and *I* didn't and this is the only way that it is possible to correct the failure of my last scream to work."

The rest of the work of this session had to do with the need this patient has to deal with the subject of separation in terms simply of the scar both on herself and mother. The part that joined the two of them is missing from both of them. This form of separation has had to be fully explored in this patient, after which there will be (as we can already see) a return to the exploration of separation in terms of anger and biting and other forms of aggression. This is where this patient knows she becomes a whole person and the mother becomes a whole person and the two of them can become separate without scars and without the maiming which this patient all her life has taken for granted, and which has played into her fantasy of being a second-class citizen because a woman.

After this hour she was able to see the possibility of a break from her analyst, each of them remaining whole and each containing something of the other, and each able to identify with the other. But these are sophisticated matters and they seem a long way just at this moment from this patient's treatment and from the present where separation means scars and gaps.

21
The Psychology of Madness:
A Contribution from Psycho-Analysis

A paper prepared for the British Psycho-Analytical Society, October 1965

The practice of psycho-analysis for thirty-five years cannot but leave its mark. For me there have come about changes in my theoretical formulation, and these I have tried to state as they consolidated themselves in my mind. Often what I have discovered had been already discovered and even better stated, either by Freud himself or by other psycho-analysts or by poets and philosophers. This does not deter me from continuing to write down (and to read when a public is available) what is my latest brain-child.

At the moment I am caught up with the idea that psycho-analytic theory has something to offer in regard to the theory of madness, that is madness that is met with clinically either in the form of a fear of madness, or as some other kind of insane manifestation. I would like to try to state this, even if I shall find that I am only stating the (psycho-analytically) obvious.

We have the only really useful formulation that exists of the way the human being psychologically develops from an absolutely dependent immature being to a relatively independent mature adult. The theory is exceedingly complex and difficult to state succinctly, and we know there are great gaps in our understanding. Nevertheless, there is the theory, and in this way psycho-analysis has made a contribution which is accepted generally but usually not acknowledged.

It was often said in reference to psycho-analytic theory that in the development of the normal child there is a period of psycho-neurosis. A more correct statement would be that at the height of the Oedipus complex phase before the onset of the latency period there is to be expected every kind of symptom in transient form. In fact normality at this age can be described in terms of this symptomatology so that abnormality becomes related to the absence of some kind of symptom or to the canalisation of the symptomatology in one direction. It is the rigidity of the defences that constitutes abnormality at this phase, not the defences themselves. The defences themselves are not abnormal, and they are being organised by the individual along with his or her emergence from dependence towards independent existence based on a sense of identity. This comes to the fore in a new and significant way in adolescence.

It is in this phase that the cultural provision as manifested in the child's immediate environment or in the family pattern alters the symptomatology although it does not of course produce the underlying drives and anxieties. What are referred to as symptoms in this context are not to be called symptoms in the description of a child because of the fact that the word symptom connotes pathology. Two side-issues from this theme can be mentioned. One that is so interesting is put forward by Erik Erikson, who shows that communities can mould what is being called here the symptomatology into directions which will eventually be valuable in the localised community.[1] The second has to do with the effect of a breakdown of the child's immediate environment at this stage so that in fact the child is not able to display the variegated symptomatology which is appropriate but must conform or take over an identification with some aspect of the environment, thereby losing personal experience.

The theme of the polymorpho-perverse symptomatology of childhood described by Paula Heimann[2] applies in this wide area of the manifestations that belong to the pre-latency period which would be called symptoms if they were to appear clinically when the individual has reached the age at which he or she would be expected to be adult. It can be understood how there came about the idea that in psychoanalytic theory all children were psycho-neurotic, but on closer scrutiny we find that this is not part of the theory. Nevertheless we are able to diagnose illness in children of this age which must be called psycho-neurotic because it is not psychotic, and we find that the basis of our diagnosis is not observation of symptomatology but a carefully considered assessment of the defence organisation, especially its generalised or localised rigidity.

With the extension of psycho-analytic theory backwards and all the new work on ego psychology and on the stage of absolute depen-

1. Erik H. Erikson, *Childhood and Society* (New York: Norton, 1950).
2. Paula Heimann, "A Contribution to the Re-evaluation of the Oedipus Complex: The Early Stages," *International Journal of Psycho-Analysis* 33 (1952); also in *New Directions in Psycho-Analysis,* by Melanie Klein and others (London: Karnac Books, 1977).

dence of infant on mother, etc., we have reached a new theme. We have reached to various theories which link psycho-analytic practice with the therapy of psychosis. By "psychosis" is meant in this context illness which has its point of origin in the stages of individual development prior to the establishment of an individual personality pattern. Obviously the ego support of the parental figures or figure is of the utmost importance at this very early stage which nevertheless can be described in terms of the individual infant unless there is distortion by environmental failure or abnormality.

Psycho-analysis now comes to the consideration of the aetiology of illness which belongs to the territory of schizophrenia (be it noted that in this context it is necessary to jump back over the problems of the aetiology of the antisocial tendency and of depression, each of which needs separate treatment).

There is very great resistance, especially among psychiatrists who are not psycho-analytically oriented, to the idea of schizophrenia as psychological, that is to say at least theoretically capable of prevention or cure. In any case psychiatrists have their own problems. Every psychiatrist has an immense load of serious cases. He is always threatened by the possibility of suicide among the patients in his immediate care, and there are heavy burdens associated with taking responsibility for certification and de-certification and with the prevention of such things as murder and the abuse of children. Moreover the psychiatrist must deal with social pressure since all those who need protection from themselves or who need to be isolated from society inevitably come under his care and in the end he cannot refuse them. He may refuse a case but this only means that someone else must take it. It can hardly be expected that psychiatry will welcome a study of the individual psychotic patient when such study seems to show that the aetiology of the illness is not entirely one of inheritance although inheritance and constitutional factors are often important.

The trend in psycho-analytic study of psychosis is nevertheless towards the theory of psychological origin. Surprisingly it appears that in the psychoses there is not only the inheritance factor but also an environmental factor operative at the very earliest stage, that is to say when dependence is absolute. In other words the internal strains and stresses that belong to life and that are inherent in living and growing seem to be typically found in the normality that relates to psycho-neurosis, psycho-neurosis being evidence of failure. By contrast, in digging down into the aetiology of the psychotic patient one comes to two types of external factor, heredity (which for the psychiatrist is an external thing) and environmental distortion at the phase of the individual's absolute dependence. In other words psychosis has to do with distortions during the phase of the formation of the personality pattern, whereas psycho-neurosis belongs to the difficulties that are experienced by individuals whose personality patterns can be taken for granted in the sense of being formed and healthy enough.

The extremely complex theory or theories of very early infantile development lead the observing public to ask a question which is similar to the question: "Are all children neurotic?" The new question is: "Is every infant mad?" This is a question which cannot be answered in a few words, but the first reply must certainly be in the negative. The theory does not involve the idea of a madness phase in infantile development. Nevertheless the door must be left open for the formulation of a theory in which some experience of madness, whatever that may mean, is universal, and this means that it is impossible to think of a child who was so well cared for in earliest infancy that there was no occasion for overstrain of the personality as it is integrated at a given moment. It must be conceded, however, that there are very roughly speaking two kinds of human being, those who do not carry around with them a significant experience of mental breakdown in earliest infancy and those who do carry around with them such an experience and who must therefore flee from it, flirt with it, fear it, and to some extent be always preoccupied with the threat of it. It could be said, and with truth, that this is not fair.

It is important to state this fact, that the psycho-analytic study of madness, whatever that means, is being done chiefly on the basis of the analysis of what are called borderline cases. The advances in the understanding of psychosis are not so likely to come from the direct study of the very severely broken down mad patient. The analysts' work therefore at the present time is open to the criticism that what is true of the borderline case is not true of the broken down case or of organised madness. Undoubtedly there will be found to be significant differences between the madness that is sometimes accessible to examination and even treatment in the borderline case and the madness of the case of total breakdown. Nevertheless for the time being work must be done that can be done and that can be a natural development of the application of the psycho-analytic technique to the more deeply disturbed aspects of the personalities of our patients.

It seems unlikely that there is such a thing as madness which belongs entirely to the present. This way of looking at madness received an important reinforcement through the work on general paralysis of the insane. This illness is caused by a physical disease of the brain and yet it is possible to see in the psychology of the patient an illness which belongs specifically to that patient and his personality and character, and the details relate to the patient's early history. In the same way a brain tumour may produce a mental illness which will be like a mental illness which was latent in that individual but which would not have become manifest had it not been for the physical disease.

Case: A boy in my care was brought to hospital because he was beginning to get bullied at school. He developed this tendency very steadily and gradually and it was this steady development that drew attention to the fact that there might be a physical cause for the illness. In a few months from the indefinite onset he became a person who provoked persecution and punishment. He was suffering from a sella tursica cyst, and as this increased in size, giving rise to intercranial pressure with papilloedema, he became a thoroughgoing paranoid case. After the removal of the cyst he gradually returned to being like he was before the onset of the illness, quite free from a paranoid tendency. The cyst could not be entirely removed and after a few years there was a return of the illness along with a new growth of the cyst.

At the present time Ronald Laing and his co-workers are drawing our attention to the way in which schizophrenia can be the normal state of an individual who is growing up or who has grown up in an environment that is dominated by persons with schizophrenic traits. His clinical material is very convincing but at the moment he fails to carry the logic of his attitude to a consideration of the same thing in terms of the infant-parent relationship at the period of absolute or near-absolute dependence. If he were to extend his work in this direction he would find what he is putting forward to be even more true and he would be getting near to making a significant statement in regard to the aetiology of schizophrenia. In the meantime he is making significant observations about certain schizophrenic patients and already his work can be applied in the field of management-treatment of some mentally ill persons who are labelled schizophrenic.

In my paper "Psychosis and Child Care," [3] which I gave in 1952, I

3. In *Collected Papers: Through Paediatrics to Psycho-Analysis* (London: Tavistock, 1958; New York: Basic Books, 1975; London: Hogarth Press, 1975).

surprised myself by saying that schizophrenia is an environmental deficiency disease, i.e. it is an illness which depends more on certain environmental abnormalities than does psycho-neurosis. It is true that there are also powerful inherited factors in some cases of schizophrenia, but it must be remembered that from the purely psychological angle inherited factors are environmental, that is, external to the life and experience of the individual psyche. In this paper I was getting near to the statement about madness that I wish to make here and now.

In my approach to my central but very simple theme I wish to bring in also the idea of the fear of madness. This is something which dominates the life of many of our patients. I have written on this subject that it may be taken as an axiom that madness that is feared has already been experienced.[4] In my opinion this statement contains an important truth and yet it is not quite true. A modification of the statement is needed, and this will take me to the heart of my communication.

To continue with the theme in these terms, a significantly large number of persons, some of whom come into analysis or into psychiatric care, live in a state of fear which can be tracked down to a fear of madness. It may take the form of a fear of incontinence or a fear of screaming in public, or there may be panics and the fear of panics which is even worse; and there may be a sense of impending doom and various other very severe fears each of which contains an element which is outside the operation of logic. A patient may, for instance, be dominated by a fear of dying which has nothing to do with the fear of death but which is entirely a matter of the fear of dying without anybody being there at the time; i.e. with nobody there who is concerned in some way that derives directly from the very early infant-parent relationship. Such patients can organise life so that they are never alone.

In trying to receive the communication that these patients attempt to make when we give them a chance, as we do especially in psychoanalysis, what we find looks like a fear of madness that will come. It is of value to us if not actually to the patient to know that the fear is not of madness to come but of madness that has already been expe-

---

4. "Classification: Is There a Psycho-Analytic Contribution to Psychiatric Classification?" (1959–1964), in *The Maturational Processes and the Facilitating Environment* (London: Hogarth Press; New York: International Universities Press, 1965). See also Chapter 18 in this volume, "Fear of Breakdown."

rienced. It is a fear of the return of madness. One might expect that an interpretation along these lines would relieve the situation, but in fact it is unlikely to produce relief except in so far as the patient gets relief from intellectual understanding of what is likely to turn up in the course of further analysis. The reason why relief is not obtained by the patient is that the patient has a stake in remembering the madness which has been experienced. In fact a great deal of time can be spent in remembering and reliving examples of madness which are like cover memories. The patient's need is to remember the original madness, but in fact the madness belongs to a very early stage before the organisation in the ego of those intellectual processes which can abstract experiences that have been catalogued and can present them for use in terms of conscious memory. In other words madness that has to be remembered can only be remembered in the reliving of it. Naturally there are very great difficulties when a patient attempts to relive madness, and one of the big difficulties is to find an analyst who will understand what is taking place. It is quite difficult in the present state of our knowledge for the analyst to remember in this kind of experience that it is the aim of the patient to reach to the madness, i.e. to be mad in the analytic setting, the nearest that the patient can ever do to remembering. In order to organise the setting for this the patient sometimes has to be mad in a more superficial way, i.e. has to organise what Dr Little calls a delusional transference,[5] and the analyst has to take the delusional transference, accept it and understand its performance.

For example, a girl who is at school brings to the analysis the idea of being given too much homework and being over-pressed at school. She brings this as very urgent material and it helps her to get to an extreme of agony with a severe headache and hours of screaming. She has been able to tell me that in fact her teacher is not over-pressing her and also that she has not been given too much homework. It is not even possible for me in making interpretations to talk about the idea of a strict teacher who over-taxes her pupil. In terms of the teacher and the homework the patient is telling me that I am over-taxing her and any word from me, even a correct interpretation, is a persecution. The point of the exercise is that without being too mad in the secondary sense this patient is able then to reach to the re-

5. Margaret I. Little, "On Delusional Transference (Transference Psychosis)," *International Journal of Psycho-Analysis* 39 (1958); also in Little, *Transference Neurosis and Transference Psychosis* (New York, London: Jason Aronson, 1981).

experiencing of the original madness, or at any rate she gets to an extreme of agony which is next door to the original madness.

In such a case any attempt on the part of the analyst to be sane or logical destroys the only route that the patient can forge back to the madness which needs to be recovered in experience because it cannot be recovered in memory. In this way the analyst has to be able to tolerate whole sessions or even periods of analysis in which logic is not applicable in any description of the transference. The patient then is under a compulsion, arising out of some *basic urge that patients have towards becoming normal,* to get to the madness; and this is slightly more powerful than the need to get away from it. For this reason there is no natural outcome apart from treatment. The individual is forever caught up in a conflict, nicely balanced between the fear of madness and the need to be mad. In some cases it is a relief when the tragic thing happens and the patient goes mad, because if a natural recovery is allowed for, the patient has to some extent "remembered" the original madness. This is, however, never quite true, but it may be true enough so that clinical relief is obtained by the fact of the breakdown. It will be seen that if in such a case the breakdown is met by a psychiatric urge to cure then the whole point of the breakdown is lost because in breaking down the patient had a positive aim and the breakdown is not so much an illness as a first step towards health.

At this point it is necessary to remember the basic assumption that belongs to the psycho-analytic theory that defences are organised around anxiety. What we see clinically when we meet an ill person is the organisation of defences and we know that we cannot cure our patient by the analysis of defences although much of our work is engaged in precisely doing this. The cure only comes if the patient can reach to the anxiety around which the defences were organised. There may be many subsequent versions of this, and the patient reaches one after another, but cure only comes if the patient reaches to the original state of breakdown.

It is now necessary to try to state what is wrong with the wording of the axiom that the fear of madness is the fear of madness that has been experienced. First it is necessary to be quite clear on one point, which is that the words "the fear of madness" ordinarily would refer to the fear that anyone might have or should have at the thought of insanity; not only the horror of the illness itself with all the mental pain involved, but also the social effect on the individual and even on the family of the fact of mental breakdown, which the community fears and therefore hates. This is the obvious meaning of the words that are being employed here, and it is necessary to point out that in this particular study the words are being used differently. These same words are being used to describe what we may discover about unconscious motivation in patients who have been in analysis for a long time, or who have become by some means or other, perhaps through the passage of time and the process of growth, able to tolerate and cope with anxieties which were unthinkable in their original setting.

Secondly, there is something wrong with the statement even in the specialised setting in which it is being given in this chapter. It is not really true to say that the patient is trying to remember madness which has been and around which defences were organised. The reason why this is so is that at the original place where the defences were organised madness was not experienced because by the nature of what is being discussed the individual was not able to experience it. A state of affairs arose involving a breakdown of defences, defences that were appropriate at the age and in the setting of the individual. The ego support of a parental figure has to be taken into consideration here in regard to its being a reliable or unreliable support. In the simplest possible case there was therefore a split second in which the threat of madness was experienced, but anxiety at this level is unthinkable. Its intensity is beyond description and new defences are organised immediately so that in fact madness was not experienced. Yet on the other hand madness was potentially a fact. In attempting to find an analogy I saw a hyacinth bulb being planted in a bowl. I thought, there is a wonderful smell locked up in that bulb; I knew of course that there is no place in the bulb where a smell is locked up. Dissection of the bulb would not give the dissector the experience of a smell of hyacinths, if the appropriate spot were to be reached. Nevertheless there is in the bulb a potential which eventually will become the characteristic smell as the flower opens. This is only an analogy but it could carry a picture of what I am trying to state. It is an important part of my thesis that the original madness or breakdown of defences if it were to be experienced would be indescribably painful. The nearest that we can get is to take what is available of psychotic anxiety such as

   a. disintegration
   b. unreality feelings
   c. lack of relatedness
   d. depersonalisation or lack of psycho-somatic cohesion
   e. split-off intellectual functioning

f. falling forever

g. E.C.T. with panic as a generalised feeling which may contain any of these.

Nevertheless we can see if we look that whenever we reach to any of these things clinically we know there is some ego-organisation able to suffer, which means to go on suffering so as to be aware of suffering. The core of madness has to be taken to be something so much worse because of the fact that it cannot be experienced by the individual who by definition has not the ego-organisation to hold it and so to experience it.

It might be valuable to use a symbol, X, and so say that the infant or small child has an ego-organisation appropriate to the stage of development and that something happens such as a reaction to an impingement (an external factor which has been allowed through by faulty environmental functioning) and that then there is a state of affairs called X. This state may result in a re-organisation of defences. Such may happen once or many times or perhaps many times in a pattern. From the organisation of the defences one gets a clinical picture and the diagnosis is made on the basis of the defence organisation. The defence organisation in turn depends for its characteristics to some extent on a contribution from the environment. What is absolutely personal to the individual is X.

I now come to an attempt to restate the original axiom. The individual who reaches these things in the course of a treatment is repeatedly reaching towards X, but of course the individual can only get as near X as the new ego strength plus ego support in the transference can make possible. The continuation of the analysis means that the patient continually reaches to new experiences in the direction towards X and in the way I have described these experiences cannot be recalled as memories. They have to be lived in the transference relationship and they appear clinically as localised madnesses. Constantly the analyst is bewildered by finding that the patient is able to be more and more mad for a few minutes or for an hour in the treatment setting, and sometimes the madness spreads out over the edges of the session. It requires a considerable experience and courage to know where one is in the circumstances and to see the value to the patient when the patient reaches nearer and nearer to the X which belongs to that individual patient. Nevertheless if the analyst is not able to look at it in this way, but out of fear or out of ignorance or out of the inconvenience of having so ill a patient on his hands he tends to waste these things that happen in the treatment, he cannot cure the patient. Constantly he finds himself correcting the delusional transference or in some way or other bringing the patient round to sanity instead of allowing the madness to become a manageable experience from which the patient can make spontaneous recovery. Looked at in this way psychiatry that is based on meeting social need and the treatment of large numbers of patients is at the present time in a phase of fighting the wrong enemy. This is brought out in the work of Ronald Laing and his collaborators. It does not matter if we find that we cannot always agree with their theory or with their presentation of their theory. At any rate my thesis in this paper compels me to welcome many of the statements of these workers in the field.

It is unfortunate that the theory that I am putting forward here, even if it is correct, certainly does not lead to an immediate step forward in affecting psychotherapy. It will not be found by those who are meeting these problems in their psycho-analytic practices that this detail of theory makes it possible for them to do better work tomorrow. In fact at its best it can give them some understanding and of course it may lead them into deeper waters. Nevertheless there are some cases where the patient goes on trying to get help from us and yet we cannot reach a satisfactory end-point, and of course these cases are of various kinds; one kind I am suggesting can be understood better on the basis of the thesis that I am putting forward, and an advantage here is that if the analyst understands what is going on he or she is able to tolerate the very considerable tensions that belong to this kind of work. Unfortunately there is only one way of avoiding these tensions and that is by better diagnosis to avoid taking on the kind of case that must inevitably lead into these deep waters. Then if we do find a method by which we may avoid taking on these cases we must be honest and admit out loud that we need even in our theory the psychiatric help which in some ways we despise because it is not based on psychology, i.e. the physical treatments. It has occurred to me, perhaps wrongly, that from a general acceptance of this idea that I am promulgating when it arrives in the literature that is read by the thinking public, there could come some relief from the idea. It is impossible to predict but it seems to me that there is a great deal of fear of breakdown, and if it could seep through that the breakdown that is feared is a breakdown that has already done its worst, there is at least the possibility that the edge of the fear of breakdown could be dulled.

22

The Concept of Trauma in Relation to the Development of the Individual within the Family

An amalgamation of two similar versions of an essay written in March and May 1965

The vast area covered by the term "the family" has been studied in many ways. Here an attempt will be made to relate the function of the family to the idea of trauma, and this must involve a study of trauma as a concept in metapsychology. The link between the two ideas is that the family gives to the growing child a *protection from trauma*.

I shall first approach the problem of trauma from the clinical angle, and then briefly discuss the theory of trauma.

A Trauma That Involved a Patient

I was engaged in the analysis and management of the case of a child, a girl coming up to the age of puberty, who had a physical disability interwoven with her emotional disturbance. I was fortunate in having this girl in good paediatric care over the period of time when adjunctive treatment along physical lines was needed. I was able to keep in intimate touch with her during the period of hospitalisation.

Because of my special position I learned from the girl that an adult pervert was visiting the children's ward in spite of the usual care taken in a good children's hospital. I found this difficult to believe and at first tended to side with the girl's suspicion that she was hallucinating. I did, however, report what I had been told by her immediately, and in the end it became clear that all that she had told me had been actually happening.

Naturally I wanted this girl to go home because, as suddenly became obvious, it is a child's family and home that best protects a child from trauma. But she herself was unable to consider either removal to her home or removal to alternative hospital surroundings. In fact the only procedure was for me first to recover from the trauma myself, and then to allow the hospital to deal with the trouble in its own way. Facts having been established, the hospital quickly got into action, and a sense of security was re-established.

The girl was producing material at the time which showed that she was at the prepubertal stage. For instance, a significant drawing showed an unsophisticated girl, in a dress of sewn leaves, being taught to dance by a black leopard. The girl's arms were outstretched, and she had two apples which she had just picked to eat, in the right hand, and she had a blue bird on the left hand. The contrast between the innocent girl and the potentially sinister leopard was striking, and this beautiful picture depicted the preview of sexuality that is to be found in this presexual phase. It was at this stage in the girl's development that the male pervert turned up in her life and all the children in the hospital ward were in jeopardy. It could be said that only this girl understood the danger; the others all treated the matter by being generally excited, becoming afraid of spooks or expecting every noise to mean that a man was climbing through the window. My patient was in a special position because of being able to report every detail to myself, and it is to be noted that she could not tell her parents (whom she certainly trusts) about what was happening. At first she could not even tell the nurses, and when she did tell a nurse the matter was taken lightly and not reported to the Sister. Even the parent of one of the other children made light of it.

It is in fact almost impossible to think of a pervert in a children's hospital ward at night. Denial is the natural reaction, or, alternatively, a frantic reactive activity. Parents leave their children in hospitals only by a process of idealisation of hospital and staff, and in my long experience of children's hospitals the doctors and nurses and auxiliary staff not only behave reliably but also do actually try to reproduce the conditions that belong to the family, conditions that are designed to protect the children from gross trauma. Alas! this protection from gross trauma does not cover protection from the more subtle traumata that may be worse for the children and the infants than these gross traumata that shock adults when they do occasionally happen. Gross trauma of the kind that occurred in this case is prevented in the family by the taboos against incest that are generally operative.

My patient made the comment "It's not fair." I could not agree more, and I said so. She could not put into words the full nature of the trauma, the fact that the sweet innocence that belongs to the phase of her emotional development, and which she quite correctly depicted in terms of ballet, was being spoiled by the premature introduction of the sexuality of a man, that is, of a second person objectively perceived. The subjective image of the leopard suddenly turns into what the girl called "a man being nasty." She was able to add that he might really be quite a human person, perhaps lonely, but he was certainly nasty in the context of the trauma and her experience of it.

I am able to add that this trauma has not spoiled this girl's "innocence," largely because of the fact that she was intimately in touch with myself, a person professionally involved, one whom she had found she could trust in both gross and subtle ways. I cannot say, however, that the other children may not have been hurt. And of course the fact that she had her own family and that she absolutely trusted all the members of this family was the constant factor that made her able to believe me and to use me.

If my patient has not been adversely affected this is also due to the fact that in her analysis it is the very subtle trauma and *not the gross trauma* that has been significant and that she has been able to use. To illustrate this I give an example of a typical session that contained forward movement:

The patient reclined on the couch as usual, and talked very softly of this and that. I needed to be (as usual with her) very close in order to be able to hear. At these moments she is very sensitive to any changes in the room, and I do avoid upsetting her by not making careless changes. In many ways the patient needs to get me in her control, and I must give full attention. I follow her needs by altering the heat of the fire exactly as she wants or by opening or closing the window, and perhaps supplying her with paper handkerchiefs or other objects she knows are available. Conditions being well-nigh perfect she begins to want me to talk, but there is no material for me to use, and I know (from past experience) that if I talk I shall upset her. I say something, it hardly matters what: "You need me to be in your control, as if a part of you, . . ."; before I have gone far she is frantically upset. She curls up and withdraws, and she is inconsolable. She cries and is clearly *deeply wounded*. There is now a

time factor involved, so that I cannot stop until I know the phase is
past; the phase must be allowed to come to a natural conclusion.

I am helped by my theoretical understanding of what Dr Margaret
Little calls the delusional transference.[1] I do not have to bring in
anything gross such as the matter of this pervert and his invasion of
the children's ward. All I need to do is to accept the role allotted to
me. In this way, within the ambit of a powerful positive transference,
the girl becomes wounded and reaches to the distress and to the
crying which she cannot reach on her own. In the end the phase
resolves itself and the patient becomes able to say: "You sounded
angry with me when you said . . ."

By now she was emerging from a paranoid episode, which had the
following pattern:

1. I was fitting in with her idea of a person who is in her omnipotent control, almost part of her.
2. I "moved" very slightly, and was immediately outside her control.
3. The next part was unconscious; she hated me.
4. She knew I was a persecutor.
5. She saw that this had been a delusion.
6. She now became able in a very small way to reach (3) to the
   hate of me (whom she trusted) for my minute excursion out of
   the area of her omnipotence.

In this experience the patient had felt real because of the distress
and the crying. She *always feels awful,* but for a quarter of an hour
she had felt awful *about something.*

It was now time for the session (prolonged on this occasion by ten
minutes) to end, and the patient prepared to go. This kind of session
with maximal distress carries some satisfaction for her, whereas other
sessions seem unreal, especially if she has allowed herself to enjoy
some activity, and to make me enjoy myself and so get a false impression that all is well with her. All is not well.

And now as she went I realised that she knew at the beginning that
all this was liable to happen. When the session started she had said:
"I wish this was one of the times when it was Mummy who was to
come for me." I knew this sign well, and I had been therefore pre-

1. Margaret I. Little, "On Delusional Transference (Transference Psychosis)," *International Journal of Psycho-Analysis* 39 (1958); also in Little, *Transference Neurosis and
Transference Psychosis* (New York, London: Jason Aronson, 1981).

pared for what would happen, though I could not tell what form this day's disillusioning would take. My job was first to co-operate with the process of her idealisation of me, and then to share the burden of the responsibility for the breakup of the idealisation by her hate, hate which would come to her as a delusion of my being angry with her. *Just a little she achieves ambivalence in this way.*

It will be noted that this work gets well behind the trouble arising out of the visits of the male pervert, except that the words: "It isn't fair" provide a link. It isn't fair for the idealised object (subjective, almost) to show its independence, its own separateness, its freedom from her omnipotent control.

If this analysis succeeds it will be because of a long series of those minute traumata *that are staged by the patient,* and that involve phases of delusional transference.

A Woman Patient's Experience of a Trauma

It would not be difficult for an analyst to find examples of such events in his or her current clinical work. Here is another example, taken from the same week of my clinical experience.

An adult woman patient has a very well-organised defence against hope. In a previous analysis and in my analysis of her nothing has ever become conscious. Whatever happens has already been foreseen by the patient. There is a despair in the whole picture which never alters, so that this potentially valuable person accepts defeat all along the line, and lives in a mildly depressed mood. She "knows the analysis cannot succeed."

This state of affairs started when an exceptionally happy early childhood ended abruptly because her father died and her mother immediately became melancholic. The mother's melancholia was clearly present in her exceptionally lively and imaginative and happy-making attitude towards this her only child, all of which lasted until the moment of her husband's death. The melancholia lasted until her own death. In the session that I am choosing to report a new thing happened: the patient found that my main *interpretation must be right* and yet she had not foreseen this; the interpretation was there-fore "traumatic," in the sense of getting behind the defences. This benign trauma reflected the patient's new feeling about the malignant trauma.

At the time I was only seeing the patient once a week. The week before this particular session the patient was to have come at a changed time. She came at her ordinary time and went away when told at the door that she had made a mistake. In the session to which I am referring (a week later) she started off telling me about this, and how she saw on the face of the person who had answered the door a look of criticism, almost: "you have been naughty."

She then went on to say how much she liked this person, who nearly always let her into my house. There followed the usual depressive material. She had been glad to get away and not to have the session. Other things were reported. The worst was as follows: her friend had reacted in a terrible way to something she had said. It had to do with an adopted child who was happy but who had not been told of being adopted. My patient had said: "Well I hope they will get on with telling the child soon," and the friend had become very angry and had put it all down to a psychiatric attitude to life engendered in people having analyses. The friend's bad mood had lasted a long time and was intolerable. This was given as absolutely devastating, but always there was this same sad mood of the patient which reduces everything to the same thing: something potentially good, even wonderful, but of course spoilt.

There were other examples of this in the patient's material. One example had to do with a new version of the incident which led up to her suicide attempt. She had gone in all good faith to ask for extra opportunity to do special work (at the university) because of an examination failure due to the burden of the mother's melancholia, and unexpectedly had been accused of claiming special privileges. This led on to a new version of the moment of the original trauma, when she went to her mother after her father's death, expecting to find the usual very happy-making mother, and instead finding a new person, one who was irritable, unreasonable, and no longer in a special relation to my patient (then a child of six).

It will be noted that (as I had come to expect in this analysis) this new material was not really new; the patient had always known all this, but on this day she had felt like giving me a clearer picture of what she had always remembered clearly.

Now came my interpretation. This was no more than a linking of these examples of trauma with the episode at the door with the person who, instead of letting her in, told her she had made a mistake. It was at this point that my patient experienced her first analytic "trauma," or "benign trauma," if the term may be permitted. She was astounded. She had not made this link herself. She could see that the link was valid but she could not immediately "take" it.

She now saw what she had not seen before, that is to say, she recognized the delusion that was at the centre of the episode at the door. In fact the person at the door had been nice. But my patient had seen the person's face as forbidding and accusatory. The reaction had been as to a persecutor. (This person stood for me in the transference, and in fact the patient had also said of me when she came to this, the following session, and when I was ordinarily understanding and certainly not angry, that for some reason or other she resented my being nice.)

It was now possible to see here the pattern, the same pattern that I have described above in my description of the young girl's session. This adult patient came with all defences down, "knowing" she would be let in. The person at the door would be within the area of her omnipotence, part of the "average expectable environment." But she was not so. Here followed unconscious hate of the person. What was conscious was a delusion of the person's criticism, from which the patient escaped with alacrity, feeling lucky to get away.

Now the patient had experienced in the "delusional transference" the persecution which is a necessary step towards experience of the hate of a good object, this being the stuff of disillusionment. Perhaps for the first time in a decade of analysis the patient had reached to a shift in the defences, defences originally organised relative to the sudden and unpredictable change in the mother that followed her father's unpredictable death.[2]

A Similar Example

Here I would add a third example that came to hand while I was writing these notes.

In a case that I am watching from outside, a woman analytic patient went as usual to her analyst and pressed the electric bell. She was in a special state which has to do with hope in this person who

2. Little, "Delusional Transference." W. R. Bion, "Attacks on Linking," *International Journal of Psycho-Analysis* 40 (1959); also in Bion, *Second Thoughts* (London: Heinemann Medical Books Ltd., 1967). Winnicott refers to the value of Little's concept in "Dependence in Infant-Care, in Child-Care and in the Psycho-Analytic Setting" (1963) in *The Maturational Processes and the Facilitating Environment* (London: Hogarth Press; New York: Universities Press, 1965).

is usually hopeless. Evidently the bell did not ring, so she pressed again, whereupon someone came and opened the door. When this patient went into her session she said: "So you were there all the time while I was waiting outside the door." (The implication was: you hate me!) The analyst did not know what was going on, and is reported (perhaps wrongly) to have said: "Do you realise what it is that you are saying?" (In effect, this was a reproof.) The patient was in despair because of this.

It is possible to look back on this material and to see that the analyst (as reported by this patient) missed interpreting along the lines of the delusional transference. She might have said nothing, or she might have said: "you hated me when the door-bell did not ring and no-one came to let you in; but you did not know about this hate of me, and what you saw was my hate of yourself."

In this instance I made the experiment of giving this patient this bit of information from outside her analysis. The result was that she remembered feeling most intense and bitter hate of her analyst as she passed her analyst's door on her way to the waiting-room. She could not have reported this because she was unaware of it, but in any case "it would have been so mad . . ." (delusional transference).

Here the same mechanism is at work as in the other cases described. In each instance there is a traumatisation, with hate appearing clinically as a delusion of being hated.

The Therapeutic Consultation

Another type of clinical experience that had made a link for me between the idea of the family and that of trauma comes out of a study that I am making of what I call the Therapeutic Consultation. I am trying to show that in a very common type of child psychiatry case there is a possibility of doing effective and deep psychotherapy by making full use of one, or a limited number, of interviews. If my thesis is correct, then it becomes urgently necessary to be able to diagnose according to the case's suitability for such treatment. In this type of case the child may well be severely disturbed, clinically.

One common denominator in these cases is the existence of a functioning family or at least a family situation. In fact, where there is severe psychiatric illness in one or other parent, or where the home has already broken or has a built-in unreliability, then it is unlikely that this type of quick therapy will work.

In other words, the main work in such cases is done by the family and within the family, and the therapist acts by making a change in the child that is qualitatively accurate and quantitatively sufficient to enable the family to function again, in respect of this child. Once stated, this idea is easily accepted. These cases are important in that they have a close link with the therapy of one or other child that is all the time being done in any family that is functioning, regardless of psychiatric or specialised professional help.

Brief Description of a Child Psychiatry Case

Phyllis was brought to me at the age of 16 years because of difficulties of personality that had not yet organised themselves into an illness pattern. In the course of a significant psychotherapeutic interview Phyllis said: "I always feel that I am standing or sitting on a church spire. As I look around I find no support anywhere, and I am just balancing."

Clearly this anxiety might be related to a fear of an unreliable feature in Phyllis's childhood experiences; it might refer to some kind of failure of holding on the part of the mother, at a time when Phyllis was immature in the sense of being dependent.

Now it happens that I had notes of this case made when Phyllis was brought to me as a small child, in fact at 1¾ years when her mother was six months pregnant. At that age her straightforward development had become interrupted, and in fact Phyllis had never properly recovered. It was at 1¾ that she reacted to being told that she was to go away to stay with her grandmother (with whom she had a good relationship) while the new baby was being born. Presumably at this age she was also physically aware of the physical changes in her mother. Two days after being given this news she reacted with a week of refusal to take food, and she screamed incessantly. After this she settled down into being nervous and irritable and somewhat of a problem of management. Thus did her illness start.

It would seem that several factors were at work here:

1. As a small child Phyllis was not able to deal with her mother's pregnancy and all that went with it. It is difficult to give information to a child of 1¾; either the child gets no message at all or else the message received is one of total change of parental attitude or of sudden disillusionment.

2. Perhaps the parents did not handle this matter well, although

these parents may be counted on in general to behave in a sensitive way.

3. To announce this change, a change already expected because of the mother's shape, in terms of: "You will be going away . . ." may have been a bad method, making it even more difficult than would be normal at this age for the little child to deal with the mother's pregnancy by an identification with the mother. In my notes I see that I reported a little later that Phyllis did make an attempt to be like her mother, in that she developed a compulsion to stick out her abdomen and to strut about, awkwardly imitating her mother.

Whatever the cause, Phyllis became highly disturbed at the time when her mother was pregnant. One must assume that she became aware of a threat of "unthinkable anxiety," the primitive or archaic anxiety that well-cared-for infants do not actually experience until they have become equipped to deal with environmental failure by self-care (introjected mothering). Such anxieties include:

falling forever;
disintegration;
depersonalisation;
disorientation.

I had known of this child's reaction to this threat at the time, and it was interesting to me to be given the 16-year-old Phyllis's sophisticated version of this awareness of the threat to her existence which belonged to the age of 1¾ years. She had all her life felt herself to be *just balancing*. The words "on the spire of a church steeple" do not add anything of general significance; but the words "standing or sitting" are possibly derived from her actual experiences on her mother's lap before her second birthday, around which date her sister was born.

It can be seen from this example that parents in building their families do have a great deal of influence on their children's emotional development. They make mistakes, but they do also plan, and they think out how to introduce ideas to small children in appropriate language, and in a thousand ways *parents protect their children from traumatisation*. In this case there was a localised traumatisation, and this had an effect on the child's personality. The parents had done all they could do to mend what happened so long ago, but they needed help. This help was given in a psychotherapeutic interview with the child, in which the child's personal problem was brought to the fore in the child's own way. This is history-taking through the child, the only way in which the details of a case-history can be actually used in the psychotherapeutic process. A full-scale treatment, with the main work done relative to the transference neurosis (or psychosis), can be said to be a prolonged history-taking.

In this case the parents had carried the burden of the girl's illness for eight years; and they were able and willing to continue to carry it, although they both had considerable personal difficulties. They did need, however, a certain amount of help, by which the girl became able to make use of that which the family had to offer through its normal functioning.

Brief Description of Another Child Psychiatry Case[3]

Here is an older girl's reaction to the birth of a sibling. This child of 8 years was able to put me in touch with her reaction that took place at 3 years at the moment of being traumatised by a concatenation of circumstances. There were reasons (which need not be given here) why her mother became physically ill and also seriously depressed at the time of her sister's birth. In fact, for a few weeks at that time this child had had to experience her very good mother's rejection of her, since the mother became temporarily deranged to the extent of hating her new baby and her child. The baby was cared for within the family setting over this period, chiefly by the father, but she did nevertheless suffer an eclipse relative to the mother.

A nightmare (given me in one therapeutic consultation when she was 8 years old) took her back to this date when she was 3. Figure 1 shows how she went towards her mother and the new baby, taking "tins of baby food" and prepared to cope with the new situation by various cross-identifications, such as being the mother, being the baby, and herself helping to make the baby grow.

The rejection that she found (because of the mother's puerperal disorder) reversed all this, and Figure 2 actually shows her at the moment of becoming a deprived child. A symptom of her state was a compulsion to steal, and at first she stole tins of baby food, for which she developed a craving.

The first drawing then illustrates the nightmare, and the second illustrates her memory of actually becoming "deprived," that is, sud-

3. Described at length as Case 17, "Ruth," in Winnicott, *Therapeutic Consultations in Child Psychiatry* (London: Hogarth Press; New York: Basic Books, 1971).

denly out of touch with her mother. The baby shrinks because of the fact that the baby-food does not reach its target; and behind the deprived child is water, poisonous water which threatens to make the baby and the mother (and herself) shrink (the opposite of growing). The water was bitter tears, tears that could not flow from the eyes in sadness, and also the water belongs to the bed-wetting that became a manifest temporary symptom.

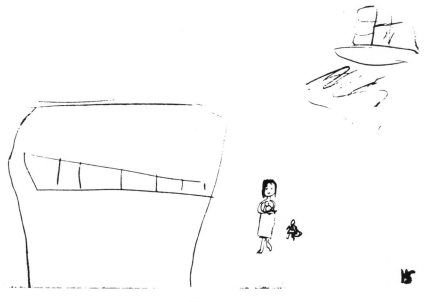

Figure 1

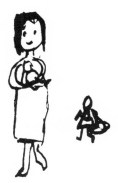

This detail from figure 1 is reproduced in the size
to which it was drawn.

The first picture, the nightmare, gives the hope, and the second picture gives the despair due to the rebuff for which the little girl was totally unprepared. Because of the mother's illness, psycho-somatic and depressive, this family failed to protect this child from trauma at the time of the birth of the baby, so that the child's capacity to identify with the mother came to grief.

In this case the family did well by the baby, and also did eventually see the girl through except for a part that needed specialised help

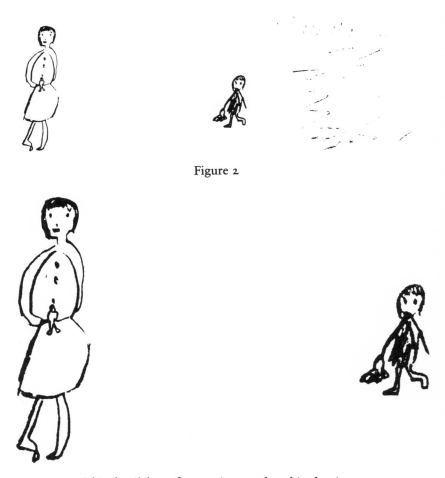

Figure 2

This detail from figure 2 is reproduced in the size
to which it was drawn.

from myself. One interview sufficed, after which the family went ahead with its function of caring for these two children and for the next one when he arrived.

General Comment

The average family is all the time preventing and clearing up the disturbances in this and that child, usually without professional help. It is surely a mistake for a psychotherapist to usurp the total family functioning except where this functioning is doomed to failure because of some inherent defect. Where the family is functioning the therapist's aim should be to enable the child that is brought for treatment to make use of that which the family can in fact do better and more economically than anyone else can do, namely the over-all mental nursing during the whole period until recovery has taken place.

Brief Description of Another Case[4]

This case illustrates the capacity of a child to state his personal problem. A boy with schizoid characteristics began to degenerate in his school work in spite of being of high intelligence. He was well tolerated at school though becoming increasingly odd. He was referred to me by his G.P. because of an increasing inability to return to school from home. When due back at school he always developed an obscure illness with fever.

His parents brought him to see me and I gave him one long psychotherapeutic consultation, in the course of which he gave me his basic problem in the form of an abstraction from an "abstract" that he had painted (Figure 3).

I interpreted to him that this was *a statement of simultaneous acceptance and refusal.* The result was like the opening of floodgates. Clinically the boy improved from the time of this very rich and rewarding (i.e. rewarding from my point of view) consultation, and he has matured in almost all respects.

The point here is that this kind of work, done in one interview, is only possible when the child's family is functioning, and in this case

4. Described at length as Case 9, "Ashton," in *Therapeutic Consultations in Child Psychiatry.*

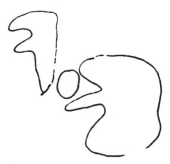

Figure 3

working in with the school. The family (helped by the school) did nearly all the work, both before and after the psychotherapeutic interview; but there was needed this one piece of enlightenment which the parents could not give, and in fact the boy would not have given them the opportunity. In one respect his mother had failed him in infancy, and then it was too late for her to do what she had failed to do at the appropriate time. She and her husband could do and did do everything else well.

Here is a positive example of a boy's confidence in his family and in each of his parents, this confidence enabling him to make use of me, and to dig deeply and immediately into his own personal problems of personality structure.

There were traumata in this boy's very early infancy which the parents could not prevent, but which did in fact nearly cause him to be a case of infantile schizophrenia. Instead he developed into a schizoid person, a person who increasingly needed to try to solve one problem. This and other similar problems would have lain hopelessly unsolved in him if he had become an infantile schizophrenia case, or perhaps one of those odd mental defectives who show patchy intellectual brilliance.

From the Abnormal to the Normal

The therapeutic consultation is effective when there is a functioning family, but professional help is needed in enabling a boy or girl to use the family which facilitates his or her maturational processes.

This links, clearly, with the work done by the functioning family in respect of its members who from time to time need and get individual attention.

It also links with that part of the family function that has to do with the Reality Principle and with the disillusioning process as (for example) the personal adjustments that relate to the arrival of siblings, etc., etc. At the peak of this is the Oedipus complex, the individual's adjustment to the fact of the triangle in interpersonal relationships.

In terms of the earlier stages of the individual's integration and other maturational processes the mother (in particular) plays her role as the one who disillusions her infant; and the basis of her work in this respect is the initial stage in which (by specialised adaptation) she gives each infant the illusion of the experience of omnipotence. The success of the mother's and the family's disillusioning function is to be measured in terms of the child's capacity for *ambivalence,* but the basis for ambivalence is this *experience of omnipotence* relative to an object. The environmental reflection of ambivalence involves the idea of trauma. This leads on to a consideration of the nature of trauma.

The Nature of Trauma

The idea of trauma involves a consideration of external factors; in other words it belongs to dependence. Trauma is a failure relative to dependence. Trauma is that which breaks up an idealisation of an object by the individual's hate, reactive to that object's failure to perform its function.[5]

Trauma therefore varies in its meaning according to the stage of the emotional development of the child. Thus:

A. At the start trauma implies a breakdown in the area of reliability in the "average expectable environment," at the stage of near-absolute dependence. The result of such breakdown shows in failure or relative failure in the establishment of personality structure and ego organisation.

B. De-adaptation is the second part of the maternal function, the first being the giving of opportunity to the infant for an *experience of omnipotence.* Normally, the mother's adaptation leads on to graduated adaptive failure. This leads on to the family's function of gradually introducing the Reality Principle to the child.

5. Winnicott, "Weaning" (1949), in *The Child, The Family and the Outside World* (Penguin, 1964; Reading, Mass.: Addison-Wesley, 1987).

A study of trauma therefore involves the investigator in a study of the natural history of the environment relative to a developing individual. The environment is adaptive and then de-adaptive; the change from adaptation to de-adaptation is related intimately to each individual's maturation and so the gradual development in the individual of the complex mental mechanisms that make possible, eventually, a move from dependence towards independence.

Thus there is a normal aspect of trauma. The mother is always "traumatising" within a framework of adaptation. In this way the infant passes from absolute to relative dependence. But the result is not as of trauma, because of the mother's ability to sense the baby's capacity, moment by moment, to employ new mental mechanisms. The infant's sense of the not-me depends on the fact of the mother's operation in this field of maternal care.[6] The parents acting together, and then the functioning of the family unit, continue this process of the disillusioning of the child.[7]

Clinically it is common to find that a mother cannot wean her child. She complains that the child "will not wean." It may well be that the mother is in a depressive phase, in which hate (both active and passive) is not available to consciousness or for use in relationships. The mother, in fact, cannot play her part in the disillusioning process, of which weaning is an expression.[8] In other words, a normal or healthy mother is able to summon up ambivalence in object-relating and to be able to use it appropriately.

The same difficulty may appear in the form of a child's school-refusal, the mother usually being unaware of the part she is playing. The child may be conscious of the fact that what he or she cannot stand is the mother's inability to deal with loss of him or her.

C. Trauma in the more popular sense of the term implies a breaking of faith. The infant or child has built up a capacity to "believe in,"[9] and environmental provision first fits into this and then fails. In this way the environment persecutes by getting through the defences. The infant's or the child's reactive hate breaks up the ideal-

6. Joan Riviere, "On the Genesis of Psychical Conflict in Earliest Infancy," *International Journal of Psycho-Analysis* 17 (1936).

7. Winnicott, "The World in Small Doses" (1949), in *The Child, The Family and the Outside World*.

8. Winnicott, "Weaning."

9. Winnicott, "Morals and Education" (1963), in *The Maturational Processes and the Facilitating Environment*.

ised object, and this is liable to be experienced in terms of a delusion of persecution by good objects. Where the reaction is one of appropriate anger or hatred the term trauma is not apposite. In other words, where there is appropriate anger the environmental failure has not been beyond the individual's capacity to cope with his or her reaction.

D. The more the child achieves integration the more severely the child can be *hurt* by being traumatised; hurt, or made to suffer, as opposed to being prevented from achieving integration. Eventually in the Oedipus complex, in inter-relationships as between three whole persons, the child needs to live through a period in which the personal reliability of the parents is experienced in order that the total equipment (projection and introjection mechanisms) may be used, and in which a personal or inner psychic reality may become established which makes fantasy an experience comparable to actual object-relating. A total presentation of this theme would need to include the concept of transitional phenomena.[10] The result of such growth in the individual is a capacity for ambivalence.

E. In the end, trauma is the destruction of the purity of individual experience by a too sudden or unpredictable intrusion of actual fact, and by the generation of hate in the individual, hate of the good object, experienced not as hate but delusionally as being hated.

The Family

It is the baby's own mother who is most likely to do what is needed environmentally for a baby, simply because of her total relationship to that baby. In the same way it is the family that is most likely to provide what corresponds to this in relation to the more sophisticated life of the child and of the adolescent. Limited social groups continue what the family has started, and in health the maturing child becomes more and more able to take part in the maintenance of group-structure and group-functioning.

Family functioning can be looked on as preventing trauma, provided that the meaning of the word "trauma" can be allowed *to change with the growth of the child from infancy to full maturity, growth from dependence towards independence.* On this basis the

10. Winnicott, "Transitional Objects and Transitional Phenomena" (1951), in *Collected Papers: Through Paediatrics to Psycho-Analysis* (London: Tavistock, 1958; New York: Basic Books, 1975; Hogarth Press, 1975).

family can be studied not only as a structured attitude of parents, near relations and siblings, but also as something that is in part *produced by the urgent needs of the children themselves,* needs arising out of dependence, and out of the fact that the individual maturational process only becomes realised in a facilitating environment.

23

Notes on Withdrawal and Regression

Written for a seminar in December 1965

In order to arrive at a Wednesday session in such a way that it can be understood I must refer to the previous day. On the Tuesday the patient was already disillusioned and becoming devoid of affect. She used two things: the formality of the doctor who was extra-ordinarily good with her in U.S.A. and an unfortunate sentence in a book by Searles. It was a feature of this hour that although she was taken up with these matters in such a way that the whole world was included, and myself also, she would from time to time emerge from her cocoon to say to me, fixing me with her eye in a way that is characteristic of her and that belongs to her good relationship to her good nurse, "You do know, don't you, that I am very fond of you indeed?" She was obviously struggling with other feelings about me which she could not get at but which she could find to some extent in relationship to the two doctors.

On Wednesday there was one of these characteristic days which certainly do alarm the inexperienced. She was a different person although I am only too familiar with what she is like when she is this different person. One could say she is indignant "with God on her side." The correct word for the Wednesday session was withdrawal. *This was the first of the points for discussion.* With this patient it is extremely important that I understand the difference between regression and withdrawal. Clinically the two states are practically the same. It will be seen, however, that there is an extreme difference between the two. In regression there is dependence and in withdrawal there is pathological independence. I have learned in the school of this analysis that withdrawal is something that I do well to allow, and in the first part of the analysis this was the important feature and resulted in there being many hours in which nothing whatever was done. The process was silent and concerned what happens in extreme dependence. When withdrawal became an alternative important feature the patient always became very angry whenever I mistook it for a regression or did not realise that withdrawal must be treated differently. More difficult is the fact that in practice one does watch the changeover from withdrawal into regression as the patient becomes able to recognise the positive in one's attitude. It will be understood that in withdrawal the expectation is of persecutory environment. In any case on this Wednesday the patient was about as withdrawn as possible, completely hidden under two rugs and wedged in between two pillows. Quite suddenly she emerged, and then she was as angry as it is possible for her to be, which is saying a lot. She went on right to the end of the hour, starting off with a criticism of me for leaving her withdrawn, going on to all the deficiencies which she can easily find and can enumerate in my technique, and finally getting up and going just about the right time saying that she was certainly not coming back to waste her time in this way.

There have been in the past more acutely wounding episodes like this but never I think one in which there was so much real feeling which the patient knew she was meaning. I did not of course defend myself in any way (or I hope I did not); I just left it that she had finished her analysis and I saw her out of the door in her car along with her nurse who comes with her and watched them go off. It was the chauffeur who waved to me in a friendly way.

This was the second point for discussion: the extreme reaction of a delusional transference and the need to just put up with it. I think that one does need a great deal of confidence in oneself to just take all this without saying anything out loud in self-defence. Fortunately in this case there was no question of suicide and so I could just think "Well if the worst comes to the worst the patient has finished with me." I knew, however, that she has no-one else to go to; but even so she might have broken down to the extent of going off to a whole series of fringe therapists, which she knows a lot about.

The next day, Thursday, brought its rewards in this instance. The patient was now back to an affectionate relationship. Her whole way of making contact with the rugs and the cushions was different. She was obviously in a state of the unconscious co-operation of the analysis being operative so that she was able to tell me dreams that had validity. Eventually she said that she had felt extremely guilty about what had happened, so much so that she was going to bring me two peaches for my weekend. *This provided the next point for discussion.*

There were two things here. Firstly, I had a discussion with her about analysts taking presents, because I knew that she is fully aware of what is written on the subject. I pointed out the difference between the neurotic and the psychotic in this respect. I reminded her that she practically does not know what psycho-neurosis is about. If a neurotic patient brings me a present I tend to refuse it because I know that I will have to pay for it in inflated currency. In the case of a psychotic, however (and here I was really meaning to include the depressive anxieties which are not fully available to this patient), I find that presents have to do with damage already done. In other words I nearly always accept, and I find there is not much difference between accepting two peaches and accepting a co-operative mood or an affectionate attitude. I was of course concerned that the two peaches symbolically represented idealised breasts, but I was contented to leave it at that and was eventually rewarded, I think.

The second thing had to do with the patient's ability at this point to talk about how awful she had been. She went over the previous hour in terms of her having been "cutting" in her remarks, and this was a correct description. She reminded me and herself that when she feels like she did she is able to lacerate anyone who is near and to really hurt them.

A dream had to do with jumping from the ninth floor of a block of flats (her parents' flat is on the ninth floor) down to my flat, without apparently coming to harm, my flat being probably on the ground floor.

The next day she came with her state of mind and her attitude continuing. Actually she brought Bittra chocolate which seemed to me to be an improvement on the peaches and the idealisation that they carry. There was another dream of jumping from a plane which apparently was rather exhibitionistic and led to no harm, and there was also a dream that there was a man somewhere and whatever she did she could not make him take any notice of her. She was determined, however, to make him notice her even if this meant wearing the modern skirt that is above the knees. Up to the present she has scorned doing anything to attract a man because if he is not already attracted the whole thing is no good.

24
New Light on Children's Thinking

Introductory lecture given at a conference for
members of the teaching profession held at
the Devon Centre for Further Education,
3 January 1965

My contribution is not so much a positive contribution to the specific subject of thinking as a comment from the child psychiatry angle on thinking as a function. I must be allowed to be ignorant of the writings of those who have made the subject of thinking especially their own. My hope is that what I have to say will help you to put the other things you hear into a relationship with the general theory of the development of the human personality, the human person. There is a general theory, which must leave room for everything, including the not yet known and the not yet envisaged, and then there are specific studies of thinking, some of which will be dealt with in your conference.

I was thinking ... you might have programmed your conference according to the ways the word is used. When I *think* what I have let myself in for I am appalled. First I find myself *thinking round* the subject, cunningly hoping to get away with it by exploiting a distraction. But then I find myself *thinking around* the meaning of the word "think." Then I start to *think up* a way of presenting the contribution that I want to make. Every now and again I *think* some words that had better remain unsaid and I make a mental note: next time *think* before you accept this sort of invitation! However, it would be *unthinkable* to get out of my obligation by excusing myself on the grounds of having flu or gout, so I plunge in, in spite of the poet's warning that to *think* is to be full of sorrow.

There is no alternative; I must *think* this thing *out*, without hoping to *think it through*. Then I shall have to take whatever will be *thought of* my effort, and take it in good part. Afterwards, of course, I shall *think of* all the things I have not *thought of*. How much better to have *thought forward* and to have predicted your criticisms.

I suppose one could look at each of these meanings of the word think and try to apply them to a child of one year.

Think—recognise (belongs to various kinds of maturity)[1]

Think round—try cunningly to circumvent (1 year & animals)

Think around—lovingly examine (6 months + or −)

Think up—creating in absence of one's muse (2 years & animals)

Think—not speak (5 years, latency)

Unthinkable—fear of superego (develops with superego formation)

Think—take a comprehensive view (develops meaning through life)

Think out—do deliberate mental dissection (ask Piaget)

Think through—complete limited thinking task (maturity)

Think of—verdict after due consideration (2 years + or −)

Think of—remember (earlier than 1 year)

Think of—recall (later than 1 year)

Think forward—predict consequences (very early)

A child of one may not *think up*, but he certainly *thinks*. He uses his brain in so far as he has one. But his spoken words are three or perhaps one only. Perhaps he thinks with the words he understands but cannot use. There is obscurity here. It would be unwise to spend time wrangling over the date at which a child thinks. Better, surely, to compare thinking with other functions that have parallel existence. We may find functions that some would name thinking and others would refrain from including in that category.

I shall not try to do original thinking here. I shall simply use ideas that have come to me before, and that I have already used in lectures and writings. I have found (not claiming originality) that we must assume that nothing is lost that has been registered, at least from the birthdate and probably from just before the birthdate. Naturally what is not registered is not under consideration (and there is a great deal to be said about the way that things or events or sensations can only be registered as they were experienced). There is such a thing as premature ego awakening, and on the other hand some babies are late in seeming to notice anything but their own sensations and functioning. Autistic children have an extreme degree of this tendency to be and to remain introverted.

I would divide what I have to say into two parts:

1. The words placed in parentheses in this list were written in by hand after the lecture had been typed.—EDS.

1. Cataloguing (in health) and
2. the mind becoming exploited in defence.

1. Cataloguing

In health it appears that everything that is registered is catalogued and categorised and collated. This is not strictly speaking thinking but it involves the electronic apparatus that is used in thinking. Presumably in thinking proper there is a deliberate directing of the mind in a specific mental task which has some limited, although perhaps short-lived, aim. It may be that the word "deliberate" needs to be restated in a phrase that allows for conscious and unconscious motivation.

I have only to look round and I find this stated better than I can state it.

> We know very little about the precognitive ordering of incipient thought, but I suspect that we could find out more about some of its features by exploring more intensively, by such techniques as electromyography, the intimate postures and expressive movements of the body. Meantime, as one would expect, the creative writers provide examples of nominally discursive statement which shows on inspection some of the characteristics of presentational symbolism and at times traces of a richer matrix, perhaps more confused, from which their words and images have emerged.[2]

A list can be made of properties of the human baby:
    Body functioning, sensori-motor
    Imaginative elaboration of body functioning (fantasy)
add: The cataloguing, categorising and collating faculty

Memories   a. not conscious ever
             b. conscious   museum
                                   gallery (private)
                                   exhibition
                                   theatre

The collation function develops its own life and enables prediction to be made. This comes into the service of the need to preserve omnipotence. Parallel with this, the elaboration of function enriched by memories passes over into creative imagination, dream and play (also serving omnipotence).

2. D. W. Harding, "The Hinterland of Thought," in *Experience into Words: Essays on Poetry* (London: Chatto and Windus, 1963).

In this way thinking comes into being as an aspect of the creative imagination. It serves the survival of the experience of omnipotence. It is an ingredient of integration.

Some babies specialise in thinking and reach out for words; others specialise in auditory, visual, or other sensuous experiences, and in memories and creative imagination of hallucinatory kind, and these latter may not reach out for words. There is no question of the one being normal and the other abnormal. Misunderstanding may occur in debate through the fact that one person talking belongs to the thinking and verbalising kind, while another belongs to the kind that hallucinates in the visual or auditory field instead of expressing the self in words. Somehow the word people tend to claim sanity, and those who see visions do not know how to defend their position when accused of insanity. Logical argument really belongs to the verbalisers. Feeling or a feeling of certainty or truth or "real" belongs to the others.

Psycho-analysis had much difficulty in adjusting to the needs of those who see and hear first and think last. Jungians, by contrast, have tended to cater for those who conceptualise without verbal juggling, and some think that Jungians are not as good at logic and shared reality.

Thus my first idea concerns the development of thinking out of cataloguing, categorising and collating, and these functions start very early indeed, even if they take time to develop full complexity.

2. Thinking as a Mother-Substitute, a Sitter-in

The second idea has to do with the way the baby's intellect can be exploited. First, the intellect is an aspect of the cataloguing, categorising and collating function, enabling memories to become available until they become lost in primary or secondary repression. Then the intellect has its own functioning, depending on the quality of the electronic apparatus and also on the way that the emotional development of the individual is taking shape.

Exploitation of the intellect can start very early, in premature ego awareness. A patient says: "When I was born I sat up and started lecturing: 'You do it this way.'" She has this pattern for life. At one year she actually said: "I will I like," and she sees her life as a follow-through of this statement of a personal philosophy.

To make my point I take a simplified picture of a baby being fed.

The baby is at a stage of very great dependence, and the mother is playing her part well, adapting to her baby's needs, being able to do so because of her ability to give herself over temporarily to this one job—the care of her baby. She is closely identified with the baby and she is able to put herself in the baby's shoes, so to speak.

Adaptation is a fact, and very close to 100 percent, but it rapidly becomes less than 100 percent according to the baby's development which allows the mother more and more freedom. What is this that develops in the baby? It is the baby's intelligence.

The baby thinks to himself (while screaming) that it is all right really because the noises off-stage indicate that something is coming that will just meet his needs. Also he has his memories. He may scream, but he is not distressed, because he has retained hope, knowing (by putting two and two together) that relief is at hand, relief from a pressing need and a sense of threat to omnipotence. This development of the baby's understanding of what is going on results in the mother's increasing ability to *fail to adapt* to her baby's needs.

One baby gets round the matter by thinking, and the other gets round it by fantasy and by enjoying the experience imaginatively before it becomes actual.

If we now take the case of a baby whose mother's failure to adapt is too rapid, we can find that the baby survives by means of the mind. The mother exploits the baby's power to think things out and to collate and to understand. If the baby has a good mental apparatus this thinking becomes a substitute for maternal care and adaptation. The baby "mothers" himself by means of understanding, understanding too much. It is a case of "Cogito, ergo in mea potestate sum."

In the extreme the mind and the baby's thinking have enabled the baby, now growing up and acquiring a developmental pattern, to do without the most important aspects of the maternal care that is needed by all human beings, namely reliability and adaptation to basic need. Like whiskey one's own understanding is more reliable than the mother-figure was.

This results in the uneasy intelligence of some whose good brains have become exploited. The intelligence is hiding a degree of deprivation. In other words, there is always for those with exploited brains a threat of a breakdown from intelligence and understanding to mental chaos or to disintegration of the personality.

Intelligence and thinking can be measured and used and appreciated but it is to be remembered that intelligence can be exploited and that it can hide such things as deprivation and threatened chaos. A partial breakdown is represented clinically by an obsessional organisation, with disorganisation always around the corner.

Forward movement in the emotional development of an individual is away from an unorganised state towards integration, away from chaos towards understanding, away from ignorance towards knowledge and the power to predict, away from dependence towards independence. Thinking is one aspect of the integrative process, going ahead of full participation.

To repeat my second idea; whereas thinking is an aspect of the individual's creative imagination, it can become exploited in the individual economy in defence against archaic anxiety and against chaos and against disintegrative tendencies or memories of disintegrative breakdown related to deprivation.

In a positive way thinking is a part of the creative impulse, but there are alternatives to thinking and these alternatives have some advantages over thinking. For instance, logical thinking takes a long time and may never get there, but the flash of intuition takes no time and it gets there immediately. Science needs both of these ways of going along. Here we are reaching out for words, thinking, and trying to be logical, and including a study of the unconscious which affords a vast extension of the range of logic. But at the same time we need to be able to reach out for symbols and to create imaginatively and in preverbal language; we need to be able to think hallucinatorily.

25

Comment on Obsessional Neurosis and "Frankie"

A written version of discussion remarks made at the Twenty-Fourth International Psycho-Analytical Congress, Amsterdam, July 1965[1]

In the discussion I made two separate comments, the one to do with the nature of obsessional neurosis and the other to do with the case under discussion.

In regard to the theory of obsessional neurosis I attempted to formulate a concept of a split-off intellectual functioning, which I believe to be an essential feature of a thorough-going obsessional neurosis case. The conflicts belonging to the personality have become localised into this split-off intellectual area. It is because of the fact of this split that there can never be any outcome in the obsessional neurotic's efforts and activities. The best that can happen is that for the time being the obsessional person has arranged a kind of order in the place of the idea of confusion. This is a never-ending alternation and has to be contrasted with the universal attempt of human beings to arrange for the experience of some kind of structurisation of the personality or of society in defence against the experience of chaos. Here there is a possibility of an outcome because the work is not being done in the split-off area of the personality.

In regard to the case, I limited my observations to a study of the beginning of the treatment of Frankie as reported with faithful detail by his child analyst.[2] I prefaced my remarks by a reminder that if we are able to discuss this case in detail we are indebted to her report and indeed the description of this analytic treatment has rightly been used for more than a decade in the teaching of the psycho-analytic

---

1. From the *International Journal of Psycho-Analysis* 47 (1966), which see for a summary of the paper discussed and further remarks. Copyright © Institute of Psycho-Analysis.

2. See Berta Bornstein, "The Analysis of a Phobic Child," in *The Psycho-Analytic Study of the Child*, vol. 3/4 (London: Imago, 1949).

technique. I made an attempt to look critically at her handling of the first interview.

> Frankie started his first session by building a hospital which was separated into a "lady department," a "baby department," and a "men's department." In the lobby, a lonely boy of 4 was seated all by himself, on a chair placed in an elevated position.

The further details of the game showed that this was a place where babies are born and the game, the analyst reports, was repeated in the analysis for many weeks. It "betrayed the intensity of the boy's fury against his mother and sister." Undoubtedly the material justified this assumption and the interpretations that followed. The detail that I picked out for discussion was that at the very beginning there was the boy "seated all by himself on a chair placed in an elevated position." I felt that one could take this detail and give it the fullest possible significance because this is what he brought to the analysis at the age of $5\frac{1}{2}$. In an atmosphere where there are mothers and babies, although he did in fact separate the newborn babies from their mothers, there was the idea of mothers (and fathers too) concerned as human beings with infants. This applies to the mother's holding of the baby in the womb and also her general post-natal care of her infant. Frankie evidently wanted to make it clear that from his point of view he was seated on a chair placed in an elevated position; in other words he was held by a thing, a contraption, or whatever one might wish to call it. This thing is a split-off function of the mother, not part of her attitude. I drew attention to the fact that this detail could have very great significance in this case, possibly being the one thing above all others that the boy wished to convey to the analyst. There is material in support of this idea because the analyst writes that

> Frankie was a planned child, that her pregnancy had been uneventful, and that she had felt happy and contented in anticipating her first baby's arrival. The delivery was normal, the child healthy, yet the very first moment she held the baby in her arms, she had felt estranged from him. The little boy's crying had given her an uncanny and uneasy feeling. She felt quite different toward her second child, a girl.

In further discussion of this there is room to think that the mother was interfered with in her first relationship to this boy by unconscious features derived from her relationship to her brother. I suggested that the whole of the case could be described around this detail, even including the basic phobia of elevators. There is nothing that a child can do about being held by a split-off function except to think of the mechanics of its working well or badly. There would be an alternation between elation (or some equivalent) and being dropped, and the description of the further analysis of this patient as a young man certainly does not contradict this idea. I went further and I said that although a great deal of good work has been done in these analyses, the cure of this man cannot be reached unless this first detail of his analysis at the age of 5½ can be met and his helplessness in respect of his being cared for by a split-off maternal function instead of by a mother reached in the transference setting.

This comment is made on the basis of the theory of the infant-mother relationship which takes into account a stage of absolute dependence, that is to say a stage before the infant has separated out the mother from the details of the infant care provision.[3] There must come a time in the history of every infant when from the infant's point of view there comes about the idea of a recognition of the mother who provides. Naturally if there is an environmental split, that is to say, a mother and some mechanical contrivance supplying the needs of infant care, then the inherent task of the infant in respect of recognising that the details of infant care are an expression of a person's love becomes not only more difficult but in fact impossible. In some way or other in the transference the analyst has the very heavy task of correcting the environmental split which in the aetiology of the case made synthesis impossible for the infant.

I recognise that in criticising these two analyses in this way I am trying to use to effect the very rich material provided by the two analysts in an attempt to make a suggestion which might prove to be constructive either in this case or in a similar case.

3. Winnicott, "The Theory of the Parent-Infant Relationship" (1960), in *The Maturational Processes and the Facilitating Environment* (London: Hogarth Press; New York: International Universities Press, 1965).

26

A Note on the Mother-Foetus Relationship

Undated; probably written in the mid-1960s

There are many ways of putting into words the relation of a mother to the baby which she carries and bears. Firstly, of course, there is the simple biological statement.

In psycho-analytic writings there are copious references to the mother's conscious and unconscious fantasies about her child. Often we find the expression "baby" equated with penis, with faeces, with money or with articles of furniture, pillows, etc. etc. We also hear of the mother's identification with her baby, and of her identification of the baby with one or other of her parents, and love, hate and fear of the baby are able to be explained along these lines.

The mother-foetus relationship can also be stated with profit in the following terms: if the biological ability of the mother to produce a real whole live baby is represented by 100 percent, her psychological ability can be stated as a rough percentage. By this I mean that no mother is 100 percent able to produce a whole live child in fantasy. Some mothers, indeed, have scarcely 50 percent capacity; and imagine their confusion, then, when they find themselves faced with a baby which they are told they have brought into the world and yet in which they do not entirely believe. It is only half human, only half alive, only half complete, or only half healthy. It may fall to pieces if not kept together by clothes and binder. Its belly may be full of wind instead of guts, or there may be nothing inside except piss and shit. Or it may have one of the well-known deformities, water on the brain, cleft palate, club foot, or the so-called stigmata of degeneration. It may be a monster.

At any rate it is not he, or she, but IT.

If a baby really *is* born with a defect or deformity the harmful effect on the mother and father may be quite startling, providing the opposite of reassurance against fears of inability to produce a 100 percent human being. I know of a case where a man's illness dated from the birth of a monster to his wife.

Breast-feeding gives the mother (and father by proxy) a second chance. Personal nursing and breast-feeding make a mother feel that a child is real, that is, if she previously doubted it owing to her less than 100 percent capacity for producing a baby in fantasy.

Miscarriages often testify to this condition. Let us say that a three months miscarriage represents a 33⅓ percent capacity. If a pregnant woman is in analysis and the analyst is unable to get in time to the interpretation of the patient's fantasies of her inside (and of insides in general) the patient may have a miscarriage almost as an act of honesty. It is as if she would be claiming what is false if she were to go through with the pregnancy and produce a whole baby. There is only hope if the analyst can bring the fantasies of the inside into the analysis, and so face the biological inside from its secondary function as a repository for consciously repudiated fantasy.

The clue to the analysis of this aspect of motherhood is the interpretation of the relation of fantasy to orgastic functioning (chiefly oral) in the transference situation. In this way the inner world of fantasy becomes felt as real, something which need not be secret, and something which can be personally owned; and at the same time the analyst witnesses the disappearance of the patient's hitherto compulsive *placing* of the post-incorporative fantasy material *inside the belly.*

Biological function can then proceed undisturbed, and the mother may bring her foetus to full term, and need not be ill even if she should have the sad experience of giving birth to a baby that is deformed.

27

Absence and Presence of a Sense of Guilt Illustrated in Two Patients

Undated; probably written in 1966[1]

I

In the course of the analytic treatment of a woman who has needed to dig very deep and into the very early phases of her life we have arrived at a stage at which my mistakes are becoming more and more significant, mistakes I do make, and I think that all analysts must make mistakes or in some way or other fail. There is no doubt that the pattern of the failure of the analyst if he is free from a set pattern of his own belongs to the pattern according to which the patient's own environment failed at a significant stage. The trouble is that in the very sensitive work which we can sometimes do over a limited period of time we may be able to give the patient something which is better than he or she got at the beginning, although of course only in token form. We do not have twenty-four-hour care of a patient, as parents have of their child or a mother has of her infant. In a way one learns to dread the endings of this period in which one has done very sensitive work adapting to the needs of the patient. The end comes with some way in which one's other interests divert one's attention so that the patient is no longer in the "only child" position, no longer one's preoccupation. Then the patient gets a shock and is torn to pieces and it is our fault. The only thing we can do is to acknowledge the fact when challenged. The difficulties arise from the very sensitive and good work that we have just done. We have raised hopes. The patient has been able to let us displace an unsatisfactory parent or parent-figure. Now of course when we fail the failure is worse because when we succeed what we did was better.

I have just reached this point with a patient and the result is very

---

1. This was found among Winnicott's papers together with his lecture "The Absence of a Sense of Guilt" (1966), now in Winnicott, *Deprivation and Delinquency* (London, New York: Tavistock, 1985).—EDS.

distressing to the patient and to me. However much I tell myself that eventually I had to be the one who fails I cannot help feeling absolutely awful because I can so easily see that the mistake that I made could have been avoided. In this particular case I allowed myself to be deceived by a moment in which the patient appeared to be almost normal and wanting to talk about my work and my life and in spite of all that I know and believe in I fell into this trap and eventually in a state of longing to have somebody to talk to about myself I made one or two references to my alternative preoccupations. At first of course the patient found this fascinating and was glad to know about my being alive and about my life and other interests. Soon, however, the reaction started, as I knew it must as soon as I had opened my mouth. In a few days' time the patient was completely destroyed and I was to blame. The agony that she went through was tremendous and if she had committed suicide on various occasions it would have been to avoid just this agony. Anyone who is not engaged in this work might think that here the matter would rest. The patient would be very angry with me for being exactly like her mother only worse because I was better to begin with. But this is not what happened. This patient went into a state in which she felt she must be loathsome. No-one could possibly do this sort of thing except in reaction to some awful quality about her which makes everybody do the worst.

It will be seen here that she has manufactured a situation in which she experiences very severe guilt feelings around which she might easily organise her life if she does not commit suicide on the basis of expiation. It could be a case of sackcloth and ashes and no outcome. As her analyst I have had opportunity to get to know this that happens to her in great detail and I am able to see that what she really cannot stand is that I may have made a mistake or failed her not because she is loathsome but because of something about me, something that she could not possibly be aware of because it is outside her sphere of influence. It is this that she cannot manage and the whole of her life is an illustration of it. If I could be allowed to simplify a little I could say that what I did wrong was exactly equivalent to what her mother did wrong in becoming pregnant and so interrupting the only-child relationship. It was managed rather badly and in any case the mother had to attend to her pregnancy rather early, that is to say, before my patient was a year old. At that tender age a baby has not got the wide range of defences and in fact has not really come to terms with there being a universe outside that of which he or she is the hub. The mother is just here in the process of introducing the child to these hard facts that are called the Reality Principle. In another way of putting it this child at one year was not able to know anything at all about the union of the parents in all its forms, something which she could have dealt with at the age of two or three by means of identifying with one or other in some form of the act of union.

My failure therefore was something that she had to try to bring within the area of her own omnipotence, and she could only do this by knowing very well about her own horrible ideas and impulses and feeling guilty and so explaining what I had done in terms of retribution. It is true that this patient has often wanted to destroy me, but this at its most real has to do with the very primitive aspects of her loving, where loving is object-relating. It is something which can develop into eating and ideas of incorporating that which is valued. What my failure had done was to sidetrack the patient from this main issue so that she now wanted to kill me not as part of loving but in reaction to my having broken up the processes of her growth. It can perhaps be seen from this illustration that this patient would feel no guilt if she were to kill me today, because I have to be killed and she is simply the agent of fate. The place where a true sense of guilt was in the process of developing was just there where she was nearly able to see that in loving me she would eat me, and that the ideas around all this would involve my destruction. She was just getting near this which feels real to her when she gets there. In failing her I did what her parents did and her mother doing this to her so early gave her a lifetime of trying to feel guilty but never succeeding.

Over and over again she had been able to work up the histrionics of remorse around compulsive destruction, but none of this ever felt real although indeed the destruction could be real enough. From here it is possible to see what a patient meant who came to me about fifteen years ago and whose first words were: "I want you to help me to find my own nastiness." This patient had had a very terrible environment from the beginning and it took years of analysis for her to be able to reach to the place where she knew about the nastiness which she would find in herself in a good environment.

II

I would like to look at a rather different kind of patient in order to try and get a new slant on the meaning of the sense of guilt. This patient is a woman who would probably be diagnosed as potentially schizophrenic. In the course of a treatment she is schizoid in recurring phases although she is also more like a psycho-neurotic much of the time. She would not like me to say this because she values her schizoid part of her personality and despises psycho-neurosis. You will understand that psycho-neurosis is very near to things like ambivalence and compromise and all the things which we call healthy. Life is only possible on the basis of compromise. The democratic method is an agreed compromise and socialisation is the same. The schizoid part of this woman's illness makes her despise compromise. There is some kind of idealisation which is essential to her well-being. One result of this is that her illness tends to make her get her own way and she is intelligent enough to be able to make this work to an amazing degree. If she gets her own way then there is no compromise and she can afford to wait. For this woman the sense of guilt can be absolutely overwhelming. It has nothing to do with society's idea of what is good or bad, and she has abandoned her religion because as presented to her the church seemed to give her a sense of values which was arbitrary. Where she feels overwhelmed with guilt is when she feels she has betrayed herself. She feels she would rather stay ill for the rest of her life than get well if that meant accepting compromise. This makes her very awkward as a person. Amongst other things this woman has had considerable sexual difficulties starting off with a conviction that if she really loved a man he would turn away from her. Gradually she has come around to being able to allow a man to fall in love with her, even one that she likes very much. There has been a long series culminating in something which could really, one would think, turn into a marriage. There has been some sexual experience between these two people. As can be imagined in this type of case there is no guilt whatever associated with having sex or not having sex. The place where this patient felt guilt of an extreme kind was when there was just the possibility that she might become pregnant. From this point she withdrew her sexual compliance and gradually began to organise the break-up of the relationship.

Her dreams showed that if she were to become pregnant this could only be with someone that she has not yet found who is exactly the right person. It has been a struggle for her to even look at the possibility that the right person will never turn up. The fact is that the right person would have been a man in the past, in ordinary circumstances her father, someone who would come into her life because of her mother's love of her man. The right man would have come into her life as a complication in a basic relationship to her mother. In her case the basic relationship to her mother was defective. The relationship between the parents was problematical, and in any case her father wanted a boy and never took much interest in her as a girl at all. On all counts, therefore, the right man did not appear, and so she is left not looking for a marriage partner but looking for what she missed, the first love affair within the family. She may not be able to find a man who is first of all willing to play the part assigned to him, being the right man, with sex under taboo, and then able and willing gradually to change around into becoming a husband in the course of time.

I am giving this in illustration of the kind of guilt sense which is very fierce and which is absolute and which belongs to the disaster of self-betrayal. As compared with this, moralistic teachings look rather feeble. The common or garden moralist could look at this woman and say that she is deficient in sense of guilt. She can be shown to be a thief, and a liar, and a wangler, and she has no sense of guilt at all about extra-marital sex. It would not occur to her to worry if a man that she was interested in was married. It turns out, however, that her whole life-pattern is determined by a sense of absolute values which makes her able to see at a glance whether an abstract painting is true or false. I like to give this as an example because I, for instance, can look at an abstract and not know how to begin to judge it because it does not touch on something that particularly belongs to me. With this patient there is no doubt, and the judgement is immediate and as it happens it corresponds very closely with the judgement of the ordinary run of highly sensitised art criticism. For this patient a false line in an abstract painting is so much worse than immoral that other language has to be found for its description or simply the picture has to be rejected. On the other hand an abstract that rings true has immense value. Along with this as can be imagined this patient can only start to exist and to feel real in an environment where the architecture and all the other aspects of the non-human environment are of a high standard. It is very awkward and difficult to find, and some of the best time my patient has had was spent in a monastery where there was nothing ugly. I suppose if she gets well she will be able to live amongst all that is sordid as most of us have to do, but it can be seen that this patient cannot look to the future and say "I want to be well" precisely because of this loss of sacred things in exchange for that which will be ugly, ill-arranged and sordid.

28
On the Split-off Male and Female Elements

On 2 February 1966, Winnicott gave a paper to a Scientific Meeting of the British Psycho-Analytical Society entitled "The Split-off Male and Female Elements to Be Found Clinically in Men and Women: Theoretical Inferences." He later included this paper as a subsection of chapter 5 in his book *Playing and Reality* (1971).

The present chapter begins with a reproduction of this paper (Section I). In Section II are three pieces of case material, the first written in 1959 and the others in 1963, which were found typed out in Winnicott's "Ideas" file. They relate to the same patient and the same subject matter as the paper, and were probably used both for teaching and in his preliminary thinking around the subject of the dissociation between the male and female elements. Further material relating to this patient can be found in Chapters 10 and 15 of this volume.

Section III contains the main part of Winnicott's answer to comments on his paper, written for *Psychoanalytic Forum*. The comments were made by Margaret Mead, Masud Khan, Richard Sterba, Herbert Rosenfeld and Decio Soares de Souza. Although both comments and answers were written in 1968–69, they appeared, together with the original paper, in *Psychoanalytic Forum* in 1972.

EDITORS

I. The Split-off Male and Female Elements to Be Found in Men and Women

A paper read to the British Psycho-Analytical Society, 2 February 1966

There is nothing new either inside or outside psycho-analysis in the idea that men and women have a "predisposition towards bisexuality."

I try here to use what I have learned about bisexuality from analyses that have gone step by step towards a certain point and have focused on one detail. No attempt will be made here to trace the steps by which an analysis comes to this kind of material. It can be said that a great deal of work usually has had to be done before this type of material has become significant and calls for priority. It is difficult to see how all this preliminary work can be avoided. The slowness of the analytic process is a manifestation of a defence the analyst must respect, as we respect all defences. While it is the patient who is all the time teaching the analyst, the analyst should be able to know, theoretically, about the matters that concern the deepest or most central features of personality, else he may fail to recognise and to meet new demands on his understanding and technique when at long last the patient is able to bring deeply buried matters into the content of the transference, thereby affording opportunity for mutative interpretation. The analyst, by interpreting, shows how much and how little of the patient's communication he is able to receive.

As a basis for the idea that I wish to give here I suggest that creativity is one of the common denominators of men and women. In another language, however, creativity is the prerogative of women, and in yet another language it is a masculine feature. It is this last of the three that concerns me in what follows here.

Clinical Data

Illustrative Case

I propose to start with a clinical example. This concerns the treatment of a man of middle age, a married man with a family, and successful in one of the professions. The analysis has proceeded along classical lines. This man has had a long analysis and I am not by any means his first psychotherapist. A great deal of work has been done by him and by each of us therapists and analysts in turn, and much change has been brought about in his personality. But there is still something he avers that makes it impossible for him to stop. He knows that what he came for he has not reached. If he cuts his losses the sacrifice is too great.

In the present phase of this analysis something has been reached which is new *for me*. It has to do with the way I am dealing with the non-masculine element in his personality.

> On a Friday the patient came and reported much as usual. The thing that struck me on this Friday was that the patient was talking about *penis envy*. I use this term advisedly, and I must invite acceptance of the fact that this term was appropriate here in view of the material, and of its presentation. Obviously this term, penis envy, is not usually applied in the description of a man.
>
> The change that belongs to this particular phase is shown in the way I handled this. On this particular occasion I said to him: "I am listening to a girl. I know perfectly well that you are a man but I am listening to a girl, and I am talking to a girl. I am telling this girl: 'You are talking about penis envy.'"
>
> I wish to emphasise that this has nothing to do with homosexuality.
>
> (It has been pointed out to me that my interpretation in each of its two parts could be thought of as related to playing, and as far as possible removed from authoritative interpretation that is next door to indoctrination.)
>
> It was clear to me, by the profound effect of this interpretation, that my remark was in some way apposite, and indeed I would not be reporting this incident in this context were it not for the fact that the work that started on this Friday did in fact break into a vicious circle. I had grown accustomed to a routine of good work, good interpretations, good immediate results, and then destruction and disillusionment that followed each time because of the patient's gradual recognition that something fundamental had remained unchanged; there was this unknown factor which had kept this man working at his own analysis for a quarter of a century. Would his

work with me suffer the same fate as his work with the other therapists?

On this occasion there was an immediate effect in the form of intellectual acceptance, and relief, and then there were more remote effects. After a pause the patient said: "If I were to tell someone about this girl I would be called mad."

The matter could have been left there, but I am glad, in view of subsequent events, that I went further. It was my next remark that surprised me, and it clinched the matter. I said: "It was not that *you* told this to anyone; it is *I* who see the girl and hear a girl talking, when actually there is a man on my couch. The mad person is *myself*."

I did not have to elaborate this point because it went home. The patient said that he now felt sane in a mad environment. In other words he was now released from a dilemma. As he said, subsequently, "I myself could never say (knowing myself to be a man) 'I am a girl.' I am not mad that way. But you said it, and you have spoken to both parts of me."

This madness which was mine enabled him to see himself as a girl *from my position*. He knows himself to be a man, and never doubts that he is a man.

Is it obvious what was happening here? For my part, I have needed to live through a deep personal experience in order to arrive at the understanding I feel I now have reached.

This complex state of affairs has a special reality for this man because he and I have been driven to the conclusion (though unable to prove it) that his mother (who is not alive now) saw a girl baby when she saw him as a baby before she came round to thinking of him as a boy. In other words this man had to fit into her idea that her baby would be and was a girl. (He was the second child, the first being a boy.) We have very good evidence from inside the analysis that in her early management of him the mother held him and dealt with him in all sorts of physical ways as if she failed to see him as a male. On the basis of this pattern he later arranged his defences, but it was the mother's "madness" that saw a girl where there was a boy, and this was brought right into the present by my having said "It is I who am mad." On this Friday he went away profoundly moved and feeling that this was the first significant shift in the analysis for a long time (although, as I have said, there had always been continuous progress in the sense of good work being done).[1]

I would like to give further details relative to this Friday incident.

1. For a detailed discussion of the mirror-role of mother in child development see "Mirror-Role of Mother and Family" (1967), in *Playing and Reality* (London: Tavistock; New York: Basic Books, 1971; Penguin, 1974).—D.W.W.

When he came on the following Monday he told me that he was ill. It was quite clear to me that he had an infection and I reminded him that his wife would have it the next day, which in fact happened. Nevertheless, he was inviting me to *interpret* this illness, which started on the Saturday, as if it were psycho-somatic. What he tried to tell me was that on the Friday night he had had a satisfactory sexual intercourse with his wife, and so he *ought* to have felt better on the Saturday, but instead of feeling better he had become ill and had felt ill. I was able to leave aside the physical disorder and talk about the incongruity of his feeling ill after the intercourse that he felt ought to have been a healing experience. (He might, indeed, have said: "I have flu, but in spite of that I feel better in myself.")

My interpretation continued along the line started up on the Friday. I said: "You feel as if you ought to be pleased that here was an interpretation of mine that had released masculine behaviour. *The girl that I was talking to, however, does not want the man released,* and indeed she is not interested in him. What she wants is full acknowledgement of herself and of her own rights over your body. Her penis envy especially includes envy of you as a male." I went on: "The feeling ill is a protest from the female self, this girl, because she has always hoped that the analysis would in fact find out that this man, yourself, is and always has been a girl (and 'being ill' is a pregenital pregnancy). The only end to the analysis that this girl can look for is the discovery that in fact you are a girl." Out of this one could begin to understand his conviction that the analysis could never end.[2]

In the subsequent weeks there was a great deal of material confirming the validity of my interpretation and my attitude, and the patient felt that he could see now that his analysis had ceased to be under doom of interminability.

Later I was able to see that the patient's resistance had now shifted to a denial of the importance of my having said "It is I who am mad." He tried to pass this off as just my way of putting things—a figure of speech that could be forgotten. I found, however, that here is one of those examples of delusional transference that puzzle patients and analysts alike, and the crux of the problem of management is just here in this interpretation, which I confess I nearly did not allow myself to make.

When I gave myself time to think over what had happened I was puzzled. Here was no new theoretical concept, here was no new prin-

2. It will be understood, I hope, that I am not suggesting that this man's very real physical illness, flu, was brought about by the emotional trends that co-existed with the physical.—D.W.W.

ciple of technique. In fact, I and my patient had been over this ground before. Yet we had here something new, new in my own attitude and new in his capacity to make use of my interpretative work. I decided to surrender myself to whatever this might mean in myself, and the result is to be found in this paper that I am presenting.

Dissociation

The first thing I noticed was that I had never before fully accepted the complete dissociation between the man (or woman) and the aspect of the personality that has the opposite sex. In the case of this man patient the dissociation was nearly complete.

Here, then, I found myself with a new edge to an old weapon, and I wondered how this would or could affect the work I was doing with other patients, both men and women, or boys and girls. I decided, therefore, to study this type of dissociation, leaving aside but not forgetting all the other types of splitting.

Male and Female Elements in Men and Women[3]

There was in this case a dissociation that was on the point of breaking down. The dissociation defence was giving way to an acceptance of bisexuality as a quality of the unit or total self. I saw that I was dealing with what could be called a *pure female element*. At first it surprised me that I could reach this only by looking at the material presented by a male patient.[4]

A further clinical observation belongs to this case. Some of the re-

3. I shall continue to use this terminology ("male and female elements") for the time being, since I know of no other suitable descriptive terms. Certainly "active" and "passive" are not correct terms, and I must continue the argument using the terms that are available.—D.W.W.

4. It would be logical here to follow up the work this man and I did together with a similar piece of work involving a girl or a woman patient. For instance, a young woman reminds me of old material belonging to her early latency when she longed to be a boy. She spent much time and energy willing herself a penis. She needed, however, a special piece of understanding, which was that she, an obvious girl, happy to be a girl, at the same time (with a 10 percent dissociated part) knew and always had known that she was a boy. Associated with this was a certainty of having been castrated and so deprived of destructive potential, and along with this was murder of mother and the whole of her masochistic defence organisation which was central in her personality structure.

Giving clinical examples here involves me in a risk of distracting the reader's attention from my main theme; also, if my ideas are true and universal, then each reader will have personal cases illustrating the place of dissociation rather than of repression related to male and female elements in men and women.—D.W.W.

lief that followed our arrival at the new platform for our work together came from the fact that we now could explain why my interpretations, made on good grounds, in respect of use of objects, oral erotic satisfactions in the transference, oral sadistic ideas in respect of the patient's interest in the analyst as part-object or as a person with breast or penis—why such interpretations were never mutative. They were accepted, but: so what? Now that the new position had been reached the patient felt a sense of relationship with me, and this was extremely vivid. It had to do with identity. The pure female split-off element found a primary unity with me as analyst, and this gave the man a feeling of having started to live. I have been affected by this detail, as will appear in my application to theory of what I have found in this case.

Addendum to the Clinical Section

It is rewarding to review one's current clinical material keeping in mind this one example of dissociation, the split-off girl element in a male patient. The subject can quickly become vast and complex, so that a few observations must be chosen for special mention.

a. One may, to one's surprise, find that one is dealing with and attempting to analyse the split-off part, while the main functioning person appears only in projected form. This is like treating a child only to find that one is treating one or other parent by proxy. Every possible variation on this theme may come one's way.

b. The other-sex element may be completely split off so that, for instance, a man may not be able to make any link at all with the split-off part. This applies especially when the personality is otherwise sane and integrated. Where the functioning personality is already organised into multiple splits there is less accent on "I am sane," and therefore less resistance against the idea "I am a girl" (in the case of a man) or "I am a boy" (in the case of a girl).

c. There may be found clinically a near-complete other-sex dissociation, organised in relation to external factors at a very early date, mixed in with later dissociations organised as a defence, based more or less on cross-identifications. The reality of this later organised defence may militate against the patient's revival in the analysis of the earlier reactive split.

(There is an axiom here, that a patient will always cling to the full exploitation of personal and *internal* factors, which give him or her a measure of omnipotent control, rather than allow the idea of a crude reaction to an environmental factor, whether distortion or failure. Environmental influence, bad or even good, comes into our work as a traumatic idea, intolerable because not operating within the area of the patient's omnipotence. Compare the melancholic's claim to be responsible for *all* evil.)

d. The split-off other-sex part of the personality tends to remain of one age, or to grow but slowly. As compared with this, the truly imaginative figures of the person's inner psychic reality mature, inter-relate, grow old and die. For instance, a man who depends on younger girls for keeping his split-off girl-self alive may gradually become able to employ for his special purpose girls of marriageable age. But should he live to ninety it is unlikely that the girls so employed will reach thirty. Yet in a man patient the girl (hiding the pure girl element of earlier formation) may have girl characteristics, may be breast-proud, experience penis envy, become pregnant, be equipped with no male external genitalia and even possess female sexual equipment and enjoy female sexual experience.

e. An important issue here is the assessment of all this in terms of psychiatric health. The man who initiates girls into sexual experience may well be one who is more identified with the girl than with himself. This gives him the capacity to go all out to wake up the girl's sex and to satisfy her. He pays for this by getting but little male satisfaction himself, and he pays also in terms of his need to seek always a new girl, this being the opposite of object-constancy.

At the other extreme is the illness of impotence. In between the two lies the whole range of relative potency mixed with dependence of various types and degrees. What is normal depends on the social expectation of any one social group at any one particular time. Could it not be said that at the patriarchal extreme of society sexual intercourse is rape, and at the matriarchal extreme the man with a split-off female element who must satisfy many women is at a premium even if in doing so he annihilates himself?

In between the extremes is bisexuality and an expectation of sexual experience which is less than optimal. This goes along with the idea that social health is mildly depressive—except for holidays.

It is interesting that the existence of this split-off female element actually prevents homosexual practice. In the case of my patient he always fled from homosexual advances at the critical moment because (as he came to see and to tell me) putting homosexuality into practice would establish his maleness which (from the split-off female element self) he never wanted to know for certain.

(In the normal, where bisexuality is a fact, homosexual ideas do not conflict in this way largely because the anal factor (which is a secondary matter) has not attained supremacy over fellatio, and in the fantasy of a fellatio union the matter of the person's biological sex is not significant.)

f. It seems that in the evolution of Greek myth the first homosexuals were men who imitated women so as to get into as close as possible a relationship with the supreme goddess. This belonged to a matriarchal era out of which a patriarchal god system appeared with Zeus as head. Zeus (symbol of the patriarchal system) initiated the idea of the boy loved sexually by man, and along with this went the relegation of women to a lower status. If this is a true statement of the history of the development of ideas, it gives the link that I need if I am to be able to join my clinical observations about the split-off female element in the case of men patients with the theory of object-relating. (The split-off male element in women patients is of equal importance in our work, but what I have to say about object-relating can be said in terms of one only of the two possible examples of dissociation.)

Summary of Preliminary Observations

In our theory it is necessary to allow for both a male and a female element in boys and men and girls and women. These elements may be split off from each other to a high degree. This idea requires of us both a study of the clinical effects of this type of dissociation and an examination of the distilled male and female elements themselves.

I have made some observations on the first of these two, the clinical effects; now I wish to examine what I am calling the distilled male and female elements (not male and female persons).

Pure Male and Pure Female Elements

Speculation about Contrast in Kinds of Object-Relating

Let us compare and contrast the unalloyed male and female elements in the context of object-relating.

I wish to say that the element that I am calling "male" does traffic in terms of active relating or passive being related to, each being backed by instinct. It is in the development of this idea that we speak of instinct drive in the baby's relation to the breast and to feeding, and subsequently in relation to all the experiences involving the main erotogenic zones, and to subsidiary drives and satisfactions. My suggestion is that, by contrast, the pure female element relates to the breast (or to the mother) in the sense of *the baby becoming the breast (or mother), in the sense that the object is the subject.* I can see no instinct drive in this.

(There is also to be remembered the use of the word "instinct" that comes from ethology; however, I doubt very much whether imprinting is a matter that affects the newborn human infant at all. I will say here and now that I believe the whole subject of imprinting is irrelevant to the study of the early object-relating of human infants. It certainly has nothing to do with the trauma of separation at two years, the very place where its prime importance has been assumed.)

The term subjective object has been used in describing the first object, the object *not yet repudiated as a not-me phenomenon.* Here in this relatedness of pure female element to "breast" is a practical application of the idea of the subjective object, and the experience of this paves the way for the objective subject—that is, the idea of a self, and the feeling of real that springs from the sense of having an identity.

However complex the psychology of the sense of self and of the establishment of an identity eventually becomes as a baby grows, no sense of self emerges except on the basis of this relating in the sense of BEING. This sense of being is something that antedates the idea of being-at-one-with, because there has not yet been anything else except identity. Two separate persons can *feel* at one, but here at the place that I am examining the baby and the object *are* one. The term "primary identification" has perhaps been used for just this that I am describing, and I am trying to show how vitally important this first experience is for the initiation of all subsequent experiences of identification.

Projective and introjective identifications both stem from this place where each is the same as the other.

In the growth of the human baby, as the ego begins to organise, this that I am calling the object-relating of the pure female element establishes what is perhaps the simplest of all experiences, the experience of *being.* Here one finds a true continuity of generations, being which is passed on from one generation to another, via the female element of men and women and of male and female infants. I think this has been said before, but always in terms of women and girls, which confuses the issue. It is a matter of the female elements in both males and females.

By contrast, the object-relating of the male element to the object presupposes separateness. As soon as there is the ego-organisation available, the baby allows the object the quality of being not-me or separate, and experiences id satisfactions that include anger relative to frustration. Drive satisfaction enhances the separation of the object from the baby, and leads to objectification of the object. Henceforth, on the male element side, identification needs to be based on complex mental mechanisms, mental mechanisms that must be given time to appear, to develop, and to become established as part of the new baby's equipment. On the female element side, however, identity requires so little mental structure that this primary identity can be a feature from very early, and the foundation for simple being can be laid (let us say) from the birth date, or before, or soon after, or from whenever the mind has become free from the handicaps to its functioning due to immaturity and to brain damage associated with the birth process.

Psycho-analysts have perhaps given special attention to this male element or drive aspect of object-relating, and yet have neglected the subject-object identity to which I am drawing attention here, which is at the basis of the capacity to be. The male element *does* while the female element (in males and females) *is*. Here would come in those males in Greek myth who tried to be at one with the supreme goddess. Here also is a way of stating a male person's very deep-seated envy of women whose female element men take for granted, sometimes in error.

It seems that frustration belongs to satisfaction-seeking. To the experience of being belongs something else, not frustration, but maiming. I wish to study this specific detail.

Identity: Child and Breast

It is not possible to state what I am calling here the female element's relation to the breast without the concept of the good-enough and the not-good-enough mother.

(Such an observation is even more true in this area than it is in the comparable area covered by the terms "transitional phenomena" and "transitional objects." The transitional object represents the mother's ability to present the world in such a way that the infant does not at first have to know that the object is not created by the infant. In our immediate context we may allow a total significance to the meaning of adaptation, the mother either giving the infant the opportunity to feel that the breast is the infant, or else not doing so. The breast here is a symbol not of doing but of being.)

This being a good-enough purveyor of female element must be a matter of very subtle details of handling, and in giving consideration to these matters one can draw on the writing of Margaret Mead and of Erik Erikson, who are able to describe the ways in which maternal care in various types of culture determines at a very early age the patterns of the defences of the individual, and also gives the blueprints for later sublimation. These are very subtle matters that we study in respect of *this* mother and *this* child.

The Nature of the Environmental Factor

I now return to the consideration of the very early stage in which the pattern is being laid down by the manner in which the mother in subtle ways handles her infant. I must refer in detail to this very special example of the environmental factor. Either the mother has a breast that *is*, so that the baby can also *be* when the baby and mother are not yet separated out in the infant's rudimentary mind; or else the mother is incapable of making this contribution, in which case the baby has to develop without the capacity to be, or with a crippled capacity to be.

(Clinically one needs to deal with the case of the baby who has to make do with an identity with a breast that is active, which is a male-element breast, but which is not satisfactory for the initial identity which needs a breast that *is*, not a breast that *does*. Instead of "being like," this baby has to "do like," or to be done to, which from our point of view here is the same thing.)

The mother who is able to do this very subtle thing that I am referring to does not produce a child whose "pure female" self is envious of the breast, since for this child the breast is the self and the self is the breast. Envy is a term that might become applicable in the experience of a tantalizing failure of the breast as something that is.

The Male and Female Elements Contrasted

These considerations have involved me then in a curious statement about the pure male and the pure female aspects of the infant boy or girl. I have arrived at a position in which I say that object-relating in terms of *this pure female element has nothing to do with drive (or instinct)*. Object-relating backed by instinct drive belongs to the male element in the personality uncontaminated by the female element. This line of argument involves me in great difficulties, and yet it seems as if in a statement of the initial stages of the emotional development of the individual it is necessary to separate out (not boys from girls but) the uncontaminated boy element from the uncontaminated girl element. The classical statement in regard to finding, using, oral erotism, oral sadism, anal stages, etc., arises out of a consideration of the life of the pure male element. Studies of identification based on introjection or on incorporation are studies of the experience of the already mixed male and female elements. Study of the pure female element leads us elsewhere.

The study of the pure distilled uncontaminated female element leads us to BEING, and this forms the only basis for self-discovery and a sense of existing (and then on to the capacity to develop an inside, to be a container, to have a capacity to use the mechanisms of projection and introjection and to relate to the world in terms of introjection and projection).

At risk of being repetitious I wish to restate: when the girl element in the boy or girl baby or patient finds the breast it is the self that has been found. If the question is asked, what does the girl baby do with the breast?—the answer must be that this girl element *is* the breast and shares the qualities of breast and mother and is desirable. In the course of time, desirable means edible and this means that the infant is in danger because of being desirable, or, in more sophisticated language, exciting. Exciting implies: liable to make someone's male element *do* something. In this way a man's penis may be an exciting female element generating male-element activity in the girl. But (it must be made clear) no girl or woman is like this; in health, there is a variable amount of girl element in a girl, and in a boy. Also, hereditary-factor elements enter in, so that it would easily be possible to find a boy with a stronger girl element than the girl standing next to him, who may have less pure-female-element potential. Add to this the variable capacity of mothers to hand on the desirability of the good breast or of that part of the maternal function that the good breast symbolises, and it can be seen that some boys and girls are doomed to grow up with a lop-sided bisexuality, loaded on the wrong side of their biological provision.

I am reminded of the question: what is the nature of the communication Shakespeare offers in his delineation of Hamlet's personality and character?

Hamlet is mainly about the awful dilemma that Hamlet found himself in, and there was no solution for him because of the dissociation that was taking place in him as a defence mechanism. It would be rewarding to hear an actor play Hamlet with this in mind. This actor would have a special way of delivering the first line of the famous soliloquy: "To be, or not to be . . ." He would say, as if trying to get to the bottom of something that cannot be fathomed, "To be, . . . or . . ." and then he would pause, because in fact the character Hamlet does not know the alternative. At last he would come in with the rather banal alternative: ". . . or not to be"; and then he would be well away on a journey that can lead nowhere. "Whether 'tis nobler in the mind to suffer / The slings and arrows of outrageous fortune, / Or to take arms against a sea of troubles, / And by opposing end them?" (Act III, Sc. 1). Here Hamlet has gone over into the sado-masochistic alternative, and he has left aside the theme he started with. The rest of the play is a long working-out of the statement of the problem. I mean: Hamlet is depicted at this stage as searching for an alternative to the idea "To be." He was searching for a way to state the dissociation that had taken place in his personality between his male and female elements, elements which had up to the time of the death of his father lived together in harmony, being but aspects of his richly endowed person. Yes, inevitably I write as if writing of a person, not a stage character.

As I see it, this difficult soliloquy is difficult because Hamlet had himself not got the clue to his dilemma—since it lay in his own changed state. Shakespeare had the clue, but Hamlet could not go to Shakespeare's play.

If the play is looked at in this way it seems possible to use Hamlet's altered attitude to Ophelia and his cruelty to her as a picture of his ruthless rejection of his own female element, now split off and handed over to her, with his unwelcome male element threatening to take over his whole personality. The cruelty to Ophelia can be a measure of his reluctance to abandon his split-off female element.

In this way it is *the play* (if Hamlet could have read it, or seen it acted) that could have shown him the nature of his dilemma. The play within the play failed to do this, and I would say that it was staged by him to bring to life his male element which was challenged to the full by the tragedy that had become interwoven with it.

It could be found that the same dilemma in Shakespeare himself provides the problem behind the content of the sonnets. But this is to ignore or even insult the main feature of the sonnets, namely, the poetry. Indeed, as Professor L. C. Knights (1946) specifically insists, it is only too easy to forget the poetry of the plays in writing of the *dramatis personae* as if they were historical persons.

Summary

1. I have examined the implications for me in my work of my new degree of recognition of the importance of dissociation in some men and women in respect of these male or female elements and the parts of their personalities that are built on these foundations.

2. I have looked at the artificially dissected male and female elements, and I have found that, for the time being, I associate impulse related to objects (also the passive voice of this) with the male element, whereas I find that the characteristic of the female element in the context of object-relating is identity, giving the child the basis for being, and then, later on, a basis for a sense of self. But I find that it is here, in the absolute dependence on maternal provision of that special quality by which the mother meets or fails to meet the earliest functioning of the female element, that we may seek the foundation for the experience of being. I wrote: "There is thus no sense in making use of the word 'id' for phenomena that are not covered and catalogued and experienced and eventually interpreted by ego functioning."[5]

Now I want to say: "After being—doing and being done to. But first, being."

Added Note on the Subject of Stealing

Stealing belongs to the male element in boys and girls. The question arises: what corresponds to this in terms of the female element in boys

5. "Ego Integration in Child Development" (1962), in *The Maturational Processes and the Facilitating Environment* (London: Hogarth Press; New York: International Universities Press, 1965).

and girls? The answer can be that in respect of this element the individual usurps the mother's position and her seat or garments, in this way deriving desirability and seductiveness stolen from the mother.

II. Clinical Material

Dated 1959

After a long weekend in which the patient had been coping with external reality he came very full of all this but his interest in these details began to wane quite soon. He said: "It seems a long time ago since the Thursday session." I said: "Yes, a long time since the idea came to you about the napkin." By this time he was right back in the Thursday session and he said that really he had not left the feeling belonging to these last three days of analysis in spite of all that had been going on. From there he continued slowly and clearly along the line initiated last week. The theme that developed was one of his exploitation of his female self. He had always known a good deal about the homosexual element and he had previously reported a great deal of compulsive fantasy about being a woman. Here, however, he came to a new aspect of this problem and one which seemed as if it might be productive. He produced some kind of idea in which there was no way out, no possibility of altering something.

In my interpretation eventually I said that if he were an infant being dealt with by a mother in the way that we reconstructed last week there was absolutely no way out for him, no alternative whatever, except for him to exploit every particle in himself of being female and wanting to be so. Anything in the way of a protest in this early stage would have been completely futile.

Gradually he could come to the idea of getting rid of his mother and of her whole attitude and of the napkin, but the important thing was that he was bringing to me an absolute helplessness. He could of course magically deal with the situation. He could leave his body and get free of the napkin that way. Physically, however, he had no choice whatever. The realisation of this was very painful to him and nevertheless had led him to be able to develop the theme of there being an element in him which feels female. In respect of all this the position of his genitals was just an awkward complication and something that he could not believe in and I reminded him of the toy pistol which he left lying on the bed downstairs in the dream while he passed by and went up into the attic.

From here we got to the relationship to his mother in terms of woman and daughter and the patient developed this theme in respect of his relationship to his present girl friend with whom his impotence is not important and in fact is as much in the way as his potency would be because the main thing in their relationship is that it is the quality of a relationship between two women.

In the second session of the three during this week the patient quickly got back to the analysis and to this new thing, an ability to consider his female self. He was rather slow at getting at the details and I made some interpretation reminding him of the alternative which was an absolute negative in a sense of there being no possibility whatever of his dealing with it. The alternative means the elimination of his mother at a very early infantile stage and he is not capable of doing this except magically which is of no use. Just for a moment the patient tried to follow me but he then said that this new position he was in in regard to his female self was tremendously important to him and he needed time to be in it and to discover what there is to be found there. Quite subtle things turned up, as for instance, he found himself not touching his chest, thinking "Oh he'll think I am fiddling with my breast." It was obvious that there was an extreme degree of the experiencing of himself as a female and that he had never allowed himself to get to this position before. Quite often he felt he must re-organise his defences or resistances and that he must get out of this curious position. At times he railed against his former analyst, a woman, who had not been able to meet this thing in him which was now found to be so important. It was not that it was really unconscious.

I allowed him the whole hour for the exploration of these phenomena, and one of the places he arrived at was a statement of something very difficult in his relationship to his wife. He had no idea when he married her that he would find that she has a perversion which exactly corresponds with what could so easily become a perversion in himself. She finds it sexually highly exciting if he shows any manifestation of his female self, as for instance overeating on holiday to get a big tummy. Here was a very great danger and the source of his fear of his wife. This was perhaps the most significant unexpected detail arising out of the experience of the hour.

The third hour was in the morning, when he came from an overnight experience at home. He had found himself to be much less frightened of his wife. Exasperating things had happened but he was less exasperated. He quickly recaptured the atmosphere of the previous two sessions and there was a pause. At this moment there came into my mind the word "mockery." I put it this way because I think that there could be a useful discussion around the sort of thing which I am now going to describe. It concerns the unconscious processes in the analyst. I was quite prepared to drop the idea of mockery but on looking round I could see exactly where it belonged. It had to do with the attitude of his wife, and therefore of his mother, in regard to his female self manifestations. I allowed this idea to disappear and then on examining the situation I found that I could come in with an interpretation of mockery. I was helped by the material, as for instance the secrecy about this aspect of himself. I allowed myself to say the interpretation that was in my mind, which was that the danger from his point of view was that his wife (or his mother) would mock him in regard to this female self.

Dated 1963

The patient came very late which is extremely unusual. He was furiously angry, full of immense hate of his wife, complete with details. Perhaps the most difficult thing was that in the middle of it all when she said: "I'm sorry I was awful" he had a sexual response which he had to hide from her and he had to get away as quickly as possible.

It seemed likely that the conflict round this was responsible for a great deal of his distress. With the girl friend he had had some play as he might with his daughter but she had interpreted hate and this had knocked him over. What he became aware of was that he had been thinking of self-destruction.

The whole hour was a muddle and no interpretation of mine was of any use. The patient was exasperated. What eventually did do some good was my interpreting that the analysis has continued in his relationship to his wife but here now, whatever it may have been at other times, he was working out his exasperation with his mother and his absolute hopelessness about dealing with her except by this method which he had now almost lost touch with but which had been so important last week, the full exploitation of his female self.

Eventually he felt that I had really met the situation when I said the home relationship is so much like your relationship to your mother that there is no man and therefore you cannot come to me because it is no use, there is no man to come to. There is no question of there being a father on whose knee you could sit looking at your mother, etc.

This was exactly what the patient needed but it took me the whole hour to get there and in the course of that time I had made many false interpretations, many of them very clever, each making me more ridiculous (mockery theme).

Incidentally, there was the curious theme that this man felt that if he had had intercourse with his wife although he would have felt satisfied and his wife would have been satisfied this could not be because it would mean that he was unfaithful to his mistress with whom, however, he has a very feeble relation as man and woman and in fact he is giving up this relationship temporarily because it is unsatisfactory and is really a relationship between two women. In the end we worked out that he was afraid to settle up everyone by responding with intercourse for fear that I would be led up a false trail. Could he trust me to know that he is not there at that point of development which would make sense of such a thing? In the transference therefore the thing is that he is dealing with his wife who is his mother and this eliminates me and makes it impossible for him to get to me as a man.

Dated 1963

The patient came and described the various neurotic disturbances which were uppermost. It seemed as if we were getting to something new, and this always pleases this patient. If I say something new or helpful or somewhat true he gains confidence in me, and this immediately produces a beneficial effect because of his inability to believe in a strong father unless he is actually experiencing something to support such a belief. It is something well known in this case that the immediate effect of any interpretation if it is at all good is much greater than would be warranted by the interpretation itself. Afterwards of course we pay for this and disillusionment sets in because of the limited improvement that has resulted from the work done. This has happened many dozens of times and both of us know all about the pattern. Here the work concerned the major symptom, or perhaps I should say the symptom which presents most clearly, his extreme embarrassment on account of putting on glasses. There is a long history to this, and the subject has been in abeyance since a great deal of work has been done on it and on the various ways in which the glasses symbolise part-objects, in particular breasts. This is the only symptom he avers that he has not told his wife about.

On this particular occasion there was reason for pointing out that the glasses in the circumstances described were a phallic symbol, and this is the first time that they had appeared in this way. They are of course also breast symbols. The hour could have proceeded along these lines and there would have been no difficulty in filling the whole time with a development of this theme. Incidentally, however, the patient today had told me a dream which made me think in another direction. He had dreamed that he was dancing on water and he wondered why none of the other people could do this. In other words, the other people would sink. He gave me this dream in such a way that it could easily have been lost in the other type of material. In making interpretations I pointed out that this was an example of the way in which all his rather obviously neurotic symptomatology came along over and over again for analysis as a defence against anxiety of quite a different kind, a defence against psychotic anxiety. I said that from my point of view the important thing of the hour was the dream which indicated a denial of falling forever down, or perhaps of drowning or of something that this symbolises.

The patient was taken aback because I had got behind his defence. At first he was annoyed but soon this turned to his being very pleased indeed because he could feel that I had said something new and important and helpful. As usual there was the exaggeration of the result because of the fact that by making an interpretation of a significant kind I proved that at least one man was alive and potent, as an analyst. He said that this was somehow connected with whiskey drinking and he could not understand if he had anxiety about disintegration and falling and depersonalisation how it could be that he produces exactly these symptoms by use of whiskey. I interpreted this as an attempt on his part to get control of all the disintegrative anxieties by producing them in an orderly way and in a well-known way by the action of the alcohol, which includes recovery from the alcoholic state.

I was unable to see the patient the next day. He was annoyed about this but this did not disturb the analysis. It may have contributed to his missing the following day, the Wednesday. On the Thursday he came and told me that it was extremely important that I had made that interpretation on the Monday. On the Tuesday he had been to some party at which there were many ghosts from the past; in other words he met significant homosexual figures that belonged to his dangerously homosexual era when he was twenty to twenty-five years old. He felt very false and awkward introducing his wife to a former homosexual partner. If I had left the interpreting of these deeper anxieties till after the meeting with these people, it is unlikely that we would have reached where we reached on Monday. It was also the other way round very important to him on the Tuesday to feel "this was dealt with on Monday by my analyst." From this we went on to a dissection of what is denied by the dream of dancing on the Blue Danube. Sinking into the water for him meant, as it worked out, giving himself over to delusions, to madness. At the stage of Thursday this meant giving himself over to knowing in a much deeper sense than he had known before that he was female. In this position he unexpectedly found himself fond of me and as near as possible in love with me. This meant that he could now love someone and it explained why it was that he had never been able to let himself go in the homosexual position before, always at a critical moment he had withdrawn himself out of homosexuality and he had made a flight into three marriages.

All this felt very real to him and he was comparing it with the work that we had done, which was also undoubtedly correct, on early infantile object relations, which had resulted just before the present phase in his arriving in rather gingerly fashion at an oral interest in the male genital. Throughout this man's analysis the idea of fellatio had been very strange and very remote from his case, something that could be spoken about but without his feeling that it had anything to do with him.

III. Answer to Comments

Written in 1968–1969

My first reaction to reading the comments on my paper is to be pleased that the matters that I raised seem to have stimulated discussion. I am grateful to the discussants for the trouble taken.

It is not my intention to attempt to reply to details because it would seem to me that it is for the reader to judge. I would like to make the following three sets of comments after reading what has been written:

A

Central to my paper is the clinical experience that was mine in this one case that I describe. Originally I had intended giving several comparable experiences illustrating these matters not only in other patients but also in patients of the other sex. It was obvious, however, that too much clinical material would detract from the main thing that I wished to say by making the paper too long.

I am of course aware of the universal acceptance of bisexuality in psycho-analytic theory. I was drawing attention to the high degree of dissociation that may be found in respect of the male and female identifications. This again has nothing new about it. The main point of my communication was the way that it was necessary, as I saw it, to deal with the environmental factor in terms of the transference. It could be said that the patient was in search of the right kind of mad analyst and that in order to meet his needs I had to assume that role. It is this special detail that I considered to be the important part of the paper, a matter of the handling of the transference and the strain on counter-transference feelings produced by acceptance of the role allotted.

B

Confusion can certainly result from my passing over from the clinical material to a theoretical discussion. As soon as one enters the field of theory one is leaving firm ground and starting up a relationship to all those who have written on the same subject, although of course one cannot pretend or hope to be in touch with the whole literature. What is needed, however, is an enumeration of the other mechanisms employed when a patient manifests sexual characteristics that are other than those that his or her biological sex justifies. There is the whole range from a high degree of sophistication to the basic phenomena including very early handling, and beyond that, heredity. Among the sophisticated mechanisms must be found a cross-identification which can be almost entirely organisation of defence. On the other hand cross-identifications may themselves be determined by expectations coming from the environment. To contribute-in in the family situation a boy or girl may need to exploit the other-than-biological sex characteristics. In my patient there was the extreme of the mother's unconscious need for a girl which determined her handling of her baby at the very early stages. The result in my patient was that although he retained his certainty of his male identity he carried with him right up to this point in the analysis that I describe the conviction that in order to have a relationship to his mother he must be a girl. In other words madness in this case was in the mother and not in the patient, although clinically the patient had felt mad and could not free himself from the psychotherapy which he was compelled to pursue but which he knew was hopeless. It happened that the striking thing was that my manipulation of the transference in terms of my being a mad analyst did free him from this terrible fixation to psychotherapy.

C

Following a consideration of these theoretical details I allowed my thoughts to carry me to the concept of male and female elements in boys and girls. I found myself greatly enriched by this way of thinking which was somewhat new to me, so that in considering this kind of problem I was now no longer thinking of boys and girls or men and women but I was thinking in terms of the male and female elements that belong to each. This made me see that the terms "active" and "passive" are not valid in this area. Active and passive are two facets of the same thing in terms of some other type of consideration which goes deeper and which is more primitive. In an attempt to formulate this I found myself in the position of comparing *being* with *doing*. At the extreme I discovered myself looking at an essential conflict of human beings, one which must be operative at a very early date; that between being the object which also has the property of being, and by contrast a confrontation with the object which involves activity and object-relating that is backed by instinct or drive.

This turned out to be a new statement of what I have tried to describe before in terms of the subjective object and the object that is objectively perceived, and I was able to re-examine for my own benefit the tremendous effect here on the immature human baby of the attitude of the mother and then of the parents in terms of adaptation to need. In other words, I found myself re-examining the movement to the reality principle from . . . what? I have never been satisfied with the use of the word "narcissistic" in this connection because the whole concept of narcissism leaves out the tremendous differences that result from the general attitude and behaviour of the mother. I was therefore left with an attempt to state in extreme form the contrast between being and doing.

The basis for this further comment was the separating out of the whole idea of boys and girls and of men and women from the idea of two basic principles, those which I call male and female elements. I suppose it is here that I cause confusion but I cannot withdraw at this stage of the argument, and I prefer to allow this half-way stage to stay. What I want to do is to explore further. I want to get right behind all the crossed-sex sophistications, cross-identifications, and even cross-expectations (where a baby or child can only contribute to a parent in terms of the other-than-biological sex), and I want to go where I find myself both drawn and driven. I want to reach in a new way a concept that no doubt has roots in the writings of other analysts.

I want to get to a statement of a basic dilemma in relatedness:

a. The baby *is* the breast (or object, or mother, etc.); the breast is the baby. This is at the extreme end of the baby's initial lack of establishment of an object as non-me, at the place where the object is 100 percent subjective, where (if the mother adapts well enough, but not otherwise) the baby *experiences* omnipotence.

b. The baby is confronted by an object (breast, etc.) and needs to come to terms with it, with limited (immature) powers of the kind that are based on the mental mechanisms of projective and introjective identifications. Here we need to note that again each child's experience is dependent on the environmental factor (mother's attitude, behaviour, etc.).

In the framework of this concept, which deals with a universal human problem, one can see that baby $\equiv$ breast is a matter of being, not of doing, while in terms of confrontation baby and breast meeting involves doing.

In psychopathology some of the greatest blocks to instinctual—or drive—involvement come when patient $\equiv$ object violently changes into patient confronts and is confronted by object, involving a change from a cosy defence to a position of anxiety of high degree and a sudden awareness of immaturity. I cannot avoid it, but just at this stage I seem to have abandoned the ladder (male and female elements) by which I climbed to the place where I experienced this vision.

29

The Concept of Clinical Regression Compared with That of Defence Organisation

A paper given at a Psychotherapy Symposium at McLean Hospital, Belmont, Massachusetts, 27 October 1967[1]

It is necessary for me to make my position clear at the outset. In this paper I am not starting from specialised clinical experience relative to the hospital management of schizophrenic patients. My clinical experience of adult cases must be assumed to be that of a psycho-analyst who, whether he likes it or not, becomes involved in the treatment of borderline patients, and those who perhaps unexpectedly become schizoid during treatment.

In my child psychiatry practice, however, I have had all types of case in my care, and have watched autism or schizophrenia of childhood develop, and this perhaps justifies me in accepting this invitation, which I feel to be an honour.

I need to be allowed to wander around in the theoretical field, unburdened by the caseload which belongs to practice rather than to the conference table. We can adopt this course, I believe, without cutting ourselves off from the source of our work, which must always be the human beings who come to us or who are brought, because of life's difficulties.

It seemed to me to be a good idea to use this opportunity to sort out a little for myself the inter-relation of two ideas, one of schizophrenia as a regression, and the other of schizophrenia as a defence organisation. It might happen that in practising my scales and arpeggios in this way I may provide material for discussion. I am not concerned either with being original or with quoting from other writers and thinkers (or even Freud).

1. Published in Eldred and Vanderpol, eds., *Psychotherapy in the Designed Therapeutic Milieu,* International Psychiatry Clinics, vol. 5, no. 1 (Boston: Little, Brown, 1968).

For the sake of those whose work takes them in the direction of the physical treatments, may I say that I shall ignore these here, simply because whatever is known or will be discovered about the biochemistry or the neuropathology or the pharmacology relative to schizophrenia, there will still be the patients there, persons like ourselves, with a history in each case of the onset of the disorder, and with a load of personal striving and suffering, and with an environment that is simply bad or good or else confusing to a degree that can be bewildering even to relate.

What I have to say, therefore, will be neither for nor against the specialist in the physical aspects of the disorder; and if I fail to refer to the work of the pure or academic psychologist, here also I must be understood to be, quite simply, busy elsewhere.

To examine the theory of schizophrenia one must have a working theory of the emotional growth of the personality. This is in itself so vast a matter that I could not possibly do it justice in a brief review. What I must do is to assume the general theory of continuity, of an inborn tendency towards growth and personal evolution, and to the theory of mental illness as a hold-up in development. This last item carries with it the idea of a dynamic towards cure—that is, if a block to development is removed then growth follows because of powerful forces belonging to the inherited tendencies in the individual human being.

Also, I can say that the statement of infantile and child development in terms of a progression of erotogenic zones, that has served us well in our treatment of psycho-neurotics, is not so useful in the context of schizophrenia as is the idea of a progression from dependence (at first near-absolute) towards independence—a subject that I have dealt with at some length in various papers.[2]

Here we pay full tribute to the environmental provision, for instance, to the nature of the mother in her presentation of the world to her infant who knows nothing else. At the beginning the environmental factor may be allowed full value, second only to the inherited tendencies of the infant. As the child acquires autonomy and acquires an identity and feels real and perceives the environment objectively as

2. See "Psychoses and Child Care" (1952) in *Collected Papers: Through Paediatrics to Psycho-Analysis* (London: Tavistock, 1958; New York: Basic Books, 1975; London: Hogarth Press, 1975); and three papers in *The Maturational Processes and the Facilitating Environment* (London: Hogarth Press; New York: International Universities Press, 1965): "The Theory of the Parent-Infant Relationship" (1960), "From Dependence Towards Independence in the Development of the Individual" (1963), and "Dependence in Infant-Care, in Child-Care and in the Psycho-Analytic Setting" (1963).

a separate phenomenon, so the environment becomes (in health) increasingly relegated to second place, except that in illness—such as schizophrenia—it always has to be remembered that *the environment may continue to be an adverse factor because of the individual's failure to obtain sufficient autonomy.*

It would not be possible to go further into the essential theory of personal development here and now, although nothing could be more relevant to the theme.

For me, the clue to the conflict that underlies illness that we label psycho-neurosis lies within the individual. The analyst of the psycho-neurotic patient is involved, as is well known, in the analysis of the patient's repressed unconscious.

By contrast, where schizophrenia lies, the analyst or whoever is treating the patient or managing the case is involved in elucidating a split in the patient's person, the extreme of a dissociation. *The split takes the place of the repressed unconscious of the psycho-neurotic.*

I have tried to clarify my ideas on this theme particularly in "Psychoses and Child Care." Here I give a diagram of my idea of the basic split in psychotic illness, but clinically the split, being sub-total, may appear in various forms of dissociation, such as True Self and False Self[3] and the intellectual life split off from psycho-somatic living.[4]

Obviously the nature of the dissociation that appears clinically may be influenced by the nature of expectations from the environment, so that a patient may be suffering from pathological expectations in the environment. The parents may have wanted a child of the other sex, for instance, or may have wanted a genius or a child that has no aggressive impulses. These pathological expectations can reinforce potential dissociations in the individual.

All this is well known and well accepted. What follows is less sure, but I shall continue to use dogmatic language.

The split in the person happened and became organised because of an environmental failure. There was a failure of the "average expectable environment." In my terms a baby is usually cared for by a "good enough" mother. Well, either the good-enough mother had to fail (perhaps she got ill) or else she was not good enough. I am not apportioning blame, only searching for aetiology.

These matters are more obviously applicable to infantile and child-

3. See "Ego Distortion in Terms of True and False Self" (1960), in *The Maturational Processes and the Facilitating Environment.*

4. See "Mind and Its Relation to the Psyche-Soma" (1949), in *Collected Papers: Through Paediatrics to Psycho-Analysis.*

hood schizophrenia, but we must find a way of applying them to the schizophrenia of adolescent and of adult persons, even when, as it seemed, things went well in early childhood, and the disorder only showed clinically at a later age. The fact is that early dependence continues to have meaning, especially in adolescence, and perhaps in a disguised way throughout life. (Example, dependence on a religious tenet might not show unless some experience should make that tenet untenable.)

For me, a good-enough mother and good-enough parents and a good-enough home do in fact give most babies and small children *the experience of not having ever been significantly let down*. In this way average children have the chance to build up a capacity to believe in themselves and the world—they build a structure on the accumulation of introjected reliability. They are blissfully unaware of their good fortune, and find it difficult to understand those of their companions who carry around with them for life experiences of unthinkable anxiety, and a deficit in the department of introjected reliability. It is among these latter persons that illness, when it occurs, tends to take a form that we label schizophrenic rather than psycho-neurotic or depressive.

I have to insert a note here, in spite of my determination to keep out everything that is not needed for the exposition of my main theme; this has to do with the fact that failures in environmental reliability at the early stages produce in the baby fractures of personal continuity, because of reactions to the unpredictable. These traumatic events carry with them unthinkable anxiety, or maximal pain.[5]

Here I come to the point where I have to confess that I did at one time think of schizophrenia and schizoid types of clinical disorder as regressions, so that I joined in the hunt for fixation points. This was a carry-over from the corresponding witch-hunt in the attempt to state the aetiology of psycho-neurosis in its various manifestations.

My attitude changed when I saw that I must think of two kinds of regression—one is simply a falling back in a direction that is the opposite to the forward movement of development. One sees regressive features appearing, and one recognises that the growth mechanisms of the individual have become blocked. The other type of regression is quite different, although it may be similar clinically. In the second

---

5. See "Ego Integration in Child Development" (1962), in *The Maturational Processes and the Facilitating Environment*.

type the patient regresses because of a new environmental provision which allows of dependence.

I am reminded of a lady, not very unusual, who kept going fairly well, in spite of much anxiety and sleeplessness, until she at last found a good reliable housekeeper; at this point she retired to bed, and luxuriated, as the saying is. Substitute "mental nurse" for "housekeeper," and then "luxuriate" becomes a "schizoid depression" plus the money to pay for it.

In other words, I found that in my study of schizoid phenomena I was using the word "regression" to mean *regression to dependence.* I did not any longer care whether the patient had stepped back in terms of erotogenic zones.

This led me to see that the patient's illness is an expression of the *healthy* elements in his or her personality, when regression is related to environmental provision. What I mean is that it is one thing if a patient simply breaks down, and it is another thing if a patient breaks down into some new environmental provision that offers reliable care. A special example is that of the schizoid patient who goes through a regressive phase because the long preparatory phase of the analysis has given him or her a sense of there being something trustworthy that can be used positively.[6] It is true that the use the patient makes of this new opportunity for dependence is complex; nevertheless the work done and the use made of the work done indicates the operation of a healthy "observing ego" element in the patient. The false self defence can be dropped and the true self can become exposed (at great risk) in the psychotic transference.

From here (and I am ashamed to have condensed what I mean to the point almost of absurdity) I began to see schizophrenia and especially the illness of the borderline case as a *sophisticated defence organisation.* Here is a direct link with Freud, and his central theme, that symptoms mean something and have value to the patient, although he was at first referring to psycho-neurotic manifestations.

Contributory to my move in this direction of theoretical understanding (a slow move it may be thought) was my wide experience of what I always called childhood schizophrenia. What we observe in children and in infants who become ill in a way that forces us to use the word "schizophrenia," although this word originally applied to

---

6. See "Metapsychological and Clinical Aspects of Regression within the Psycho-Analytical Set-Up" (1954), in *Collected Papers: Through Paediatrics to Psycho-Analysis.*

adolescents and adults, what we see very clearly is an *organisation towards invulnerability*. Differences must be expected according to the stage of the emotional development of the adult or child or baby who becomes ill. What is common to all cases is this, that the baby, child, adolescent or adult *must never again experience* the unthinkable anxiety that is at the root of schizoid illness. This unthinkable anxiety was experienced initially in a moment of failure of reliability on the part of the environmental provision when the immature personality was at the stage of absolute dependence.

The autistic child who has travelled almost all the way to mental defect is not suffering any longer; invulnerability has almost been reached. Suffering belongs to the parents. The organisation towards invulnerability has been successful, and it is this that shows clinically along with regressive features that are not in fact essential to the picture.

It will be appreciated that this theory includes the idea of trauma, by which I mean an experience against which the ego defences were inadequate at the stage of emotional development of the individual at the time, or in the state of the patient at the time. Trauma is an impingement from the environment and from the individual's reaction to the impingement that occurs prior to the individual's development of the mechanisms that make the unpredictable predictable.

Following traumatic experiences new defences are quickly organised, but in the split-second before this can take place the individual has had the continuous line of his or her existence (as recorded in the personal computer) broken, broken by automatic reaction to the environmental failure.

Elsewhere[7] I have indicated the varieties of experience of "unthinkable" or "psychotic" anxiety. They can be classified in terms of the amount of integration that survives the disaster:

No integration retained	Disintegration
Some integration retained	Falling for ever
	Going off in all directions
	Somatic split; head & body
	Absence of orientation
	Loss of directed relating to objects
Integration retained	Unpredictable physical environment instead of "average expectable"

7. "Ego Integration in Child Development."

The result of trauma must be some degree of distortion of development. It will be seen how normal and healthy anger would be in comparison with such awfulness. Anger would imply survival of the ego and a retention of the idea of an alternative experience in which the "let-down" did not occur. Clinically the state which is called "panic" easily becomes a feature. Direct study of panic is unproductive because panic is itself a defence. It is of value to look on panic as an organised awfulness arranged around a phobic situation whose aim (in the defence organisation) is to protect the individual from new examples of the unpredictable. Good-enough mothering is that which enables a baby not to have to meet the unpredictable until able to allow for environmental failures.

An important corollary is one that affects all who engage in the psychotherapy of schizophrenia in patients of whatever age. We give help by providing reliability which the patient can use in the sense that he or she can undo the defences that have been built up against unpredictability and the dire consequences in terms of the awfulness to be experienced.

If we are successful we enable the patient *to abandon invulnerability and to become a sufferer.* If we succeed life becomes precarious to one who was beginning to know a kind of stability and a freedom from pain, even if this meant non-participation in life and perhaps mental defect.

At the start we seem to see clinical improvement, but as we proceed and the patient achieves dependence on us in a big way, *then our mistakes and failures become new traumata.* We learn to expect increasing sensitivity on the part of the patient, and we begin to wonder whether it is kindness or cruelty that motivates us. We find that our inevitable specific and limited failures, often brought about by the patient, give opportunity for the patient to feel and express anger with us. Instead of cumulative trauma[8] we get cumulative angry experiences in which the object (the therapist and his room) survive the patient's anger. No treatment of borderline cases can be free from suffering, both of patient and therapist.

8. See M. Masud R. Khan, "The Concept of Cumulative Trauma," in *The Psycho-Analytic Study of the Child*, vol. 18 (London: Hogarth Press, 1963); also in Khan, *The Privacy of the Self* (London: Hogarth Press, 1974).

30

Addendum to "The Location of Cultural Experience"

Dated 18 December 1967

Since writing the paper "The Location of Cultural Experience"[1] I have gradually come to an unexpected need for something corresponding to the cultural experience but located inside instead of outside. It is on material presented by patients that I have based the writing of this addendum to my previous paper. Nevertheless I am drawing on my personal experience in trying to illustrate what I mean. It is perhaps worth recording that I found myself very much needing to sleep sitting on the floor in my room facing the dark end of the room. This was while I was trying to find out what it was that I wished to formulate. I went to sleep thinking that I would perhaps wake up finding that a certain case would properly illustrate the squiggle game, and I was surprised with what turned up. The dream told me what it was that I was trying to formulate and when I woke before I opened my eyes I knew for certain that I was facing the window; yet of course I also knew, as soon as I began to think, that I was the other way round. I gave myself a long time to get the full sensation of this mirror experience. Eventually when I felt I had had enough of it and I knew for certain by feeling that if I opened my eyes I would see the window, I gave myself the luxury of the full experience of waking up and finding myself facing the other way with my back to the window.

I went straight into the other room to dictate something which would formulate what I had in mind, now quite clear what it had to do with.

In the previous paper I stated that there is a need for some potential space for the location of playing and cultural experience in general. The impression given deliberately was that this potential space if it existed would be outside the line that divides inner from outer. I now

1. "The Location of Cultural Experience" (1967), in *Playing and Reality* (London: Travistock; New York: Basic Books, 1971; Penguin, 1974).

want to refer to a potential space that is on the inside of this line.

In the dream that was very intensely occupying me during my sleep I was having an experience in an area that I call my club. This is something that I have discovered fairly recently. It suddenly dawned on me a few years ago that I had been living for many years in a kind of a community that was just on the dream side of waking and yet which was not dream material. Once I had remembered this kind of dreaming I was able to go right back to its beginning although till the time that I started to remember it I had never brought it into consciousness.

It started perhaps thirty to forty years ago and I call it my club because of two things. One is that at that time I resigned from the Athenaeum and the other is that the kind of dreaming I am referring to has always been about a club. I remembered the time when I was dreaming and I went down towards the south coast and there discovered, probably amongst the hills of the south downs, a large house which seemed to be empty or at any rate not accessible to me. Very gradually in the course of years of dreaming this place became some community into which I gained entry. The people in it grew and developed their relationships and they changed and altogether this club has given me a tremendous sense of stability corresponding very much to the use that people do make of a club such as the Athenaeum.

I have never tried to make use of this material except to refer to it sometimes humourously when I have been asked "What were you dreaming about?" and I said: "I have been to my club." In the experience that I had just before dictating these words I had an extremely vivid adventure which had to do with emerging with friends of all kinds from the club in order to visit some place away from the club. I had had a dream during the previous night in which we went in several groups using the various cars to visit another club where I was supposed to be giving a lecture. It was not pleasant when I found that we were late and that we were expected to wear evening clothes and the hostess complained about my shabby appearance.

Life in and around the club is not usually unpleasant but on this occasion I was very glad to wake as my lecture might not even be a good one because of the confusion surrounding the arrangements for it. The very vivid excursion from the club that I experienced just before deciding to write about it was a continuation to some extent of the club life of the night before.

When I give thought to the matter I can see that it has some sort of relationship to deep dreaming, rather like that which we usually call fantasying of children, especially because it is to some extent manipulated, and it is certain that it will never contain the major excitements and anxieties that belong to the true dream.

In this kind of dreaming there is a very definite continuity in time, and in regard to placing it I must put it just on the sleep side of the line between waking and dreaming. There is undoubtedly a relationship between this and the developing fantasy world of a novelist.

It is as if I know from this experience what it would be like to be John Galsworthy with the *Forsyte Saga* making a continuous development in the course of a few years in his mind, the characters having definite personalities and characteristics and even illnesses. And I could well understand the need that an author could have to get these experiences written down and published in novel form. The mind boggles at the thought of what kind of a club or whatever corresponded to a club there must have been going on in the mind of a Tolstoy and what a need such a man would have to get things written down so that the characters can grow up and evolve and die off and not in fact become a tremendous block in the mental life of the author.

In my case there is no particular richness and nothing worth trying to write down and yet this story by its very continuity and by the surprising things that happen in it gives me a permanent novel that I am able to read without reading or that I am able to write without writing. I have noticed that an excess of tea or coffee very much increases the liability for me to be living in this area while asleep, by which I mean that the sleep which is just possible but threatened by sleeplessness is the place where I live in relation to all the people in my club, and I am very glad to have it. I do know, however, that I must allow for the dream material that only comes in truly deep sleep when the mind does not have to be active and creative and in control, in the way that caffeine helps it to be.

I think that this idea is not of particular importance to the analyst except that it may enable him to avoid doing the analysis of this kind of dream as it gets reported, just as in child analysis one avoids doing the analysis of fantasying and of the child's infinite capacity for writing comics. So one knows that one has to wait for material that comes from a deeper layer before using the material as a communication from the unconscious.

31

Playing and Culture

A talk given to the Imago Group, 12 March 1968

The idea that I have is that a satisfactory statement relating to experience in cultural matters has not been made by psycho-analysts. Possibly there has not even been a direct attempt to tackle this particular problem. It will be of importance to me if I can be given references to any such attempts that have been made, whether in the psychoanalytic or in allied literature. A very great deal indeed has been written about psychic reality as experienced by the individual who is alive. Similarly a great deal has been written on object-relating and the whole relationship of the human being to the environment or to external shared reality.

There is some attempt to get towards that which concerns me here in the observations relating to affection as compared with instinctually driven object-relating. In the negative "the affectionless child" is a term which draws attention to the importance of the capacity for affectionate feeling quality. The concept of sublimation brings the analyst towards that which I am trying to study. Also it can be said that playing is as near as possible to the subject of my research. In regard to playing, however, there is in the psycho-analytic literature a close tie-up with instinct modified by displacement, etc.

It may be considered that the orthodox approach has taken the student of metapsychology to a complete statement of the human being and of living experience. My thesis is that for some reason (which can be studied as a subject in itself) no place for cultural experience has been given in the statement of human existence by psycho-analysts. I am making an assumption here that cultural experience comes about as a direct extension from the playing of children and indeed of babies from the age of birth, and perhaps earlier.

There is obviously a close association between playing and the idea of fantasy and dream. Playing also relates to the playing of games and such things as active imagination where a deliberate attempt is made to make use of surprising elements that the imagination brings about.

When I go to a concert and meet a psycho-analytic colleague at the same concert I sometimes wonder whether we know as much as we would like to know about the experience we are both having. There is certainly an inherent difference between going to a concert and dreaming; also there is no doubt that neither of us goes to the concert simply to sit next to someone or because we are in love with the pianist. We are in a living experience which has a right to be considered as a thing in itself. We can extend this observation to the question, what do you live for? What is the basic motivation?

It is possible that we may find that it is in this area of cultural experience that many of us live most of our time when we are awake, and if we transfer this idea to childhood we can see immediately that we are talking about playing.

Undoubtedly the concept of the transitional object and of transitional phenomena brought me to my wish to study this intermediate area which has to do with living experience and which is neither dream nor object-relating. At the same time that it is neither the one nor the other of these two it is also both. This is the essential paradox, and in my paper on transitional phenomena the most important part (in my opinion) is my claim that we need to *accept the paradox,* not to resolve it. Transitional objects and phenomena are universal and protean. The study of transitional phenomena provides a valuable research ground for the student of human growth and development not only because it introduces the student to the infinity of variability in human beings but also because it has its own limits, and there are resemblances between elements, and these can be classified. In other words, it has some of the qualities of playing in that the child who is playing is using materials of external or shared reality for the expression of dream material. The personal dream is there, but two children may build similar houses because of the common denominator in the building materials and also because of archetypal elements in the dreaming. No two children can be alike, even identical twins, if the personal psychic reality be included beneath the surface markings of the personality. Nevertheless children can resemble each other and in any case they do resemble each other in that usually there are two eyes and a nose and a mouth, etc.

I suggest that if we look at philosophy and for the moment ignore the immensely significant details of content, we can see operating a dynamic which I would call a non-acceptance of the inherent paradox. For me the paradox is inherent. In terms of the transitional object it is that although the object was there to be found it was created by the baby. One could refer here to the Ronald Knox limerick, and in theology the same thing appears in the interminable discussion around the question: is there a God? If God is a projection, even so is there a God who created me in such a way that I have the material in me for such a projection? Aetiologically, if I may use a word here that usually refers to disease, the paradox must be accepted, not resolved. The important thing for me must be, have I got it in me to have the idea of God?—if not, then the idea of God is of no value to me (except superstitiously).

This problem goes right to the heart of the difficulty that some of us have in regard to Melanie Klein's root concept, though some of Bion's statements tend to make way for a resolution of an awkward conflict over basic tenets. It is possible to use Melanie Klein's emphasis on projection and introjection if at base there is allowed the individual's creative element that must be fundamental for the individual, but which need not be fundamental for the observer. Aetiologically, whatever the baby achieves arises out of the baby's aliveness, including the matter of brain function. It is here that the idea of absolute dependence has value, since the potential for creative activity in the baby does not become actual unless (in subtle ways, changing with the baby's developing capacities) the mother figure receives and can give back the projections. The projections do not take place unless there is that there to take the projections.

In dealing with this, which has interested me for two decades, I have postulated a potential space between baby and mother figure which is the location of play. This potential space only comes to have significance as a result of a baby's living experience. It is not inherited—what is inherited may or may not result in the achievement of a place for play experience in the case of any one *live* baby.

To my surprise I found that play and playing and the transitional phenomena form the basis for cultural experience in general, and that therefore what I was looking at concerned the greater part of our lives. Even here now we are in this potential space, and without good-enough mothering we should have found this discussion to be alien to us.

In my statement of playing therefore I have made it my main point that:

Play is always exciting.

It is exciting *not* because of the background of instinct, but because of the precariousness that is inherent in it, since it always deals with the knife-edge between the subjective and that which is objectively perceived.

What holds for play also holds for the St. Matthew Passion at which I am almost certain to find colleagues when I go to the Festival Hall in a few weeks' time.

32

Interpretation in Psycho-Analysis

Dated 19 February 1968

It is important from time to time to look at the basic principles of the psycho-analytic technique and to attempt to reassess the importance of the various elements that the classical technique comprises. It would be generally conceded that an important part of psycho-analytic technique is interpretation, and it is my purpose here to study once more this particular part of what we do.

The word "interpretation" implies that we are using words, and there is a further implication which is that material supplied by the patient is verbalised. In its simplest form there is the basic rule, which still has force, although many analysts never instruct their patients even on this detail. By this time, after more than half a century of psycho-analysis, patients know that they are expected to say what comes to their minds and not to withhold. It is also generally recognised now that a great deal of communication takes place from patient to analyst that is not verbalised.

This may have been noticed first in terms of the nuances of speech and the various ways in which speech certainly involved a great deal more than the meaning of the words used. Gradually analysts found themselves interpreting silences and movements and a whole host of behavioural details which were outside the realm of verbalisation. Nevertheless there were always analysts who very much preferred to stick to the verbalised material offered by the patient. When this works it has obvious advantages in that the patient does not feel persecuted by the observer's eyes.

With a silent patient, a man of 25 years, I once interpreted the movement of his fingers as his hands lay clasped across his chest. He said to me: "If you start interpreting that sort of thing then I shall have to transfer that sort of activity to something else which does not show." In other words, he was pointing out to me that unless he had verbalised his communication it was not for me to make comment.

There is also the vast subject which can be explored of the analyst's communications that are not conveyed in direct verbalisation or even in errors of verbalisation. There is no need to develop this theme, because it is obvious, but it starts off with the analyst's tone of voice and the way in which, for instance, a moralistic attitude may or may not show in a statement which by itself could be said to be nothing more than an interpretation. Interpretative comments have been explored and have certainly been discussed at great length in innumerable supervisory hours. There is perhaps no need to make a further study along these lines at the present time.

The purpose of interpretation must include a feeling that the analyst has that a communication has been made which needs acknowledgement. This is perhaps the important part of an interpretation, but this very simple purpose is often hidden amongst a lot of other matters such as instruction in regard to the use of symbols. As an example of this one could take an interpretation like "the two white objects in the dream are breasts," etc. etc. As soon as the analyst has embarked on this kind of interpretation he has left solid ground and is now in a dangerous area where he is using his own ideas and these may be wrong from the point of view of the patient at the moment.

In the simplest form the analyst gives back to the patient what the patient has communicated. It may easily happen that the analyst feels that this is a futile occupation because if the patient has communicated something what is the point of saying it back except of course for the purpose of letting the patient know that what has been said has been heard and that the analyst is trying to get the meaning correctly.

Giving an interpretation back gives the patient opportunity to correct the misunderstandings. There are analysts who accept such corrections but there are also analysts who in their interpretative role assume a position which is almost unassailable so that if the patient attempts to make a correction the analyst tends rather to think in terms of the patient's resistance than in terms of the possibility that the communication has been wrongly or inadequately received.

Here one is already discussing varieties of psycho-analyst, of which there are many, and undoubtedly one of the tasks of being an analysand is to get to know what the analyst is like and what the analyst expects and what language the analyst talks and what kind of dreams the analyst can use, etc. etc. This is not entirely unnatural because it is rather like that with a child who has to get to know what kind of parents there are to be used as parents. Nevertheless in a discussion among analysts it would tend to be taken for granted that many patients are unable to make use of analysts who require the patient to do more than a certain amount of adapting; or to put it the other way round, to make use of analysts who are not able or willing to do more than a certain amount of adapting to the needs of the patient.

The principle that I am enunciating at this moment is that the analyst reflects back what the patient has communicated. This very simple statement about interpretation may be important by the very fact that it is simple and that it avoids the tremendous complications that arise when one thinks of all the possibilities that can be classified under the interpretative urge. If this very simple principle is enunciated it immediately needs elaboration. I suggest it needs elaboration of the following kind. In the limited area of today's transference the patient has an accurate knowledge of a detail or of a set of details. It is as if there is a dissociation belonging to the place that the analysis has reached today. It is helpful to remember that in this limited way or from this limited position the patient can be giving the analyst a sample of the truth; that is to say of something that is absolutely true for the patient, and that when the analyst gives this back the interpretation is received by the patient who has already emerged to some extent from this limited area or dissociated condition. In other words, the interpretation may even be given to the whole person, whereas the material for the interpretation was derived from only a part of the whole person. As a whole person the patient would not have been able to have given the material for the interpretation.

In this way the interpretations are part of a building up of insight. An important detail is that the interpretation has been given within a certain number of minutes or even seconds of the very insightful material presented. Certainly it is given in the same analytic hour. The right interpretation given tomorrow after a supervision is of no use because of this very powerful operation of a time factor. In other words, from a limited area the patient has insight and gives material for an interpretation. The analyst takes this information and gives it back to the patient and the patient that he gives it back to is now no longer in the area of insight in regard to this particular psychoanalytic element or constellation.

With this principle in mind it is possible to feel that the reflection back to the patient of what the patient has already said or conveyed is not a waste of time but it may indeed be the best thing that the analyst can do in the analysis of that patient on that particular day.

There is a certain amount of opposition to this way of looking at things because analysts enjoy exercising the skills that they have acquired and they have a very great deal that they can say about anything that turns up. For example, a rather silent patient tells the analyst, in response to a question, a good deal about one of his main interests, which has to do with shooting pigeons and the organisation of this kind of sport. It is extremely tempting for the analyst at this point to use this material, which is more than he often gets in two or three weeks, and undoubtedly he could talk about the killing of all the unborn babies, the patient being an only child, and he could talk about the unconscious destructive fantasies in the mother, the patient's mother having been a depressive case and having committed suicide. What the analyst knew, however, was that the whole material came from a question and that it would not have come if the analyst had not invited the material, perhaps simply out of feeling that he was getting out of touch with the patient. The material therefore was not material for interpretation and the analyst had to hold back all that he could imagine in regard to the symbolic meaning of the activity which the patient was describing. After a while the analysis settled back into being a silent one and it is the patient's silence which contains the essential communication. The clues to this silence are only slowly emerging and there is nothing directly that this analyst can do to make the patient talk.

It need hardly be mentioned that often the patient produces material which the analyst can usefully interpret in another sense. It is as if the analyst can use the intellectual processes, both his own and those of the patient, to go ahead a little. The main thing is the reflection back to the patient of the material presented, perhaps a dream. Nevertheless the two together can play at using the dream for a deeper insight. There is great danger here because the interplay can be pleasurable and even exciting and can make both the patient and the analyst feel very gratified. Nevertheless there is only a certain distance that the analyst can safely take the patient beyond the place where the patient already is.

An example would be as follows: A patient gives a recurring dream, one which has dominated her life. She is starving and she is left with an orange, but she sees that the orange has been nibbled at by a rat. She has a rat phobia and the fact that the rat has touched the orange makes her unable to use the orange. The distress is extreme. It is a dream that she has been liable to all her life. Diagnostically she comes into the category of deprived child. The analyst need not do anything about this dream because the work has already been done in the dreaming and then in the remembering and in the reporting. The remembering and the reporting are results of work already done in the treatment and are of the nature of a bonus resulting from increased trust. The matter can be left there and the analyst can wait for more material to turn up. In this particular case that I am describing there was an external reason why the analyst could not afford to wait because there was not going to be an opportunity for further sessions. He therefore made the interpretation, thereby running the risk of spoiling the work that had already been done but also opening up the possibility that the patient might get further immediately. This is a matter of judgement and the analyst here felt that the degree of trust was such that he could proceed and even make a mistake. He said: The orange is the breast of the mother who was a good mother from your point of view but the mother that you lost. The rats represent both your attack on the breast and the breast's attack on you. The dream has to do with the fact that without help you are stuck because although you are still in touch with the original breast that seemed good you cannot make use of it unless you can be helped through the next stage in which you excitedly attack the breast to eat it as you would eat an orange.

It happened that in this case the patient was able to use this interpretation immediately, and she produced two examples; one of them illustrated her relationship to her mother before she lost her, and the other was a memory of the time of the actual losing of the mother. In this way the patient obtained emotional release and there was a marked clinical change for the better.

Any analyst can give innumerable examples of interpretations which patients were able to use and which took the patient further than they had reached when they were presenting the material specific to the session. Nevertheless this particular example highlights in a simple way the essential dynamics of the interpretation that goes beyond reflecting back the material presented.

It cannot be too strongly emphasised, however, in the teaching of students, that it is better to stick to the principle of the reflecting back of material presented rather than to go to the other extreme of clever interpretations which, even if accurate, may nevertheless take the patient further than the transference confidence allows, so that when the patient leaves the analyst the almost miraculous revelation that the interpretation represents suddenly becomes a threat because it is in touch with a stage of emotional development that the patient has not yet reached, at least as a total personality.

33
Thinking and Symbol-Formation

Undated; probably written in 1968

Our attention has been drawn recently to the process of thinking as it is related to psycho-analytic metapsychology, notably by Bion.[1]

Here I wish to look at one aspect of this vast subject, and in doing so I shall set aside many aspects of thinking, that are closely related to my chosen theme. My theme is the relationship between thinking and symbol-formation.

A statement on the ontological origin of thinking is already contained in a previous paper of my own, "Mind and Its Relation to the Psyche-Soma" (1949).[2] I stated in this paper the idea that thinking starts as a personal way that the infant has for dealing with the mother's graduated failure of adaptation. Thinking is part of the mechanism by which the infant tolerates both failure of adaptation to ego-need and frustration of instinct producing tension-tension, particularly the former.

There is a pathology of this process which I also tried to indicate in this paper, as when there is tantalising adaptation and failure of adaptation (due to an inadequacy in the mother's attitude) so that the need for thinking becomes stepped up; and indeed this need for thinking escalates (to use a modern term) so that thinking becomes strained as a function, or acquires a new function. I wrote: "... we find *mental functioning becoming a thing in itself,* practically replacing the good mother and making her unnecessary." I added: "Clinically, this can go along with dependence on the actual mother and a false personal growth on a compliance basis."

It will be seen from this that in my view thinking or mental functioning needs *in these cases* to be studied in its psycho-pathology, namely as something that has lost its place as a specialised aspect of

1. See Wilfred Bion, *Second Thoughts* (London: Heinemann Medical Books Ltd., 1967).
2. In *Collected Papers: Through Paediatrics to Psycho-Analysis* (London: Tavistock, 1958; New York: Basic Books, 1975; London: Hogarth Press, 1975).

the functioning of the psyche (cf. the psyche-soma), and as something that has acquired a new or secondary function.

In the cases to which I am referring thinking has become split off from the psyche-soma partnership, and has taken over a part of the role of the mother. Dependence has shifted. Dependence on the mother has proved relatively unsatisfactory, and dependence on the mind and on thinking has taken the place of reliance on the good-enough mother. Beyond this there is an extreme degree of split (or hopelessness about integration) which makes for an absence of any relationship between thinking and the good-enough-mothering function. Even thinking has failed.

In this paper I am further exploring the area in which there is retained some degree of success of this defence, in which thinking acts as a substitute for mother-care, and in which there develops a false self in the shape of an exploited intellect. The defence has not entirely failed.

In the article referred to ("Mind and Its Relation to the Psyche-Soma") I gave the case of a child who was developing along these lines and who had an idea of an ideal state: to become mentally defective. The implication is that all the time there is a strain in the infant economy even when the intellectual defence has some success; the individual longs for an alternative, and not being able to find the alternative in maternal care and dependence, there must come into existence in the economics of the mind of such a child a tendency towards the alternative of a loss of intellectual power, or a loss of mind and mental functioning.

(It will be seen that here is an example of a primary "castration" based on the loss of an ego function. Better known is for true castration anxiety to find secondary expression in the idea of loss of intellect.) (cf. Jones' APHANISIS).[3]

The basis of my further study, then, is the way in which normally the developing infant thinks and allows for adaptive failures, and the way in which a tantalising or not-quite-good-enough environmental provision exploits the infant's thinking and even makes this thinking take the place of some element of the average expectable environment.

3. See Ernest Jones, "Early Development of Female Sexuality" (1927), in *Papers on Psycho-Analysis* (London: Balliere, Tindall and Cox, 1950).

Introductory Clinical Material

The case that has led me to wish to link thinking with symbol-formation is that of a woman who is nearing the end of a long and tedious analysis by an analyst who is a colleague, I myself being involved in a way that is ancillary. The patient, a woman teacher, was dealing with a summer break in her analysis by taking a refresher course in pottery. Her reaction to the break had two aspects:

a. Successful pottery activities.

b. Hopelessness about planning for next term's teaching responsibilities. Her complaint was that *she could not think.* This was not a new feature, indeed at one time an inability to use her very good intellect was the major problem.

It is possible to describe this teacher's holiday state in a precise way because of an incident which she felt was really part of her analysis although it happened when she was away staying with someone (X).

The patient was having breakfast in bed. She got up to take the tray to the kitchen and upset everything on the floor, breaking valuable china and making a mess everywhere. She felt an extreme of exasperation, and the incident upset her profoundly.

She could find herself complaining (but only with me there, because she knew she was employing a series of delusions):

1. It was Y's fault, because Y gave X the tray, and the tray was a slippery one.

2. She screamed and X did not hear because she was out of the house.

3. In any case, X ought to have been there looking after her and then the accident wouldn't have happened.

4. If the patient's analyst had come at the moment of the accident and had taken over and had consoled her, then the whole incident would have become part of the analysis and would not have been a wasted experience.

5. A good analyst would have been there, caring for her, and taking the tray away, and there would have been no incident.

But the woman was not mad and she could *think,* and could explain to herself:

1. It would be absurd to expect an analyst to care for a patient in a holiday (analyst's holiday).

2. In any case the analyst would not be likely to have turned up at exactly the right minute.

3. If she had turned up she perhaps would have cleared up the mess and would have consoled the patient, or at any rate she would have verbalised the patient's need to have this sort of experience which would have corrected the pattern of expected experience belonging to the patient's infancy.

4. A really good analyst would have been there, giving the patient special care, and then there would have been no untoward incident. In such a case the patient would have been able to feel confidence in her environment and in herself, to a degree which would have enabled her to become angry at the failure element in the pattern of the environment of her infancy and early childhood.

In fact, this is what was actually happening, since the patient felt that the whole event was part of the analysis, and belonged to the holiday from an analysis which is beginning to succeed.

This case gives rise to the general consideration that success in analysis must include the delusion of failure, the patient's reaction to the analysis as a failure. This paradox needs to be allowed. The analyst must be able to accept this role of failing analyst as he accepts all other roles that arise out of the patient's transference neuroses and psychoses. Many an analysis has failed at the end because the analyst could not allow a delusional failure, due to his personal need to prove the truth of psycho-analytic theory through the cure of a patient. Psycho-analysis does not cure, though it is true that a patient may make use of psycho-analysis, and may achieve with adjunctive process a degree of integration and socialisation and self-discovery which he would not or could not have achieved without it.

34
On "The Use of an Object"

This chapter contains material relating to "the use of an object," a concept developed by Winnicott towards the end of his life. He made his main statement of it in a lecture given on 12 November 1968 to the New York Psychoanalytic Society: subsequently this appeared in the *International Journal of Psycho-Analysis* 50 (1969), and then in a slightly modified version in his posthumously published book *Playing and Reality* (1971). For the convenience of the reader this last version is reproduced here as Section I.

The rest of the chapter consists in such writing as belongs explicitly to the development of Winnicott's concept as well as a late paper that employs it. Most of this writing is previously unpublished; the exception is Section III, which contains some of the notes that Winnicott made in 1965 in the train on his way home from Dartington Hall, where he had been thinking and talking about the subject of freedom and control in progressive schools. We include these notes, even though they have already been published in *Deprivation and Delinquency* (1984), because they contain the first reference that we can find to "the use of an object" as such. It is obvious, however, from Winnicott's account of a dream dating from 1963, and from his letter to a colleague that accompanied it (both in Section II), that certain aspects of his concept had become explicit even earlier. He connected the dream with the writing of his review of Jung's book *Memories, Dreams, Reflections:* for the review itself, see Chapter 57 of this volume. Section IV contains a short paper, "The Use of the Word 'Use'," which was written in February 1968, and to which Winnicott attached some importance, as it had a place in the lists of papers he made in 1968 with a view to publication. Section V is a clinical illustration used by Winnicott for his 1968 lecture in New York, and this is followed by "Comments on My Paper 'The Use of an Object,'" Section VI. The comments were made in answer to the discussion at the end of the same lecture, and in particular to a remark by Dr. Bernard Fine to the effect that Winnicott had overlooked the importance of the "libidinal component of the instinctual drives and their ability to help the object to survive." Written in December of 1968, when Winnicott was just recovering from the illness that had overtaken him in New York after he gave his lecture, they were only partly typed and then finished by hand, and it is likely that had he intended them for publication he would have done some polishing. The last section of the chapter contains the unfinished and also virtually unedited paper "The Use of an Object in the Context of *Moses and Monotheism*," which was written in January 1969. Here Winnicott's concept is linked to the writing of Freud, and this allows him to bring the father into the foreground of the infant's life in a way that is rarely found elsewhere in his theoretical work.

Two more papers which are not included here could be said to belong, at least in part, to the same group. One is a talk entitled "Breastfeeding As a Communication," read in Winnicott's absence (owing to his illness) at a National Childbirth Trust conference on 28 November 1968, and now published in his book *Babies and Their Mothers* (1987). This contains a description of the value to the baby of breastfeeding in terms of survival of the breast. The other paper is "The Place of the Monarchy," written in 1970, which discusses the monarchy also in terms of its survival value. This is to be found in the collection by Winnicott entitled *Home Is Where We Start From* (1985).

EDITORS

I. The Use of an Object and Relating through Identifications

Based on a paper read to the New York Psychoanalytic Society, 12 November 1968

In this chapter I propose to put forward for discussion the idea of the use of an object. The allied subject of relating to objects seems to me to have had our full attention. The idea of the use of an object has not, however, been so much examined, and it may not even have been specifically studied.

This work on the use of an object arises out of my clinical experience and is in the direct line of development that is peculiarly mine. I cannot assume, of course, that the way in which my ideas have devel-

oped has been followed by others, but I should like to point out that
there has been a sequence, and the order that there may be in the
sequence belongs to the evolution of my work.

What I have to say in this present chapter is extremely simple. Although it comes out of my psycho-analytical experience I would not
say that it could have come out of my psycho-analytical experience of
two decades ago, because I would not then have had the technique to
make possible the transference movements that I wish to describe. For
instance, it is only in recent years that I have become able to wait and
wait for the natural evolution of the transference arising out of the
patient's growing trust in the psycho-analytic technique and setting,
and to avoid breaking up this natural process by making interpretations. It will be noticed that I am talking about the making of interpretations and not about interpretations as such. It appals me to think
how much deep change I have prevented or delayed in patients *in a
certain classification category* by my personal need to interpret. If
only we can wait, the patient arrives at understanding creatively and
with immense joy, and I now enjoy this joy more than I used to enjoy
the sense of having been clever. I think I interpret mainly to let the
patient know the limits of my understanding. The principle is that it
is the patient and only the patient who has the answers. We may or
may not enable him or her to encompass what is known or become
aware of it with acceptance.

By contrast with this comes the interpretative work that the analyst
must do, which distinguishes analysis from self-analysis. This interpreting by the analyst, if it is to have effect, must be related to the
patient's ability *to place the analyst outside the area of subjective phenomena.* What is then involved is the patient's ability to use the analyst, which is the subject of this paper. In teaching, as in the feeding
of a child, the capacity to use objects is taken for granted, but in our
work it is necessary for us to be concerned with the development and
establishment of the capacity to use objects and to recognise a patient's inability to use objects, where this is a fact.

It is in the analysis of the borderline type of case that one has the
chance to observe the delicate phenomena that give pointers to an
understanding of truly schizophrenic states. By the term "a borderline
case" I mean the kind of case in which the core of the patient's disturbance is psychotic, but the patient has enough psycho-neurotic organisation always to be able to present psycho-neurosis or psycho-
somatic disorder when the central psychotic anxiety threatens to

break through in crude form. In such cases the psycho-analyst may collude for years with the patient's need to be psycho-neurotic (as opposed to mad) and to be treated as psycho-neurotic. The analysis goes well, and everyone is pleased. The only drawback is that the analysis never ends. It can be terminated, and the patient may even mobilise a psycho-neurotic false self for the purpose of finishing and expressing gratitude. But, in fact, the patient knows that there has been no change in the underlying (psychotic) state and that the analyst and the patient have succeeded in colluding to bring about a failure. Even this failure may have value if both analyst and patient acknowledge the failure. The patient is older and the opportunities for death by accident or disease have increased, so that actual suicide *may* be avoided. Moreover, it has been fun while it lasted. If psycho-analysis could be a way of life, then such a treatment might be said to have done what it was supposed to do. But psycho-analysis is no way of life. We all hope that our patients will finish with us and forget us, and that they will find living itself to be the therapy that makes sense. Although we write papers about these borderline cases we are inwardly troubled when the madness that is there remains undiscovered and unmet. I have tried to state this in a broader way in a paper on classification.[1]

It is perhaps necessary to prevaricate a little longer to give my own view on the difference between object-relating and object-usage. In object-relating the subject allows certain alterations in the self to take place, of a kind that has caused us to invent the term "cathexis." The object has become meaningful. Projection mechanisms and identifications have been operating, and the subject is depleted to the extent that something of the subject is found in the object, though enriched by feeling. Accompanying these changes is some degree of physical involvement (however slight) towards excitement, in the direction of the functional climax of an orgasm. (In this context I deliberately omit reference to the aspect of relating that is an exercise in cross-identifications. This must be omitted here because it belongs to a phase of development that is subsequent to and not prior to the phase of development with which I am concerned in this paper, that is to say, the move away from self-containment and relating to subjective objects into the realm of object-usage.)

Object-relating is an experience of the subject that can be described

1. 1959–1964; in *The Maturational Processes and the Facilitating Environment* (London: Hogarth Press; New York: International Universities Press, 1965).

in terms of the subject as an isolate. When I speak of the use of an object, however, I take object-relating for granted, and add new features that involve the nature and the behaviour of the object. For instance, the object, if it is to be used, must necessarily be real in the sense of being part of shared reality, not a bundle of projections. It is this, I think, that makes for the world of difference that there is between relating and usage.

If I am right in this, then it follows that discussion of the subject of relating is a much easier exercise for analysts than is the discussion of usage, since relating may be examined as a phenomenon of the subject, and psycho-analysis always likes to be able to eliminate all factors that are environmental, except in so far as the environment can be thought of in terms of projective mechanisms. But in examining usage there is no escape: the analyst must take into account the nature of the object, not as a projection, but as a thing in itself.

For the time being may I leave it at that, that relating can be described in terms of the individual subject, and that usage cannot be described except in terms of acceptance of the object's independent existence, its property of having been there all the time. You will see that it is just these problems that concern us when we look at the area that I have tried to draw attention to in my work on what I have called transitional phenomena.

But this change does not come about automatically, by maturational process alone. It is this detail that I am concerned with.

In clinical terms: two babies are feeding at the breast. One is feeding on the self, since the breast and the baby have not yet become (for the baby) separate phenomena. The other is feeding from an other-than-me source, or an object that can be given cavalier treatment without effect on the baby unless it retaliates. Mothers, like analysts, can be good or not good enough; some can and some cannot carry the baby over from relating to usage.

I should like to put in a reminder here that the essential feature in the concept of transitional objects and phenomena (according to my presentation of the subject) is *the paradox, and the acceptance of the paradox:* the baby creates the object, but the object was there waiting to be created and to become a cathected object. I tried to draw attention to this aspect of transitional phenomena by claiming that in the rules of the game we all know that we will never challenge the baby to elicit an answer to the question: did you create that or did you find it?

I am now ready to go straight to the statement of my thesis. It seems I am afraid to get there, as if I fear that once the thesis is stated the purpose of my communication is at an end, because it is so very simple.

To use an object the subject must have developed a *capacity* to use objects. This is part of the change to the reality principle.

This capacity cannot be said to be inborn, nor can its development in an individual be taken for granted. The development of a capacity to use an object is another example of the maturational process as something that depends on a facilitating environment.[2]

In the sequence one can say that first there is object-relating, then in the end there is object-use; in between, however, is the most difficult thing, perhaps, in human development; or the most irksome of all the early failures that come for mending. This thing that there is in between relating and use is the subject's placing of the object outside the area of the subject's omnipotent control; that is, the subject's perception of the object as an external phenomenon, not as a projective entity, in fact recognition of it as an entity in its own right.[3]

This change (from relating to usage) means that the subject destroys the object. From here it could be argued by an armchair philosopher that there is therefore no such thing in practice as the use of an object: if the object is external, then the object is destroyed by the subject. Should the philosopher come out of his chair and sit on the floor with his patient, however, he will find that there is an intermediate position. In other words, he will find that after "subject relates to object" comes "subject destroys object" (as it becomes external); and then may come "*object survives* destruction by the subject." But there may or may not be survival. A new feature thus arrives in the theory of object-relating. The subject says to the object: "I destroyed you," and the object is there to receive the communication. From now on the subject says: "Hullo object!" "I destroyed you." "I love you." "You have value for me because of your survival of my destruction of you." "While I am loving you I am all the time destroying you in (unconscious) *fantasy.*" Here fantasy begins for the individual. The subject can now *use* the object that has survived. It is important to

2. In choosing *The Maturational Processes and the Facilitating Environment* as the title of my book in the International Psycho-Analytic Library (1965), I was showing how much I was influenced by Dr Phyllis Greenacre (1960) at the Edinburgh Congress. Unfortunately, I failed to put into the book an acknowledgement of this fact.—D.W.W.

3. I was influenced in my understanding of this point by W. Clifford M. Scott (personal communication, ca. 1940).—D.W.W.

note that it is not only that the subject destroys the object because the object is placed outside the area of omnipotent control. It is equally significant to state this the other way round and to say that it is the destruction of the object that places the object outside the area of the subject's omnipotent control. In these ways the object develops its own autonomy and life, and (if it survives) contributes in to the subject, according to its own properties.

In other words, because of the survival of the object, the subject may now have started to live a life in the world of objects, and so the subject stands to gain immeasurably; but the price has to be paid in acceptance of the ongoing destruction in unconscious fantasy relative to object-relating.

Let me repeat. This is a position that can be arrived at by the individual in early stages of emotional growth only through the actual survival of cathected objects that are at the time in process of becoming destroyed because real, becoming real because destroyed (being destructible and expendable).

From now on, this stage having been reached, projective mechanisms assist in the act of *noticing what is there,* but they are not *the reason why the object is there.* In my opinion this is a departure from theory which tends to a conception of external reality only in terms of the individual's projective mechanisms.

I have now nearly made my whole statement. Not quite, however, because it is not possible for me to take for granted an acceptance of the fact that the first impulse in the subject's relation to the object (objectively perceived, not subjective) is destructive. (Earlier I used the word "cavalier," in an attempt to give the reader a chance to imagine something at that point without too clearly pointing the way.)

The central postulate in this thesis is that, whereas the subject does not destroy the subjective object (projection material), destruction turns up and becomes a central feature so far as the object is objectively perceived, has autonomy, and belongs to "shared" reality. This is the difficult part of my thesis, at least for me.

It is generally understood that the reality principle involves the individual in anger and reactive destruction, but my thesis is that the destruction plays its part in making the reality, placing the object outside the self. For this to happen, favourable conditions are necessary.

This is simply a matter of examining the reality principle under high power. As I see it, we are familiar with the change whereby projection mechanisms enable the subject to take cognizance of the object. This is not the same as claiming that the object exists for the subject because of the operation of the subject's projection mechanisms. At first the observer uses words that seem to apply to both ideas at one and the same time, but under scrutiny we see that the two ideas are by no means identical. It is exactly here that we direct our study.

At the point of development that is under survey the subject is creating the object in the sense of finding externality itself, and it has to be added that this experience depends on the object's capacity to survive. (It is important that "survive," in this context, means "not retaliate.") If it is in an analysis that these matters are taking place, then the analyst, the analytic technique, and the analytic setting all come in as surviving or not surviving the patient's destructive attacks. This destructive activity is the patient's attempt to place the analyst outside the area of omnipotent control, that is, out in the world. Without the experience of maximum destructiveness (object not protected) the subject never places the analyst outside and therefore can never do more than experience a kind of self-analysis, using the analyst as a projection of a part of the self. In terms of feeding, the patient, then, can feed only on the self and cannot use the breast for getting fat. The patient may even enjoy the analytic experience but will not fundamentally change.

And if the analyst is a subjective phenomenon, what about waste-disposal? A further statement is needed in terms of output.[4]

In psycho-analytic practice the positive changes that come about in this area can be profound. They do not depend on interpretative work. They depend on the analyst's survival of the attacks, which involves and includes the idea of the absence of a quality change to retaliation. These attacks may be very difficult for the analyst to stand,[5] especially when they are expressed in terms of delusion, or through manipulation which makes the analyst actually do things that are technically bad. (I refer to such a thing as being unreliable at moments when reliability is all that matters, as well as to survival in terms of keeping alive and of absence of the quality of retaliation.)

The analyst feels like interpreting, but this can spoil the process, and for the patient can seem like a kind of self-defence, the analyst

4. The next task for a worker in the field of transitional phenomena is to restate the problem in terms of disposal.—D.W.W.

5. When the analyst knows that the patient carries a revolver, then, it seems to me, this work cannot be done.—D.W.W.

parrying the patient's attack. Better to wait till after the phase is over, and then discuss with the patient what has been happening. This is surely legitimate, for as analyst one has one's own needs; but verbal interpretation at this point is not the essential feature and brings its own dangers. The essential feature is the analyst's survival and the intactness of the psycho-analytic technique. Imagine how traumatic can be the actual death of the analyst when this kind of work is in process, although even the actual death of the analyst is not as bad as the development in the analyst of a change of attitude towards retaliation. These are risks that simply must be taken by the patient. Usually the analyst lives through these phases of movement in the transference, and after each phase there comes reward in terms of love, reinforced by the fact of the backcloth of unconscious destruction.

It appears to me that the idea of a developmental phase essentially involving survival of object does affect the theory of the roots of aggression. It is no good saying that a baby of a few days old envies the breast. It is legitimate, however, to say that at whatever age a baby begins to allow the breast an external position (outside the area of projection), then this means that destruction of the breast has become a feature. I mean the actual impulse to destroy. It is an important part of what a mother does, to be the first person to take the baby through this first version of the many that will be encountered, of attack that is survived. This is the right moment in the child's development, because of the child's relative feebleness, so that destruction can fairly easily be survived. However, even so it is a tricky matter; it is only too easy for a mother to react moralistically when her baby bites and hurts.[6] But this language involving "the breast" is jargon. The whole area of development and management is involved, in which adaptation is related to dependence.

It will be seen that, although destruction is the word I am using, this actual destruction belongs to the object's failure to survive. Without this failure, destruction remains potential. The word "destruction" is needed, not because of the baby's impulse to destroy, but because of the object's liability not to survive, which also means to suffer change in quality, in attitude.

The way of looking at things that belongs to my presentation of this chapter makes possible a new approach to the whole subject of

6. In fact, the baby's development is immensely complicated if he or she should happen to be born with a tooth, so that the gum's attack on the breast can never be tried out.— D.W.W.

the roots of aggression. For instance, it is not necessary to give inborn aggression more than that which is its due in company with everything else that is inborn. Undoubtedly inborn aggression must be variable in a quantitative sense in the same way that everything else that is inherited is variable as between individuals. By contrast, the variations are great that arise out of the differences in the experiences of various newborn babies according to whether they are or are not carried through this very difficult phase. Such variations in the field of experience are indeed immense. Moreover, the babies that have been seen through this phase well are likely to be more aggressive *clinically* than the ones who have not been seen through the phase well, and for whom aggression is something that cannot be encompassed, or something that can be retained only in the form of a liability to be an object of attack.

This involves a rewriting of the theory of the roots of aggression, since most of that which has already been written by analysts has been formulated without reference to that which is being discussed in this chapter. The assumption is always there, in orthodox theory, that aggression is reactive to the encounter with the reality principle, whereas here it is the destructive drive that creates the quality of externality. This is central in the structure of my argument.

Let me look for a moment at the exact place of this attack and survival in the hierarchy of relationships. More primitive and quite different is annihilation. Annihilation means "no hope"; cathexis withers up because no result completes the reflex to produce conditioning. On the other hand, attack in anger relative to the encounter with the reality principle is a more sophisticated concept, postdating the destruction that I postulate here. *There is no anger* in the destruction of the object to which I am referring, though there could be said to be joy at the object's survival. From this moment, or arising out of this phase, the object is *in fantasy* always being destroyed. This quality of "always being destroyed" makes the reality of the surviving object felt as such, strengthens the feeling tone, and contributes to object-constancy. The object can now be used.

I wish to conclude with a note on using and usage. By "use" I do not mean "exploitation." As analysts, we know what it is like to be used, which means that we can see the end of the treatment, be it several years away. Many of our patients come with this problem already solved—they can use objects and they can use us and can use analysis, just as they have used their parents and their siblings and their homes. However, there are many patients who need us to be able to give them a capacity to use us. This for them is the analytic task. In meeting the needs of such patients, we shall need to know what I am saying here about our survival of their destructiveness. A backcloth of unconscious destruction of the analyst is set up and we survive it or, alternatively, here is yet another analysis interminable.

Summary

Object-relating can be described in terms of the experience of the subject. Description of object-usage involves consideration of the nature of the object. I am offering for discussion the reasons why, in my opinion, a capacity to use an object is more sophisticated than a capacity to relate to objects; and relating may be to a subjective object, but usage implies that the object is part of external reality.

This sequence can be observed: (1) Subject *relates* to object. (2) Object is in process of being found instead of placed by the subject in the world. (3) Subject *destroys* object. (4) Object survives destruction. (5) Subject can *use* object.

The object is always being destroyed. This destruction becomes the unconscious backcloth for love of a real object: that is, an object outside the area of the subject's omnipotent control.

Study of this problem involves a statement of the positive value of destructiveness. The destructiveness, plus the object's survival of the destruction, places the object outside the area of objects set up by the subject's projective mental mechanisms. In this way a world of shared reality is created which the subject can use and which can feed back other-than-me substance into the subject.

II. D.W.W.'s Dream Related to Reviewing Jung

*An account enclosed in a letter to a colleague,
written on 29 December 1963*

This was one in the long line of significant dreams that I have had
before, during and after analysis. These dreams appear as a result of
work done, and they each cash in on new ego growth or new enlightenment. This dream had special importance for me because it cleared
up the mystery of an element of my psychology that analysis could
not reach, namely, the feeling that I would be all right if someone
would split my head open (front to back) and take out something
(tumour, abscess, sinus, suppuration) that exists and makes itself felt
right in the centre behind the root of the nose.

The dream took a long while to dream, certainly twenty minutes,
and it and its analysis occupied about two hours of the night. It was
not a nightmare because it never threatened my ego's capacity to
stand strain.

There is an immense amount of detail that is personal and that can
be ignored. I can describe the dream in terms of its metapsychology
without losing anything because once the dream was dreamed and
accepted it had done its job, so to speak, and the result is permanently
with me.

The dream can be given in its three parts:

1. There was absolute destruction, and I was part of the world and
of all people, and therefore I was being destroyed. (The important
thing in the early stages was the way in which in the dream the pure
destruction got free from all the mollifications, such as object-
relating, cruelty, sensuality, sado-masochism, etc.)

2. Then there was absolute destruction, and I was the destructive
agent. Here then was a problem for the ego, how to integrate these
two aspects of destruction?

3. Part three now appeared and *in the dream* I awakened. As I
awakened I knew I had dreamed both (1) and (2). I had therefore
solved the problem, by using the difference between the waking and
sleeping states. Here was I awake, in the dream, and I knew I had

dreamed of being destroyed and of being the destroying agent. There was no dissociation, so the three I's were altogether in touch with each other. I remembered dreaming I(2) and I(1). This felt to be immensely satisfactory although the work done had made tremendous demands on me.

I now began to wake up.

What I first knew was that I had a *very severe headache*. I could see my head split right through, with a black gap between the right and left halves. I found the words "splitting headache" coming and waking me up, and I caught on to the appropriateness of the description; this allowed me gradually to come round to being awake, and in the course of a half hour the headache left me. While I lay enduring the headache the whole dream came to me, and along with this the feeling that I now knew an important meaning of the number three. I had these three essential selves, I(3) that could remember dreaming in turn of being I(2) and I(1). Without I(3) I must remain split, solving the problem alternately in sadism and masochism, using object-relating, that is, relating to objectively perceived objects.

I had an acute awareness in the third part of the dream and when awake that destructiveness belongs to relating to objects that are outside the subjective world or the area of omnipotence. In other words, first there is the creativeness that belongs to being alive, and the world is only a subjective world. Then there is the objectively perceived world and absolute destruction of it and all its details.

I was also aware as the dream flowed over me before I quite became awake that I was dreaming a dream for Jung and for some of my patients, as well as for myself. Jung seems to have no contact with his own primitive destructive impulses, and he gives support to this idea in his writing. When playing as a small child he built and then destroyed, over and over again; he does not describe himself playing constructively in relation to *having* (in unconscious fantasy) *destroyed*. In my review I had related this to a difficulty Jung may have had in being cared for by a depressed mother (if this be true).

An Extract from the Letter Accompanying the Dream

I enclose my Dream.

It refers to a deep layer of destructiveness, yet to a somewhat sophisticated (ego-wise) coping with destructiveness.

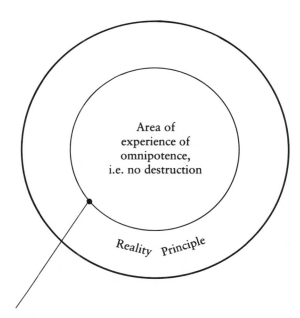

This line is between operating in the area of omnipotence, and outside it. If it's a simple journey over the line then the line is the place for destruction 100 percent.

In health the infant is helped by being given (by ordinary devoted Mum) areas of experience of omnipotence while experimenting with excursions over the line into the wasteland of destroyed reality. The wasteland turns out to have features in its own right, or survival value, etc., and surprisingly the individual child finds total destruction does not mean total destruction.

III. Notes Made on the Train, Part 2

Written in April 1965

Development of Theme of Control

Axiom. It is not profitable to discuss control apart from a statement on the diagnosis of the child or adult who may possibly come under control.

When considering the question of diagnosis of those subject to control an important factor will be the (relative) maturity of the individual as seen in the history and quality of the relationship to the primary love object that he or she has established. I suggest that we might profitably speculate in the following way:

What can a human being do with an object? At the beginning the relation is to a subjective object. Gradually subject and object become separated out, and then there is the relation to the objectively perceived object. Subject destroys object.

This splits up into: (1) subject preserves object; (2) subject *uses* object; (3) subject *destroys* object.

1. This is idealisation.

2. Use of object: this is a sophisticated idea, an achievement of healthy emotional growth, not attained except in health and in the course of time.

Meanwhile there appears

3. which appears clinically as a rendering down of the object from perfection towards some kind of badness. (Denigration, dirtying, tearing, etc.) This protects the object because it is only the perfect object that is worthy of destruction. This is not idealisation but denigration.

In the course of the individual's growth it becomes possible for the destruction to have adequate representation in the (unconscious) fantasy that is an elaboration of body functioning and instinctual experiences of all kinds.

This aspect of growth enables the individual to become concerned about the destruction that goes with object-relating, and to experience guilt relative to the destructive ideas that go with loving. On the basis of this the individual finds the motivation for constructive effort and for giving and for mending (Klein's reparation and restitution).

The practical issue here arises out of the distinction between

1. spoiling the good object to render it less good and so less under attack, and

2. the destruction that is at the root of object-relating and that becomes (in health) channelled off into the destruction that takes place in the unconscious, in the individual's inner psychic reality, in the individual's dream life and play activities, and in creative expression.

The latter does not need control; what is needed here is the provision of conditions that allow for the emotional growth of the individual, continuous from earliest infancy until the time when the complexities of fantasy and displacement become available to the individual in his or her search for a personal solution.

By contrast, the compulsive denigration, messing and destruction that belong to the former, an alteration of the object aimed at making it less exciting and less worthy of destruction, this needs society's attention. For example: the antisocial person who enters an art gallery and slashes a picture by an old master is not activated by love of the painting and in fact is not being as destructive as the art-lover is when preserving the picture and using it fully and in unconscious fantasy destroying it over and over again. Nevertheless the vandal's one act of vandalism affects society, and society must protect itself. This rather crude example may serve to show the existence of a wide difference between the destructiveness that is inherent in object-relating, and the destructiveness that stems from an individual's immaturity.

In the same way, compulsive heterosexual behaviour has a complex aetiology, and is a very long way away from the capacity of a man and woman to love each other in a sexual way when they have decided to set up together a home for possible children. In the former case there is included the element of the spoiling of what is perfect or of being spoiled, and no longer perfect, in an effort to lessen anxiety. In the latter case, relatively mature persons have dealt with destruction, with concern and with the sense of guilt within themselves, and have become free to plan to use sex constructively, not denying the crude elements that hang around in the total sex fantasy.

It is a matter for surprise when one discovers how little the romantic lover, and how very little the teenage heterosexual, knows *about the total sex fantasy,* conscious and unconscious, with its competitiveness, its cruelty, its pregenital elements of crude destruction and its dangers.

Those who wave the Progressive Flag in education do need to study these things, otherwise they too easily mistake heterosexuality for health, and find it convenient when violence does not appear, or only shows as the irrational reactive pacifism of adolescence which bears but little relation to the crude realities of the actual world which one day these adolescents will enter as competitive adults.

IV. The Use of the Word "Use"

Dated 5 February 1968

I

We get so used to words through using them and become so dulled to their usage that we need from time to time to take each one and to look at it, and to determine in so far as we are able not only how the word came into being through the poetry of etymology, but also the ways in which we are using the word now.

I have chosen to look at the word "use" because I want to see what it is that I meant when I ended a public lecture with the words: "and it is perhaps the greatest compliment we may receive if we are both found and used".[7]

In saying this I was talking generally, but by the context it could be seen that I was referring specifically to the use the patient may make of an analyst, and also I was referring to the prototype, the use the baby makes of the mother in a healthy experience of the nursing couple.

One can truly say in description of a long psycho-analytic treatment that the patient has used the analyst all the time, especially if we include "wasting" in with the word "using." Nevertheless, with cer-

7. "Communication between Infant and Mother, and Mother and Infant, Compared and Contrasted" (1968), in Winnicott, *Babies and Their Mothers* (Reading, Mass.: Addison-Wesley, 1987).

tain patients, there comes a moment or a place in the analysis when one can say that whereas up to now the patient has in some sense not used the analyst, now and from now on the patient is using the analyst. Something has happened in the patient which makes this change of language right. Closely following this there is the corresponding alteration in the experience of the patient, who now finds himself or herself being used. This can give great satisfaction to the patient and can be a reward for the years of blind groping which analysis can seem to be.

I have allowed for the fact that with many patients these matters are not highly significant, whereas for others this change is the very change which was being sought after. As is so often true when we discuss a psycho-analytic mechanism, it is a matter of diagnosis; and if we were better at diagnosis we would save ourselves and our patients a lot of time and despair.

II

It is pertinent to ask at this point: what is the state which came before use, before the analysand used the analyst? Is it possible to describe not only the dragonfly, but also the process of metamorphosis and, indeed, the chrysalis itself? That would indeed be good.

Is it not so that before the change-over into usage the patient (subject) protects the analyst (object) from being used? In the extreme the subject is left with an ideal object, or an object idealised, perfect, and unattainable.

In sophistication there is usage by wastage, that is to say, hate can be expressed in terms of waste. But the sense of waste is something that is felt by the object that is protected. It is for the observer to decide whether an example of non-use carries hate feeling, and at this stage of my exposition I am concerned only with non-use as arising automatically out of the subject's protection of the object.

Here is the subject and there is the object, but in the experience of the subject there can be no use of the object. In practice, the analysand cannot use the analyst, so that the principle task of the analyst is to enable the analysand to become able to use, with the corollary, to become able to be used.

Obviously the most glaring illustrations of this state of affairs must be those innumerable cases that are never encountered, because the symptom of the patient precludes any making use of an analyst.

Alongside this we see many treatments which are an infinite extension of non-use, kept going indefinitely by the fear of confrontation with the trouble itself—which is an inability to use and be used. Analysts must share with such patients the responsibility for treatments that belong to this category of discomforts.

Often it happens that we study extremes in order to get insight into the common problems which indeed become acute and even dominant at certain times or in certain phases of a treatment, but which do need to be weighed up with many other factors when the person is being described who is the subject in a case-history. Relatively healthy patients may come to a time of crisis in their treatment at which it can be said that nothing else matters other than the resolution of just this problem: how can the subject come to be able to use the object, and to be used?

V. Clinical Illustration of "The Use of an Object"

*Presented to the New York Psychoanalytic Society,
12 November 1968*

I refer to a married man of 50, an erudite person held in high esteem in academic circles. He is very sensitive and no doubt is not very satisfactory as a husband at physical level. There is a very good understanding, however, between him and his wife, who share their home, their family and cultural pursuits.

This man is extremely unaggressive and is all the time liable to find that it is his own fault when things go wrong. Along with his lack of aggression is a stubbornness which has provided an alternative so that in fact he has a high position in his work. He knows about his lack of aggressiveness but he likes himself as he is. It would be no good for anyone to tell him to be aggressive. On the other hand he has certain symptoms which bother him a good deal. The two main symptoms, which are inter-related, are:

1. He knows that he is capable of being highly creative in his own particular field, but he has achieved only a little, certainly very much

less than he is capable of achieving. He is liable to fill his time with administration so as not to notice the painful fact that he is not being creative. He is a well-known person, however, on account of the small area in which he has been able to function well at an earlier stage.

2. He is bothered by unpredictable compulsions which take the form of blasphemy. It is as if he must think of whatever is sacred or holy or pure and spit over it or soil it. He is very much a victim of the phobia of the sin against the Holy Ghost.

As the analysis of this man goes deeper and deeper one finds that he is suffering from a reaction to an environmental pattern in which the inadequacy was of the nature of a weak father and a strong mother. The control of aggression was not forthcoming from his father, and the mother had to supply it and he had to use his mother's fierceness but with the result that he was cut off from using his mother as a refuge. The symptom of that in the present day is sleeplessness.

When one comes to give this man help it very easily feels to him that the analyst and psycho-analysis through its theory is inviting him to become aggressive, which he does not want to become. He is very liable to misunderstand interpretations and to reconstruct what has been said in terms of an invitation toward actual aggression. Gradually a change is coming about because of the ability of the man to dream and in the dream to reach to aggressiveness rather than to masochism.

On the day which I have chosen for a slightly more detailed description he comes apologising because he has not done any homework. This I know means that he will find that he has done homework but unconsciously and that he has not had to use his ready defence of conscious or deliberate working away at dreams and the integration of past analytic sessions by the use of his very fine intellect.

There is usually a position soon reached which has to do with his unwillingness to make himself be aggressive as if that is what the analyst was wanting him to do. He quoted from Blake: "I fear the fury of my wind." And he discussed the way in which Blake had all these primitive fears of aggression towards the mother figure but how he managed to sublimate perhaps the very wind that he was so afraid of. This led on to the patient's statement that he thought he had better leave off trying to do the analysis of his troubles and how it would be better if he, like Blake, could find a way of using life by which to solve his personal problem in so far as a man of his age could be expected to solve it. How could he possibly get back to the primitive impulses and fears of early infancy? This led on to a discussion of the God of the average man of the seventeenth century as compared with the God of the present day.

Here followed a description of Cromwell and his social setting and of the very real nature of the God of Cromwell's time. He mentioned the case of a man who thought a wicked thought and a bird dropped excrement over his head which stank so badly that the man died within three days. Here for this man in Cromwell's era God could be used as a substitute for the absence of a fierce father, but at the present time the idea of a fierce God could only be seen as a subjective phenomenon and therefore this was of no use. All he could do was to come back to the sad fact that the father was a weak man and that the fierceness lay with the mother. He could therefore never come to terms with the father that he had hated. He felt hopeless about all this.

We were now in the position in which we had been before. Here was Blake or a man like Blake. There are two alternatives. One is that he never breaks wind. He therefore retains the belief that his wind is infinitely powerful and destructive, that is to say productive of a retaliatory environment. The alternative this Blake man could not achieve. He could not break wind, taking the risks involved and perhaps finding that the world and the immediate people around had not altered.

My patient is in this position that he always protects the mother because he must preserve her in order to be able to have any rest or relaxation at all. He therefore has no knowledge that his mother might survive his impulsive act. A strong father enables the child to take the risk because the father stands in the way or is there to mend matters or to prevent by his fierceness.

The result in my patient, as is usual in these cases, was that he had to adopt self-control of impulse at a very early stage before he was ready to do so on the basis of an introjected father-figure. This meant that he became inhibited. The inhibition had to be of all spontaneity and impulse in case some particle of the impulse might be destructive. The massive inhibition necessarily involved his creative gesture, so that he was left inhibited, unaggressive and uncreative.

After this I looked round and there of course I saw this man's homework. He had brought a dream without knowing it; had he known it this would have been too deliberate and too conscious and too intellectual. What he had done was quite by chance, almost as if it was part of a friendly discussion that belongs to the beginning of some sessions, this story of Cromwell. Taken as a dream, Cromwell was a fierce man who in fact cut off the head of the father figure, of the King. The patient, who knows a great deal about history, was able to fill out the whole story of Cromwell, showing how well it expressed the dream which he did not know that he had brought in which he, as Cromwell, had met the fierce father figure (actually in the shape of the God of the seventeenth century and the headmaster of his school) and how he had castrated the father figure in terms of the execution of the King. In history the result was not so good from Cromwell's point of view although it is likely that taken by and large Cromwell's act was beneficial as a political move and that it was not a clear case of destructive motivation. In the case of my patient there is still this to be worked through which is represented by the survival of the monarchy or at any rate the survival of the political system perhaps improved by the unbridled aggressiveness of Cromwell.

My patient is still working in the direction of the dream in which he himself will be in the Cromwell position instead of these awkward compulsive acts of provocation which can never produce an avenging God for a man in the twentieth century who is an agnostic and which can never alter the fact that his father, a loveable man, was in fact the weak member of the parental team.

VI. Comments on My Paper "The Use of an Object"

Dated 5 December 1968

Comment I

In my view the main idea incorporated in this paper necessitates a rewriting of an important area in psycho-analytic theory. I will state this in the following way.

Dr Fine referred to the libidinal theory, clearly stated in Hartmann-Kris-Loewenstein terms and in Anna Freud's *Mechanisms of Defence*, etc. We go on teaching about libidinal stages and erotogenic zones because of the truth of this part of our theory. Also we teach that in health there comes about a *fusion* of libidinal and aggressive drives (though here we can get into trouble because at the start aggressive drives are associated with muscle erotism and not with anger or hate).

My careful research, using many long cases and a truly large amount of short child-psychiatry material, shows me that the fusion part of our theory is not only right but is also wrong. It is at the place where it is wrong that I am trying to make a contribution.

There is a phase prior to that which makes sense of the concept of fusion. In the individual's early development it is not a case of fusion, because what is there in the activity that characterises the baby's aliveness starts off as a unit or unity. To get quickly to the idea that I have in mind one could profitably use the idea of the fire from the dragon's mouth. I quote from Pliny who (in paying tribute to fire) writes, "Who can say whether in essence fire is constructive or destructive?"[8] Indeed the physiological basis for what I am referring to is the first and subsequent breaths, out-breathing.

The paper I have presented gives psycho-analysis a chance to re-think this subject. In this vitally important early stage the "destructive" (fire-air or other) aliveness of the individual is simply a symptom of being alive, and has nothing to do with an individual's anger at the frustrations that belong to meeting the reality principle.

As I have tried to state, the drive is destructive. Survival of the object leads on to object-use, and this leads on to the separation of two phenomena

1. fantasy   and

2. actual placing of the object outside the area of projections.

Therefore this very early destructive urge has a vital positive function (when, by survival of the object, it works), namely the objectivisation of the object (the analyst in the transference). This task is bypassed in the schizoid personality or borderline case, and presumably in schizophrenic illness (see Comment II).

I see that all this may have some flaw in it, but if I am able to make my point clear then at any rate it can be discussed.

In practice the result could be of great importance, throwing light even on the adolescent characteristic by which the good is not that which is handed down by parental benignity but that which is forced into being by individual adolescent destructiveness. The parental task

8. See B. Farrington, *Greek Science* (London: Pelican Books, 1953).

and society's task here is (as with mother and baby) one of survival, and this includes survival with the quality of non-retaliation, that is, a containment of what the individual adolescent brings without becoming provoked even under provocation. But this is an application of my new (as I believe) principle of the capacity to use an object arrived at by the subject through the experiences involving survival of the object.

Comment II

I realise that it is this idea of a destructive first impulse that is difficult to grasp. It is this that needs attention and discussion. To help I wish to point out that I am referring to such things as *eagerness*. I need to include such things as expiration, salivation, burning, and certain sensory experiences such as the extreme sensory sensitivity that belongs to the minutes immediately following birth, and special features of smell, phenomena that are intolerably real, or almost intolerably so, for the baby, even under good-enough conditions of holding and handling. Just here one must allow obscurity to have a value that is superior to false clarification.

It seems likely that Rilke, by using *Raum* and *Welt*, gives this same idea in environmental terms. *Raum* is an infinite space in which the individual can operate without passing through the risky experience of destruction and survival of the object; *Welt* is by contrast the world in so far as it has, by survival, become objectified by the individual, and to be used.

VII. The Use of an Object in the Context of *Moses and Monotheism*

Dated 16 January 1969

In "Analysis Terminable and Interminable," a late masterpiece of clear and undogmatic statement, Freud seems to me to be struggling to use what he knows to be true, because of his analytic experiences, to cover what he does not know. I almost wrote, what he does not yet know, since it is so difficult for us to believe that he has left us to carry on with the researches that his invention of psycho-analysis makes possible, and yet he cannot participate when we make a step forward.

The first part of *Moses and Monotheism* is a beautiful example of an idea put forward with strength, clarity and conviction, yet without propaganda and indeed with humility. In the last part, Freud can be seen to be reaffirming the belief in repression and (as it would seem to me) overreaching himself in his formulation of monotheism as important because of the universal truth of the loved father and the repression of this in its original and stark (id) form. But the reader knows that the argument does not bear close examination. It is not that Freud is wrong about the father and the libidinal tie that becomes repressed. But it has to be noted that a proportion of persons in the world do not reach to the Oedipus complex. They never get so far in their emotional development, and therefore for them repression of the libidinised father figure has but little relevance. If one looks at religious people it is certainly not true to say that monotheistic tenets only belong to those who reached the Oedipus complex. A great deal of religion is tied up with near-psychosis and with the personal problems that stem from the big area of baby life that is important before the attainment of a three-body relationship as between whole persons.[9]

Freud was labouring under a disadvantage. He could only use psycho-analysis as far as it had gone at the time when he was writing. No-one would blame him for this especially as Freud was always prepared to let a poet or a philosopher or his own intuition open up the way for phenomena that had not been covered by the metapsychology of the time.

Freud came to an expression of his own dissatisfactions near the end of "Analysis Terminable and Interminable" while expressing satisfaction in a generous way with the writings of Empedocles. This remarkable man (born ca. 495 B.C.) of a remarkable period in the birth and growth of science in Greece formulated a "love-strife" state both for man and for the universe, and this is as near as may be to Freud's life-death instinct formulation. Freud is pleased.

It is my purpose to put forward the idea that Empedocles the Greek may have got just one step ahead of Freud, at least in one important

9. Melanie Klein tried to get round this difficulty by using the whole Oedipus complex terminology in description of internal struggles for power, as between elements that have not acquired human form. This helped but did not come as we must do when considering these matters to a statement that Freud was labouring under a disadvantage.—D.W.W.

respect. (To warn the reader I should say that I have never been in love with the death instinct and it would give me happiness if I could relieve Freud of the burden of carrying it forever on his Atlas shoulders. To start with, the development of the theory from a statement of the fact that organic matter tends to return to the inorganic carries very small weight in terms of logic. There is no clear relationship between the two sets of ideas. Also, biology has never been happy about this part of metapsychology while on the whole there is room for mutuality between biology and psycho-analysis all along the line, up to the point of the death instinct.)

It is always possible that the death instinct formulation was one of the places where Freud was near to a comprehensive statement but could not make it because, while he knew all we know about human psychology back to repression of the id in relation to cathected objects, he did not know what borderline cases and schizophrenics were going to teach us in the three decades after his death. Psycho-analysis was to learn that a great deal happens in babies associated with need, and apart from wish, and apart from (pregenital) id-representatives clamouring for satisfaction.

In other words, Freud did not know in the framework of his own well-disciplined mental functioning that we now have to deal with such a problem as this: what is there in the actual presence of the father, and the part he plays in the experience of the relationship between him and the child and between the child and him? What does this do for the baby? For there is a difference according to whether the father is there or not, is able to make a relationship or not, is sane or insane, is free or rigid in personality.

If the father dies this is significant, and when exactly in the baby's life he dies, and there is a great deal too to be taken into account that has to do with the imago of the father in the mother's inner reality and its fate there. We now find all these matters coming along for revival and correction in the transference relationship, matters which are not so much for interpretation as for experiencing.

Now, one thing in all this has very special relevance. This has to do with the immature ego—rendered strong by the mother's adapting well enough to the baby's *needs*. (This is not to be lost in the concept of her satisfaction of the baby's instinctual drives.)

As the baby moves from ego strengthening due to its being reinforced by mother's ego to having an identity of his or her own—that is, as the inherited tendency to integration carries the baby forward in the good-enough or average expectable environment—the third person plays or seems to me to play a big part. The father may or may not have been a mother-substitute, but at some time he begins to be felt to be there in a different role, and it is here I suggest that the baby is likely to make use of the father as a blue-print for his or her own integration when just becoming at times a unit. If the father is not there the baby must make the same development but more arduously, or using some other fairly stable relationship to a whole person.

In this way one can see that the father can be the first glimpse for the child of integration and of personal wholeness. It is easy to go from this interplay between introjection and projection to the important concept in the world's history of a one god, a monotheism, not a one god for me and another one god for you.[10]

It is easy to make the assumption that because the mother starts as a part object or as a conglomeration of part objects the father comes into ego-grasp in the same way. But I suggest that in a favourable case the father starts off whole (i.e. as father, not as mother surrogate) and later becomes endowed with a significant part object, that he starts off as an integrate in the ego's organisation and in the mental conceptualisation of the baby.

Could it not be said that "poetically" Freud was ready for this idea, not that monotheism had its root in the repressed idea of the father but that the two ideas of having a father and of monotheism represented the world's first attempts to recognise the individuality of man, of woman, of every individual? (Remember, the Greeks had slaves, which diminishes our regard for the amazing insights of their great thinkers, especially of the centuries around the birth date of Empedocles. Science had to wait some centuries before restarting on the basis of the universal right to be a free or an integrated autonomous individual.)[11]

I can support my thesis by quoting from Freud who wrote that, according to Empedocles, the love power *"strives to agglomerate the primal particles of the elements"* (of universe and man), *"of the four elements into a single unity"*; while the strife power "seeks to undo, etc. etc." Here then is the idea of the ego activity *agglomerating*, which is not object-relating. Presently I shall try to carry my argument

10. See *Moses and Monotheism*, Standard Edition, vol. 22, p. 128.
11. Farrington, *Greek Science*.

further by a contribution that I feel needs to be made in regard to this dualism, *philia* (love) and *neikos* (strife).[12] I believe a step further could now be made.

Before I describe this new detail I wish to refer to a footnote of Freud's. I am somewhat addicted to his footnotes and quotations which he perhaps allows to go further than he can go in terms of theory as it obtains at the time of his writing.

I refer to: "Breasted (1906) calls him (Amenophis) 'the first individual in human history.'"[13] Here, for me, is Freud stating the thesis that I am striving to present in my own laboured way. Freud was not, one feels, able to bring this up into the text because he could not deal with it in terms of repression and the mechanisms of defence and of the interplay of id, ego and superego. I feel Freud would welcome new work that makes sense of Breasted's comment in terms of a universal in the emotional development of the individual, namely, the integrative tendency that can bring the individual to unit status.

I am now free to make the contribution that I feel does possibly go in advance of Freud's position. This that I wish to put forward is a culmination of a trend in my thinking, and I can now see evidence of this trend in my papers of a decade ago. (See, for instance, "Roots of Aggression" in *The Child, the Family and the Outside World*. This is the only new chapter in the book. It is also implied in the cumbersome title of my book *The Maturational Processes and the Facilitating Environment*.)

I have recently tried to give my ideas life in a paper read to the New York Psychoanalytic Society (12 November 1968), but from the papers of the discussants (Jacobsen, Ritvo and Fine) I learned that I had by no means made myself clear, so that the idea as presented there and then was unacceptable at the time. I have revised this paper.[14] I gave the paper the name "The Use of an Object," and I wanted to state that in the emotional development of any baby there is a time of *dependence* when the *behaviour of the environment* is part and parcel of the child's development, and that this cannot be omitted. That is to say, there is no statement of the development of a baby, dependent on ego support from a mother figure or parent figure, that leaves out of account the environmental factors. This is simply saying that it is

12. See "Analysis Terminable and Interminable," Standard Edition, vol. 23, p. 246.
13. *Moses and Monotheism*, p. 21.
14. See Section I of this chapter.—EDS.

true that at the beginning the baby has not himself or herself achieved a perception, recognition and repudiation of the NOT-ME. This is something I must believe because of my clinical work.

To illustrate my meaning I looked at the early stage of drives in the individual baby. I drew a sharp distinction between the fate (in terms of personality pattern) of a baby whose first strivings were accepted and of a baby whose first strivings were reacted to. This is a statement reminiscent of Klein's paranoid position, but with this difference, that it is given in terms of environment running *pari passu* with individual life pulses. Retaliation takes the place of talion fears.

It is necessary here to rethink something that we have come to accept (to accept because in analysis of "analysable" cases it is so true), namely that one of the integrating phenomena in development is the fusion of what I will here allow myself to call life and death instincts (love and strife: Empedocles). The crux of my argument is that the first drive is itself *one* thing, something that I call "destruction," but I could have called it a combined love-strife drive. This unity is primary. This is what turns up in the baby by natural maturational process.

The fate of this unity of drive cannot be stated without reference to the environment. The drive is potentially "destructive" but whether it *is* destructive or not depends on what the object is like; does the object *survive,* that is, does it retain its character, or does it *react?* If the former, then there is no destruction, or not much, and there is a next moment when the baby can become and does gradually become aware of a cathected object plus the *fantasy* of having destroyed, hurt, damaged, or provoked the object. The baby in this extreme of environmental provision goes on in a pattern of developing personal aggressiveness that provides the backcloth of a continuous (unconscious) fantasy of destruction. Here we may use Klein's reparation concept, which links constructive play and work with this (unconscious) *fantasy backcloth* of destruction or provocation (perhaps the right word has not been found). But destruction of an object that survives, has not reacted or disappeared, leads on to use.

The baby at the other extreme that meets a pattern of environmental reaction or retaliation goes forward in quite a different way. This baby finds the reaction from the environment to be the reality of what should be his or her own provocative (or aggressive or destructive) impulse. This kind of baby can never experience or own or be moved by this personal root for aggression or destructive fantasy, and can therefore never convert it into the unconscious *fantasy* destruction of the libidinised object.

It will be seen that I am trying to rewrite one limited part of our theory. This provocative

> destructive
>
> aggressive
>
> envious (Klein)

urge is not a pleasure-pain principle phenomenon. *It has nothing to do with anger at the inevitable frustrations associated with the reality principle.* It precedes this set of phenomena that are true of neurotics but that are not true of psychotics.[15]

To make progress towards a workable theory of psychosis, analysts must abandon the whole idea of schizophrenia and paranoia as seen in terms of regression from the Oedipus Complex. The aetiology of these disorders takes us *inevitably* to stages that precede the three-body relationship. The strange corollary is that there is at the root of psychosis an *external factor*.[16] It is difficult for psycho-analysts to admit this after all the work they have done drawing attention to the internal factors in examining the aetiology of psycho-neurosis.

15. Here I can turn to Bettelheim for support. I find him difficult to read simply because he says everything and there is nothing to be said that one could be certain has not been said by him. But one must read him because he can be exactly right, or more nearly right than other writers. This applies especially to his opening chapters in *The Empty Fortress* (New York: Free Press, 1967; London: Collier-Macmillan Ltd., 1967).—D.W.W.

16. See Winnicott, "Psychoses and Child Care" (1952), in *Collected Papers: Through Paediatrics to Psycho-Analysis* (London: Tavistock, 1958; New York: Basic Books, 1975; London: Hogarth Press, 1975).

35

Development of the Theme of the Mother's Unconscious as Discovered in Psycho-Analytic Practice

Written in June 1969[1]

In this communication I wish to follow up the idea contained in my 1948 paper "Reparation in Respect of Mother's Organised Defence against Depression." The basis of that paper was Melanie Klein's formulation of the depressive position in the development of the individual. I have found this concept to be valid and useful and I eventually wrote a paper in 1954, "The Depressive Position in Normal Emotional Development," giving my own view of what Mrs Klein intended. This paper was commented on favourably by Mrs Klein.[2]

In the first of these two papers I drew attention to the common clinical observation that could be made in child psychiatry practice whereby a child in the clinic seems to be rather especially alive, delightful, nicely dressed, keen to display skill and what seemed to be creative ability, all this making for happiness in the clinic so that one could find oneself looking forward to the arrival of such a child. Nevertheless in the background was a depression or a sort of paralysis or helplessness which was the main symptomatology at home and which indicated that there was something wrong somewhere from the mother's point of view.

It took me some years to realise that these children were entertaining me as they felt they must also entertain their mothers, to deal with the mother's depressed mood. They dealt with or prevented my depression or what might be boredom in the clinic; while waiting for me they drew lovely coloured pictures or even wrote poems to add to my collection. I have no doubt that I was taken in by many such cases

1. This paper was written for the *International Journal of Psycho-Analysis;* it was not, in fact, published.—EDS.
2. Both the papers mentioned appear in *Collected Papers: Through Paediatrics to Psycho-Analysis* (London, Tavistock, 1958; New York: Basic Books, 1975; London: Hogarth Press, 1975).

before I eventually realised that the children were ill and were showing me a false self organisation and that at home the mother had to
deal with the other side of this, namely the child's inability to keep up
counteracting the mother's mood all of the twenty-four hours.

Indeed the mother had to endure the hatred belonging to the child's
sense of having been exploited and of having lost identity. The typical
case fitting in with the description above is that of a girl. By contrast
the corresponding illness in terms of the boy child makes it more
likely that he will turn up in a clinic regressed and unmanly, thumb-
sucking, mother-bound. There are various kinds of clinical picture
but in all cases there is the false self organisation, the best the child
can do in keeping contact with a mother who is liable to a depressed
mood.

I wrote that these children are always trying to get to the starting
point and always by the time they reach the starting point, which
means the place where mother is not depressed, they are exhausted
and need to rest so that they cannot get on with their own lives. I
came to find that although these children were often highly creative
this tended to fizzle out in the course of the child's development and
did not form the root for adolescent ambition and adult career or
achievement.

To get a stage further in the understanding of these children it was
necessary for me to find out in a more intimate way the distortion of
the depressive position that belongs to such cases. In brief what I
stated was that these children are making reparation in respect not of
their own destructiveness and of their own tendencies of destruction
but in respect of the mother's destructive tendencies. Achievement for
these children is the achievement of mending something wrong in the
mother and achievement therefore leaves them always without any
personal advancement. They were like the Danaides in Greek myth
who were doomed to carry water in buckets that had holes in them.
In the analyses of these children it is necessary to reach to something
new, which is to the destructiveness in the inner psychic reality of the
individual child, destructiveness actually belonging to the child and
not to the mother. In other words it is necessary to reach to the child's
innate guilt sense and so to the child's own relief at the use of constructive play and work and of creative activity which then in a favourable case becomes directly related to personal aggressiveness, hatred, destruction, and ambivalence.

The next stage in the development of these ideas came from the actual analyses of children and adults and from the difficulties that belong to the transference and countertransference in such cases. In passing I made a note that if one examines the material of a session or a phase in which a patient reaches a highly charged example of destruction (which must be considered an achievement), then one can see that prior to this the material presented contained an example of constructive activity. One can either say that the patient reached to the constructive, knowing without being aware that destruction was due to appear, or else one can say that because of the arrival at the constructive moment the patient became able to reach to the destructive moment. I have tried elsewhere to give illustrations from my clinical work.[3]

Of greater significance is the patient's gradual discovery that all constructive effort including the reconstruction of the self and the effort to reach personal health does not in fact result in a sense of achievement. This is something which is puzzling for the analyst as well as disheartening for the patient. Always it seems that success, instead of bringing the patient to a new position, simply brings him or her to the starting point, and there is no question of further progress because the patient is exhausted by the effort of getting to the place from which a start might be made. It is essential in these cases to remember that one of the factors may be that all effort towards recovery is being made to deal with someone else's hate, notably the mother's. It is necessary of course for the analyst to be in the position of the mother in the transference when these matters are ripe for interpretation. The analyst finds that genuinely wanting the patient to get well only acts as reassurance over a limited time or over a limited area. Eventually the patient knows delusionally that the analyst wishes to push the patient back in emotional development or back into the inside into the unborn state or in some way or other to destroy the growing points of the patient.

These phases in an analysis are difficult and the patient needs great confidence in the mechanical side of the analytic procedure in order to reach to the delusional state in which the analyst is hostile. In favourable cases the patient can use other figures in the environment. A child may come complaining of a persecuting teacher and school and one may even know from enquiry that the teacher is in fact ordinarily

---

3. See especially "Aggression, Guilt and Reparation" (1960), in Winnicott, *Home Is Where We Start From* (New York: Norton; London: Penguin, 1986).

permissive. The patient may be able to work up a tremendous sense of persecution in this way and so communicate with the analyst without being too mad. The same thing done in direct terms of the delusion that the analyst is antagonistic becomes intolerable to the patient because of its madness.

It can be imagined that many patients do their very best to provoke the analyst into hating them, so that they may arrive at this state, with the delusion carefully wrapped up in correct observation, and the patient will use the technical mistakes of the analyst and exploit them in a big way in order to arrive at being persecuted without losing the sense of being sane. There is every possible degree of this to be encountered in our work, in which the patient needs to reach to what in its simplest form is the mother's hate. What becomes very clear is the very great difference that exists as to whether it is the mother's hate or the mother's repressed and unconscious hate that is under consideration. In other words children seem to be able to deal with being hated and this of course is simply a way of saying that they can meet and make use of the ambivalence which the mother feels and shows. What they cannot ever satisfactorily use in their emotional development is the mother's repressed unconscious hate which they only meet in their living experiences in the form of reaction formations. At the moment that the mother hates she shows special tenderness. There is no way a child can deal with this phenomenon.

36

The Mother-Infant Experience of Mutuality

Written in 1969[1]

Whereas it is generally known that there is almost infinite subtlety in a mother's management of her baby, it took a long time for psychoanalytic theory to reach to this area of living experience. It is not difficult to see some of the reasons for the delay. Psycho-analysis, in its beginnings, had to emphasise the powerfulness of feelings and of conflicting feelings and had to explore the defences against them. In terms of childhood, psycho-analysis occupied itself for several decades with the Oedipus complex and all the complications that arise out of the feelings of boys and girls who have become whole persons related to whole persons.

Psycho-analysis gradually began to encroach on the experiences of younger children and explored the conflicts within the psyche and developed the concepts covered by words and moods and the persecutions from within and without. The psycho-analyst was always fighting the battle for the individual against those who ascribed troubles to environmental influence.

Gradually the inevitable happened and psycho-analysts, carrying with them their unique belief in the significance of details, had to start to look at dependence, that is to say, the early stages of the development of the human child when dependence is so great that the behaviour of those representing the environment could no longer be ignored.

We are now right in the study of these very early mutual influences. We must expect resistance to the work we do, this time not because of the operation of repression and of anxiety in those who meet our work, but resistance that belongs to the feeling that a sacred area is being encroached upon. It is as if a work of art were being subjected to an analytic process. Can one be sure that the capacity to appreciate the work of art fully will not be destroyed by the search-light that is

1. Published in Anthony and Benedek, eds., *Parenthood: Its Psychology and Psychopathology* (Boston: Little, Brown; London: J. and A. Churchill, 1970).

played upon the picture? It could indeed be well argued that these very early phenomena ought to be left alone, and I who have found myself making a study of them could not but insist that what we think we know about these intimacies is not useful reading material for artists or for young mothers. The sort of thing that can be discussed when we look at these early phenomena cannot be taught. It is remarkable, however, that certain people, even fathers and mothers, do like to read about these things after they have been through the experiences.

For our part as psychiatrists we have another reason why we must go ahead in our work with the examination of the subtleties of the parent-infant relationship. We have to take into consideration that this is an area of research which can throw light on the aetiology of the group of disorders that are labelled psychotic or schizoid, that is to say that are not the affective disorders or those that are called psycho-neurotic. In fact, if in our psycho-analytic work or in any other kind of psychotherapy we find ourselves temporarily involved with schizoid processes in our patients, we know that we shall be dealing in our consulting rooms with the same phenomena that characterise the experiences of mothers and infants. We shall be caught up in the immense needs of the dependent infant and in the counter-transference with the massive responsive processes which show us to some extent what is happening to parents when they have a child. As psychiatrists, therefore, we are left with no alternative but to go ahead and try to describe something of what we find, taking care not to put our views forward in the form of advice to mothers and fathers and child-minders, but to keep what we say in reserve for the use of colleagues who must find themselves involved from time to time with patients who develop dependence that is near absolute.

It is a relief that psycho-analysis has nearly come through the phase, which lasted a half-century, in which, when analysts referred to babies, they could only speak in terms of the baby's erotic and aggressive drives. It was all a matter of pregenital instinct, of oral and anal eroticism and reactions to frustration, with some rather wild additions in terms of natural aggressive behavior and destructive ideas, *agressivité*. Work of this kind had its value and continues to have value; but it is necessary now for analysts who refer to the nature of the baby to see what else is there to be seen. There are some shocks in store for the orthodox analyst if he looks further.

The Subjective Object

In order to study the way in which the human infant achieves the capacity to objectify, it is necessary to accept that at first there is no such capacity. To allow for this the theorist needs to be able to give up some tenets of which he has rightly been proud in all the years since Freud gave us the concept of the Oedipus complex, the idea of infantile sexuality, and the psycho-analytic technique for investigation that is the same as the psycho-analytic technique for therapy.

In this new area, the idea of the individual rather than of the environment (a major psycho-analytic contribution) needs to be modified or even dropped. When it is said that a baby is dependent, and at the beginning absolutely dependent, and this is really meant, then it follows that what the environment is like has significance because it is a part of the baby.

A baby is not what one may postulate by assessing that baby's potential. A baby is a complex phenomenon that includes the baby's potential *plus* the environment. To understand this idea we may look at a child of two. We may say: This child has not been the same since the new baby was born. In many cases we may diagnose illness patterns, and these illness patterns (shown as rigidity of defence organisations) call for treatment. The existence of illness patterns must not be allowed to obscure the reality that the child in question is a child *with a younger brother or sister.* With the same potential, this child would be different if he or she were the youngest child or the only child, or if a baby had been born but had died. No one would object to this idea in terms of a two-year-old, which of course does not alter the fact that it is possible to give effective psychotherapy in respect of the child's psychopathology. Psychopathology, however, is a different thing from health and from the effect on the child of the innumerable environmental features that belong to the child who is not far from absolute dependence and is but a short way along the path toward independence.

To carry the argument back to the very early stages, the significance of the environment for the baby when there is near-absolute dependence is such that *we cannot describe the baby without describing the environment.*

The stage of absolute dependence or near-absolute dependence belongs to the state of the baby at the beginning who has not yet separated a NOT-ME from what is ME, of the baby who is not yet equipped to perform this task. In other words, the object is a subjective object, not objectively perceived. Even if it is repudiated, put over there, the object is still an aspect of the baby.

How does the next stage come about? Its development and establishment are not due to the operation of the child's inherited tendencies (toward integration, object-seeking, psycho-somatic collusion, etc.). In any one case it may never happen in spite of perfectly good inherited tendencies in the baby. This development takes place *because of the baby's experiences of the mother's* (or mother substitute's) *adaptive behaviour*. The mother's adaptive behaviour makes it possible for the baby to find outside the self that which is needed and expected. By means of the *experience* of good-enough mothering the baby goes over into objective perception, having inherited the tendency to do this *and* having been given the perceptual equipment and opportunity.

In order to understand the part played by the mother it is necessary to have a concept such as the one that I have described in "Primary Maternal Preoccupation."[2] I have tried to show that we may expect good-enough mothering from the mothers of the world, and of the past ages, because of something that happens to women during pregnancy, something that lasts for some weeks after the baby's birth unless a psychiatric disturbance in the mother prevents this temporary change in her nature from occurring.

In addition, it is necessary to be able to think of a baby as beginning to have some capacity for objectivity, and yet being generally unable to objectify, with a forward and backward movement in this area of development.

Communication

In order to clarify our concepts we can usefully bring ourselves to think in terms of communication. To explain how this can help I wish to give an example.

From birth a baby can be seen to take food. Let us say that the baby finds the breast and sucks and ingests a quantity sufficient for satisfaction of instinct and for growth. This can be the same whether the baby has a brain that will one day develop as a good one or

2. In *Collected Papers: Through Paediatrics to Psycho-Analysis* (London: Tavistock, 1958; New York: Basic Books, 1975; London: Hogarth Press, 1975).

whether the baby's brain is in fact defective or damaged. What we need to know about is the communication that goes or does not go with the feeding process. It is difficult to be sure of such matters by the instrument of infant-observation, though it does seem that some babies watch the mother's face in a meaningful way even in the first weeks. At 12 weeks, however, babies can give us information from which we can do more than guess that communication is a fact.

> *Illustration 1.* Although normal babies vary considerably in their rate of development (especially as measured by observable phenomena), it can be said that at 12 weeks they are capable of play such as this: Settled in for a (breast) feed, the baby looks at the mother's face and his or her hand reaches up so that in play the baby is feeding the mother by means of a finger in her mouth.

It may be that the mother has played a part in the establishment of this play detail, but even though this is true it does not invalidate the conclusion that I draw from the fact that this kind of playing can happen.[3]

I draw the conclusion from this that, whereas all babies take in food, there does not exist a communication between the baby and the mother except in so far as there develops a mutual feeding situation. The baby feeds and the baby's experience includes the idea that the mother knows what it is like to be fed.

If this happens for all to see at 12 weeks, then in some way or other it can (but need not) be true in some obscure way at an earlier date.

In this way we actually witness a *mutuality* which is the beginning of a communication between two people; this (in the baby) is a developmental achievement, one that is dependent on the baby's inherited processes leading toward emotional growth and likewise dependent on the mother and her attitude and her capacity to make real what the baby is ready to reach out for, to discover, to create.[4]

Babies feed, and this may mean much to the mother, and the ingestion of food may give the baby gratification in terms of drive satisfactions. Another thing, however, is the communication between the baby and the mother, something that is a matter of experience and that depends on the mutuality that results from cross-identifications.

3. See "Getting to Know Your Baby" (1944), in *The Child, the Family and the Outside World*.

4. This has a direct relationship to Sechehaye's term "symbolic realization," which means enabling a real thing to become a meaningful symbol of mutuality in a specialised setting. See M. A. Sechehaye, *Symbolic Realization* (New York: International Universities Press, 1951).—D.W.W.

Melanie Klein has done full justice to the subject of projective and introjective identifications, and it is on the basis of her development of Freud's ideas of this kind that we are able to build this part of theory in which communication has significance greater than that which is usually called "object-relating."[5]

In giving this illustration, I have remained close to the familiar framework of psycho-analytic statements concerning object-relating because I wish to keep open the bridges that lead from older theory to newer theory. Nevertheless, I am obviously near to Fairbairn's statement made in 1944 that psycho-analytic theory was emphasising drive-satisfaction at the expense of what Fairbairn called "object-seeking." And Fairbairn was working, as I am here, on the ways in which psycho-analytic theory needed to be developed or modified if the analyst could hope to become able to cope with schizoid phenomena in the treatment of patients.[6]

At this point it is necessary to interpolate a reference to the obvious fact that the mother and the baby come to the point of mutuality in different ways. The mother has been a cared-for baby; also she has played at babies and at mothers; she has perhaps experienced the arrival of siblings, cared for younger babies in her own family or in other families; and she has perhaps learned or read about baby care and she may have strong views of her own on what is right and wrong in baby management.

The baby, on the other hand, is being a baby for the first time, has never been a mother, and has certainly received no instruction. The only passport the baby brings to the customs barrier is the sum of the inherited features and inborn tendencies toward growth and development.

Consequently, whereas the mother can identify with the baby, even with a baby unborn or in process of being born, and in a highly sophisticated way, the baby brings to the situation only a developing capacity to achieve cross-identifications in the *experience of mutuality* that is made a fact. This mutuality belongs to the mother's capacity to adapt to the baby's needs.[7]

5. Melanie Klein, *The Psycho-Analysis of Children* (London: Hogarth Press, 1954).

6. See W. R. D. Fairbairn, *Psycho-Analytic Studies of the Personality* (London: Tavistock, 1952), page 88: "since it is only ego structures that can *seek* relationships with objects" (my italics).—D.W.W.

7. The word "need" has significance here just as "drive" has significance in the area of satisfaction of instinct. The word "wish" is out of place as it belongs to sophistication that is not to be assumed at this stage of immaturity that is under consideration.—D.W.W.

Mutuality Unrelated to Drives

It is possible now to enter the deep waters of mutuality that does not directly relate to drives or to instinct tension. Travelling towards this, another example may be given.

Like so much of what we know of these very early babyhood experiences, this example derives from the work that has to be done in the analysis of older children or of adults when the patient is in a phase, long or short, in which regression to dependence is the main characteristic of the transference. Work of this kind always has two aspects, the first being the positive discovery in the transference of early types of experience that were missed out or distorted in the patient's own historical past, in the very early relationship to the mother; and the second being the patient's use of the therapist's failures in technique. These failures produce anger, and this has value because the anger brings the past into the present. At the time of the initial failure (or relative failure) the baby's ego-organisation was not organised sufficiently for so complex a matter as anger about a specific matter.

Analysts with a rigid analytic morality that does not allow touch miss a great deal of that which is now being described. One thing they never know, for instance, is that the analyst makes a little twitch whenever he or she goes to sleep for a moment or even wanders over in the mind (as may well happen) to some fantasy of his or her own. This twitch is the equivalent of a failure to hold in terms of mother and baby. The mind has dropped the patient. (These cases put a strain on us. There are long periods of quiescence, sometimes at a room temperature that is higher than the analyst would choose to work in.)

Illustration 2.[8] A boy of 6 years was able to give me accurate information in a one-session therapeutic consultation about the way his mother went to sleep while holding him when he was 14 months old.

This was the nearest he could get to giving me the information that his mother had a depressive illness at that date which started with her developing a tendency to go to sleep.

In the language of this paper, the boy experienced a series of fail-

---

8. Described at length as Case 4, "Bob," in *Therapeutic Consultations in Child Psychiatry* (London: Hogarth Press; New York: Basic Books, 1971); also in the *International Journal of Psycho-Analysis* 46 (1965) under the title "A Clinical Study of the Effect of a Failure of the Average Expectable Environment on a Child's Mental Functioning."

ures of communication at the points at which the mother became withdrawn.

My understanding of the child's communication in this one session enabled the boy to go forward in his development. A year later when I saw him, he was a normal boyish boy who brought his younger brother to see me. This was his own idea. He remembered the work that we had done together

Illustration 3. This example is taken from the analysis of a woman of 40 years (married, two children) who had failed to make full recovery in a six-year analysis with a woman colleague. I agreed with my colleague to see what analysis with a man might produce, and so started a second treatment.

The detail I have chosen for description has to do with the absolute need this patient had, from time to time, to be in contact with me. (She had feared to make this step with a woman analyst because of the homosexual implications.)

A variety of intimacies were tried out, chiefly those that belong to infant feeding and management. There were violent episodes. Eventually it came about that she and I were together with her head in my hands.

Without deliberate action on the part of either of us there developed a rocking rhythm. The rhythm was rather a rapid one, about 70 per minute (c.f. heartbeat), and I had to do some work to adapt to this rate. Nevertheless, there we were with *mutuality* expressed in terms of a slight but persistent rocking movement. We were *communicating* with each other without words. This was taking place at a level of development that did not require the patient to have maturity in advance of that which she found herself possessing in the regression to dependence of the phase of her analysis.

This experience, often repeated, was crucial to the therapy, and the violence that had led up to it was only now seen to be a preparation and a complex test of the analyst's capacity to meet the various communicating techniques of early infancy.

This shared rocking experience illustrates what I wish to refer to in the early stages of baby care. The baby's instinctual drives are not specifically involved. The main thing is a communication between the baby and the mother in terms of the anatomy and physiology of live bodies. The subject can easily be elaborated, and the significant phenomena will be the crude evidences of life, such as the heartbeat, breathing movements, breath warmth, movements that indicate a need for change of position, etc.

Basic Care

These primitive techniques that have intercommunication as a by-product lead naturally to still more primitive or fundamental inter-actions that are of the nature of silent communications; that is to say, the communication only becomes noisy when it fails.

Here I am in the area covered, I think, by Hartmann's phrase, "the average expectable environment," though I cannot be sure that Hart-mann intended to refer to these very early silent communications.

What I have to say here is covered by the term "holding." A wide extension of "holding" allows this one term to describe all that a mother does in the physical care of her baby, even including putting the baby down when a moment has come for the impersonal experi-ence of being held by suitable non-human materials.

In giving consideration to these matters, it is necessary to postulate a state of the mother who is (temporarily) identified with her baby so that she knows without thinking about it more or less what the baby needs. She does this, in health, without losing her own identity.[9]

I have tried elsewhere to develop the theme of the developmental processes in the baby that need, for their becoming actual, the moth-er's holding. The "silent" communication is one of reliability which, in fact, protects the baby from *automatic reactions* to impingement from external reality, these reactions breaking the baby's line of life and constituting traumata. A trauma is that against which an individ-ual has no organised defence so that a confusional state supervenes, followed perhaps by a reorganisation of defences, defences of a more primitive kind than those which were good enough before the occur-rence of the trauma.[10]

Examination of the baby being held shows that communication is either silent (reliability taken for granted) or else traumatic (produc-ing the experience of unthinkable or archaic anxiety).

This divides the world of babies into two categories:

---

9. In psychopathology she may be so much identified with the baby that she loses her maternal capacity and, if she retains some sanity, she hands the baby over to the care of a nurse. In this way she vicariously gets well held, and one can see in this a natural seeking for that which the patient may get in the analytic transference in phases of regression to dependence.—D.W.W.

10. Masud Khan has developed this aspect of trauma; see M. M. R. Khan, "Ego Distor-tion, Cumulative Trauma, and the Role of Reconstruction in the Analytic Situation," *Inter-national Journal of Psycho-Analysis* 45 (1964); also in *The Privacy of the Self* (London: Hogarth Press, 1974).—D.W.W.

1. Babies who have not been significantly "let down" in infancy, and whose belief in reliability leads towards the acquisition of a personal reliability which is an important ingredient of the state which may be termed "towards independence." These babies have a line of life and retain a capacity to move forward and backward (developmentally) and become able to take all the risks because of being well insured.

2. Babies who have been significantly "let down" once or in a pattern of environmental failures (related to the psychopathologic state of the mother or mother-substitute). These babies carry with them the experience of unthinkable or archaic anxiety. They know what it is to be in a state of acute confusion or the agony of disintegration. They know what it is like to be dropped, to fall forever, or to become split into psycho-somatic disunion.

In other words, they have experienced trauma, and their personalities have to be built round the reorganisation of defences following traumata, defences that must needs retain primitive features such as personality splitting.[11]

Of course, the world of human beings is not made up of examples of these two extremes. Those who are started off well, as most babies surely are, may be let down at later stages and suffer traumata of a kind; and *per contra* babies who have been badly let down in early stages may be almost "cured" of their disastrous beginnings by therapeutic care at later stages.

Nevertheless, it is valuable for the student of human nature to keep in mind the two extremes. Especially is it valuable for the psychiatrist and the psychotherapist to know of these matters, since a study of the aetiology and psychopathology of the schizoid states and of the special features of the schizoid or psychotic transference leads right back to the reorganisation of defences of primitive quality following the experienced acute confusional states of early infancy; these follow traumas in the area in which the baby (for healthy development) must be able to take reliability for granted, the area that is almost covered by an extended use of the term "holding." But reliable holding of a baby is something that needs to be communicated, and this is a matter of the baby's experiences. Just here psychology involves communication in physical terms, the language of which is mutuality in experience.

11. Phobic states are loose organisations in defence against defence failures.—D. W. W.

37
On the Basis for Self in Body

I. Basis for Self in Body

Written in 1970[1]

My intention in writing this article is to explore clinical material that throws light on the inter-relationship between the growing child and his or her body. The subject is obviously a very wide one, and a specialisation in one area leads automatically to neglect in other areas. Nevertheless, it is possible for me to take the word "personalisation" which I have used in another context and to see how it becomes illustrated in detailed clinical work in child psychiatry and psychoanalysis. I adopted the term "personalisation" as a kind of positive form of depersonalisation, which is a term that has been used and discussed fairly fully. Various meanings are given to the word "depersonalisation," but on the whole they involve the child's or the patient's loss of contact with the body and body functioning, and this implies the existence of some other aspect of the personality. The term "personalisation" was intended to draw attention to the fact that the indwelling of this other part of the personality in the body, and a firm link between whatever is there which we call psyche, in developmental terms represents an achievement in health. This is an achievement which becomes gradually established, and it is not unhealthy, but indeed a sign of health, that the child can use relationships in which there is maximal trust, and in such a relationship at times disintegrate, depersonalise and even for a moment abandon the almost fundamental urge to exist and to feel existent. The two things go together, therefore, in healthy development: the sense of security in a relationship maintaining opportunity for restful undoing of integrative processes, while at the same time facilitating the general inherited tendency that the child has towards integration and, as I am stressing

---

1. Published in the *Nouvelle Revue de Psychanalyse* (Spring 1971) and in the *International Journal of Child Psychotherapy* (1972).

in this paper, in the matter of in-dwelling or the inhabitation of the body and the body functioning.

Forward development is very much associated with in-dwelling as with other aspects of integration, but forward development is in all respects frightening to the individual concerned if there is not left open the way back to total dependence. And this is particularly true in the clinical field, from the years 2 to 5, after which in terms of clinical experience the return to dependence becomes obscured in a whole series of sophistications. At adolescence there is a new period in which, because of the vast implications of the new and rapid advance in terms of meeting and coping with the world, there recurs a need to keep open a way back to dependence. Clinically, this is liable to be manifest at the pre-puberty phase when the adolescent is 12 to 14 years old, after which the dependence may very easily become absorbed in the natural dependence that is free from regressive elements relative to the parents, and that already looks towards the adult status, and that is called being in love, and in the experiences of every possible kind that surround such a state.

The term "personalisation" which I have used for my own benefit may not be acceptable in a general way, but it has enabled me to gather together the examples in my clinical work that are relevant to this aspect of achievement in human development. An important case from my point of view is one that I do not propose to give in detail in this context. I have published the case in detail elsewhere.[2] Here, I wish to refer to the case in my own language.

Case History

I refer to a significant interview with a boy, Iiro, 9 years 9 months. I have often described this interview as an illustration of communication with a child because there was no common language between the boy and myself. We exchanged drawings on the basis of the squiggle game and we had an interpreter. In spite of these handicaps, the boy communicated to me his special need, which belonged both to his own development and to a complication in his mother's attitude towards his disability. In fact, Iiro was under almost constant treatment in the Orthopaedic Department because of a condition of syndactele.

2. Case 1, "Iiro," in *Therapeutic Consultations in Child Psychiatry* (London: Hogarth Press; New York: Basic Books, 1971).

The surgeon said that this boy co-operated almost too well. He wondered why this could be. The boy had had innumerable operations on his hands and feet. In this condition, the fingers and toes are joined together and there is no clear indication for the surgeon who would like to create fingers and toes out of the chaotic state that exists. This is an hereditary disease, and Iiro, in the middle of a fairly large family, was the only one who had inherited the disorder. Some of the urgency in the use of the orthopaedic surgeon's skill came from the fact that the mother had the same condition and she could only accept this boy on the basis of doing everything possible to cure him of a deformity for which she felt responsible. On the basis of having everything possible done for him, she had found herself more fond of this boy than of any of her other children. Here was a clear situation, therefore, of a boy brought to see me from the orthopaedic ward, a happy, likeable and intelligent boy, who nevertheless, along with his mother, was constantly in search of further orthopaedic help, asking indeed for better plastic surgery than the surgeon was capable of putting into practice.

The interest of the case lies in the fact that at a deeper level this boy communicated something else other than his need to be made normal so that he could play the flute. What he indicated was that it made sense to have everything possible done by surgery (although he did not know, of course, of his mother's tremendous sense of guilt); but he needed one thing, which was this: he must be certain that first of all he was loved as he was when he was born, or at some theoretical start to his existence. If accepted as deformed, which implied that it would be normal to be born with feet and hands like his, then he could go forward with any amount of co-operation with his mother and the surgeon. He communicated this without conscious motivation, but in terms of his great love of ducks, and the first drawing he saw as the webbed foot of a duck. Further on in the interview he was able to use an eel as symbolical of his early state—that is to say, before the question of arms and legs or of fingers and toes became relevant. Several points of theoretical interest follow an examination of this case. Obviously a child does not know about a disparity like this at the beginning. Gradually, in the course of time, the child has to recognise the fact of the deformity. It is possible that he never recognised this fact until the interview with me, when he was 9 years and 9 months old. What the boy must be able to adjust to is the attitude of his mother and of other people towards his deformity, and eventually it becomes necessary for him to see himself as abnormal. At the start, however, the normality for the child must be his own somatic shape and function. As he starts so he must be accepted. So he must be loved. It is a matter of being loved without sanctions.

It is very easy to carry these observations over to an examination of the needs of children who are not deformed. Being loved at the beginning means being accepted, and it is a distortion from the child's point of view if the mother-figure has an attitude of: "I love you if you are good, if you are clean, if you smile, if you drink it all up," etc., etc. These sanctions can come later, but at the beginning the child has a blueprint for normality which is largely a matter of the shape and functioning of his or her own body. It may be thought that surely these matters belong to a later age, when the child has become a relatively sophisticated person. The observation cannot be neglected, however, that these are matters of the very earliest days of the child's life. It is truly at the beginning that the child needs to be accepted as such, and benefits from such acceptance. A corollary would be that almost every child has been accepted in the last stages before birth: that is to say, when there is a readiness for birth—but love is shown in terms of the physical care which is usually, but not always, adequate when it is a matter of the foetus in the womb. In these terms, the basis for what I call personalisation, or an absence of a special liability to depersonalisation, starts even before the child's birth, and is certainly very much a matter of significance once the child has to be held by people whose emotional involvement needs to be taken into account, as well as their physiological responses. The beginning of that part of the baby's development, which I am calling personalisation, or which can be described as an in-dwelling of the psyche in the soma, is to be found in the mother or mother-figure's ability to join up her emotional involvement, which originally is physical and physiological.

In the development of this theme one could take many diverse paths. My method will be to use another clinical example, chosen because of its availability in my mind.

I am reminded of a consultation that a girl, Jill, aged 17, had with me in 1968. She used this consultation in a positive way, and in fact it made her able to go forward with her development, which had become held up. From her mother's letter which I received before the consultation, I learnt this:

Jill has been feeling a bit lost. It might seem as though her problems were mainly social or educational. Her overt and articulate complaints are chiefly about herself "vis à vis the world." She does not make friends readily. She feels stupid and lacks a sense of purpose. I feel that these complaints of hers may be masking a deeper resentment against her family, or lack of one, or against me, for various reasons she cannot express. It is "they" surely who have somehow failed to equip her with self-confidence, so that instead of joining in with her contemporaries' battle for freedom, she is, as it were, stuck in the doorway, possibly still hoping to make up on what she has missed before she can move on.

And the mother added a biographical note:

She was born in 1950: breast-fed for nine months, and though small, a satisfactory greedy infant. When she was 3 her father (who was of *my* father's generation) died. I do not think the impact of his death was blurred or blunted for her. For a long time afterwards she spoke of it and of its effect on both of us. She would make drawings representing the two different situations: hers and mine. She had, and still has, a grandfather and several uncles, but in her day-to-day life there has not been any consistently available or really important male figure.

She gave the impression of being an ordinarily happy, often rather gay, small child. She had good resources in the way of imaginative play. When she was 12, I had a breakdown (severe depression) and went to a mental hospital for ten months. She has never talked much about this time. Once, when asked, she said: "I knew you would come back, of course."

Interview

The following is my description of the interview, dictated from notes within hours after the interview.

Jill, aged 17 years. Consultation: 7.2.68.

First and only child. The father died when she was 3. Addition to the family: Tommy (adopted), whom I once saw in consultation. He was then 6 and she was 8. The father was thirty years older than the mother.

Jill came alone. She was a very slight person, dressed in a grey corduroy frock. She might have been 13. One of the first things that she said was that she was nearly 18. Evidently she was rather self-conscious about seeming to be so slight.

At first there was a rather sticky period in which it was not certain how we could use each other. I went through the ordinary preliminaries about her coming. Did she come because of being sent or because of wanting help? She said that it was only at school that there was trouble and her work worried her there. She had a mental block when she wrote essays and this made her very depressed. In greater detail she described the way in which if she collected material for an essay and then came to put it together, she soon reached a place where she could not proceed. She would like to go to university but she felt bound to fail in her application because she was not sure of wanting to go there, where after all it would be simply a continuation of everything that happened at school.

In other words, she would be held up again by the block in her mental functioning.

She did not have many friends, although attending the high school. She seemed to feel that the subjects that she was studying were not really worthwhile studying. One of them was art, and she was obsessed with the question: What sort of art is any good?

I talked a little bit about herself and her setting, where I told her that I knew she was living with her mother, with no father, and I let her know also that the mother had told me about her own (the mother's) depressions, and the fact that Jill's life was disturbed by the mother's breakdown when Jill was 12 (ten months in hospital).

There was something Jill was trying to tell me which was that she always felt things were all right really in her life, until some incident, probably an accident, since which time she had felt a lack of confidence in an ultimate outcome that could be satisfactory. She began to describe this. She said that she had always felt that she could curl up and that this would be a successful defence, but since the accident she no longer felt that this defence could be relied upon. We talked about this, and it seemed clear that she felt that some part of herself sticking out was in danger from the environment, but that if curled up then this part would not be in danger. Naturally, one thought of the idea of a penis with castration anxiety, but this seemed to be too crude a language to describe what was happening in this girl's mind. I could explore around this area without harm, and I was left with the idea that this was not a good enough way of describing her anxiety. At some point we transferred over to the squiggle game. I felt that she would be more at ease with something that we were doing together, and certainly it seemed to work out that way. So we went ahead as if we were children together, and it all seemed quite natural.

   1. My first squiggle she turned into a sort of swan.

2. Her first squiggle I transformed into a girl's head, with a length of hair like Jill's.

3. My next squiggle she changed very imaginatively into a dog, seen at a curious angle from behind.

4. Her next squiggle I turned into what she called a colt.

5. My next she could do nothing with. She said, "There is too much in it already." This corresponded with something she had already said about life—how complex it can be at any one moment, with all sorts of possibilities crowding in.

6. Her next I turned into a vase. She agreed that it was a recognisable shape for a glass vase and seemed relieved that we had got to something more simple and circumscribed.

7. Of my next she simply said, "That's a modern chair."

8. I made her next into some kind of little dog. This led to the fact that Jill's family had a border terrier for a pet.

9. She changed my next into architecture—a concert hall of a very modern variety. She had worked in an architect's office for a few months doing menial jobs, but she evidently liked the idea of architecture as a job.

10. Her next I turned into a pair of glasses like mine.

Somewhere while all this was going on we were talking together. She said about her dreams that they were not nice. It was something like falling in the street or downstairs. Her legs gave way, etc. She told me that her left leg was actually a centimetre shorter than her right one: a fact which was not apparent, although she was wearing a very short mini-skirt, but evidently it had great meaning for herself.

She mentioned the idea that in a dream she felt as if there was a limb missing. When we returned to the subject of not being able to concentrate, I said that in considering her own self she was feeling that if she gathered together all the bits and had a look in order to see how she could put them all together, there would be something missing, like when she gathered material for an essay. I joined this up with the undoubted fact that she had had to live her life without having a father. It appeared that there was no feeling at all about the death of her father, except that she was irritated when people who knew him talked about him so that she felt very much left out. It was something they knew about and she did not.

This was where she told me about the way that her defence (curling up) had broken down following a street accident. She also had an accident in which she broke her front teeth, and she was very self-conscious about this which made her lisp. She said how stupid it was. She was emptying a wheelbarrow, with the dog on a lead, because the rabbit was loose. The dog was scared and she turned round to be angry with the dog but the handle of the wheelbarrow jumped up and broke her teeth. She said: "It's ironical. I was being angry with the dog, and I was the one to get hurt." The accident gave her considerable shock and undoubtedly upset her mother, too, because it altered her appearance. In this I recognised the existence of a truly external factor, like the death of her father when she was 3. She talked about her father being very old anyway.

For the time being we discussed her feelings about being a boy or a girl. She very much wanted to be a boy from the time Tommy came, when she was 7 or 8, right up till she was 10; now she probably would prefer to be a girl. I fished around for envy of Tommy's penis, but she simply said that she knew all about the differences between boys and girls before Tommy came. It has to be remarked that Tommy was always a very difficult boy. Jill went on to say that when she was 12 her mother became ill. I asked about dreams in which she was a boy, and her answer was definitely that she did not have that dream. She had some friends, perhaps three girls.

Now came the significant part of the consultation. This was her drawing of the broken-off limb in the dream, the thing that she always felt about herself. She went back to it afterwards and talked about the colour of it. It was like the stump of a leg. Its flesh was pale and mauve, like the flesh of a dogfish (biology dissection). It was a dead colour. In talking about it, she said that she was able to think of it more as a limb bitten off by a wild animal rather than as something hurt in an accident. This reminded me of the dog in the accident in which "ironically" it was her own teeth that got knocked out.

Eventually I made an interpretation, saying that I thought that this was the nearest she could get to her reaction to her father's death. She did not remember him as a person and she did not mourn his loss. Nevertheless, when he died a bit of her life died with him, so that there was something missing. At the same time, it could be said that she bit off something of him because we had to remember the importance of her teeth which she had discussed in connection with the accident with the wheelbarrow. I talked about the way in which little children of 3 would play with their father's fingers or watch-chains or something of his, and would bite around it, and it could be fairly certainly assumed that she was liable to play in this way with her father. His death and removal then would feel to her as if she had really bitten instead of playing at biting, this resulting in a fantasy of severance of the finger or whatever it might be.

She was able to take this as something for consideration.

In the end, she expressed a certain amount of astonishment at the drawing of the limb which was there for us to look at and which had brought this central theme so much into the foreground: that is, her feeling that in any examination of herself there would be found to be something missing. It turned out that the limb that was torn off in this way was the left one which was her short one.

We made some sort of résumé at the end and discussed the possible value of such an interview and also the possibility that she might be disturbed by it. Finally, she was quite positive. She quite simply said: "I am glad I came. Goodbye." And she went in a state of friendliness.

My comment to her was that the appropriate word was "sad." If she could get away from the anxiety about there being something missing, then she might be able to find that the appropriate statement was that it was very sad for a girl when her father died when she was 3 years old.

Comment

This case could be taken to illustrate the way in which, although a small child would not know that one limb was shorter than the other, there would come a time when she would find that the attitude of parents and doctors, and particularly of her mother, with hypochondriacal anxieties occasionally consolidating into a depressive illness, make it necessary to accept the fact that there is something wrong somewhere. In this case, the deformity was so slight that it could have been ignored completely.

Nevertheless, when Jill came to arrange herself and her personality around the fact of not having a father and the detail of having lost him at the age of 3 when, according to the family saga, she was very fond of him, she elaborated this insignificant fact into the dream of a leg bitten off by a wild animal. The same mechanism was at work in her mental life, and until the consultation she was unable to go forward in her emotional or intellectual growth. It happened that she was able to resume her development following the consultation, and the follow-up has shown that effectual psychotherapy was in fact achieved.

Integration in the developing human being takes a wide variety of forms, one of which is the development of a satisfactory working arrangement between the psyche and the soma. This starts prior to the time when it is necessary to add the concepts of intellect and verbalisation.

The basis of a self forms on the fact of the body which, being alive, not only has shape, but which also functions. Observations relevant to this (which I have called personalisation in order to link it up with the disorder called depersonalisation)[3] are made primarily in direct study of infants and their mothers interacting naturally. As a useful adjunct to such observations I draw attention to the help that can be derived from a study of children with physical abnormalities. In this paper there was room only for two examples, but these may suffice to illustrate the way in which clinical details may throw light on such complex phenomena. Many physical abnormalities are not of such a nature that a baby could be aware of them as abnormalities. In fact, the baby tends to assume that what is there is normal. Normal is what is there. It is often a fact that the baby or child becomes aware of deformity or abnormality through perception of unexplained facts, as in the attitude of those, or of some of those, in the immediate environment.

A very complex example would be provided by the fact of mental defect, where the apparatus for dealing with complex perceptions is itself crippled by the same deformity that is causing the environmental distortion. I have not discussed such a case here. It will be possible, I think, to extract one principle from these cases which has almost universal application, and I can use the message given me by Iiro, chosen for my first case. In effect, what he said in discussing his congenital syndactele was, "I will co-operate with anyone who can help to mend my abnormality, provided I am first of all accepted and loved as I am." Being accepted and loved "as I am" meant to Iiro "as I knew myself through knowing my own body before I found people saw me as abnormal; and they were right because, as I gradually came to see and understand, I am deformed."

In this way, even a deformed baby can grow up into a healthy child with a self that is not deformed and a sense of self that is based on the experience of living as an accepted person. Distortions of the ego

3. "Primitive Emotional Development" (1945) and "Mind and Its Relation to the Psyche-Soma" (1949), in *Collected Papers: Through Paediatrics to Psycho-Analysis* (London: Tavistock, 1958; New York: Basic Books, 1975; London: Hogarth Press, 1975).

may come from distortions of the attitude of those who care for the child. A mother with a baby is constantly introducing and re-introducing the baby's body and psyche to each other, and it can readily be seen that this easy but important task becomes difficult if the baby has an abnormality that makes the mother feel ashamed, guilty, frightened, excited, hopeless. Under such circumstances she can do her best, and no more.

A corollary is that the psychotherapist need not say: this child cannot be helped because of the physical abnormality. The self, the sense of self and the child's ego-organisation may all be intact because of being based on a body that was normal for the child in the formative period.

In regard to this article, the main thing has to do with the word "self." I did wonder if I could write something out about this word, but of course as soon as I came to do it I found that there is much uncertainty even in my own mind about my own meaning. I found I had written the following: For me the self, which is not the ego, is the person who is me, who is only me, who has a totality based on the operation of the maturational process. At the same time the self has parts, and in fact is constituted of these parts. These parts agglutinate from a direction interior-exterior in the course of the operation of the maturational process, aided as it must be (maximally at the beginning) by the human environment which holds and handles and in a live way facilitates. The self finds itself naturally placed in the body, but may in certain circumstances become dissociated from the body or the body from it. The self essentially recognises itself in the eyes and facial expression of the mother and in the mirror which can come to represent the mother's face. Eventually the self arrives at a significant relationship between the child and the sum of the identifications which (after enough of incorporation and introjection of mental representations) become organised in the shape of an internal psychic living reality. The relationship between the boy or girl and his or her own internal psychic organisation becomes modified according to the expectations that are displayed by the father and mother and those who have become significant in the external life of the individual. It is the self and the life of the self that alone makes sense of action or of living from the point of view of the individual who has grown so far and who is continuing to grow from dependence and immaturity towards independence, and the capacity to identify with mature love objects without loss of individual identity.

II. Two Further Clinical Examples

Undated; probably written in 1970[4]

These clinical examples and the theoretical considerations to which they give rise make me think of two other cases, which may suitably broaden out the subject of personalisation and of psycho-somatic in-dwelling. One concerns a young woman with a severe disability, and the other a healthy girl who happened to have a dark skin. With these two cases this contribution must end, although the elucidation of the general problem is only just beginning.

Hannah, Aged 18 Years

Hannah was referred to me by an organisation in the voluntary social services. The principal social worker wrote:

> Born with slight spina bifida, i.e. some swelling at bottom of spine about the size of a nut, this has grown with the years; feet and legs affected, had a dislocated hip but no hydrocephalus. Hannah seems to have had no treatment until the age of 4 years when she was admitted to hospital—she went up thinking she was going for a routine operation appointment and neither she nor her mother had any idea that she would be kept in. Mother feels many of Hannah's difficulties have stemmed from this. Had illeostomy at age of 10. Both parents and child much affected; mother not sufficiently pre-pared for what was to happen. On return home, when Hannah went to see the private doctor he remarked in front of her, "You are like a boy now aren't you Hannah but you have got it in the wrong place." Had a good deal of trouble with soiling following operation which the hospital dealt with by ordering daily enemas to be done by district nurse—this continued for months until parents protested.
>
> 1961, 1962 and 1963 further in-patient treatment for legs and feet. January 1964 Hannah admitted, at *her* request, to hospital for removal of the lump on her spine which she felt had grown too large

---

4. These examples were found together with the foregoing article in Winnicott's pa-pers.—EDS.

to enable her to wear a tight skirt. At this stage Hannah was very conscious of wanting to be perfect in her body, for this reason she had undergone intensive treatment for her legs and feet and now wished to get her back right. The operation was a major one lasting two hours and Hannah was very ill afterwards. Unfortunately she has not had complete success through these operations. She has been advised that she should wear calipers but refuses to do this. She recently asked her surgeon if he would amputate both her legs so that she could then have perfect looking artificial ones but this was refused. She has since had a new type of caliper fitting over the leg to look like a leg but as these are jointed at the knee and ankle and only reach to just above the knees they have not really fitted the bill. Hannah still feels very much that she is crippled, has talked at length to her mother about this saying that it is worse for her than someone who is more handicapped because people expect her to be normal. She still feels very badly about her legs and tries to hide them by wearing long boots, trousers, etc. She also, I feel, has not resolved her feelings about illeostomy and has herself expressed a wish to talk to a psychiatrist.

Our social work organisation has kept in close touch with Hannah's mother and at one time was giving her very intensive support. She has been a wonderful mother to the child and allows her to talk over her feelings but, as she remarked the other day, she feels that Hannah really needs somebody other than herself with whom she can talk.

Here follows an account of Hannah's interview with me, dictated from notes made at the time.

Consultation 10/1/68

Hannah came alone to see me, the consultation being arranged by the voluntary social work agency.

Family intact.

Hannah: 18 years.

Sister: 24 years.

We discussed odd items. She had come straight from art school.

Father: a stores manager. He had been a draughtsman and this may have influenced Hannah in her choice of going to art school.

Before settling down to work with Hannah, I raised the question of the motivation. I said that she may have simply come because pushed to come, or she may have wanted to come on her own. After thinking it out she said: "Well, both."

After a pause I saw that she was looking at the picture on my wall so I introduced the subject of painting and drawing. I suppose she had not noticed that she looked at the picture, because she said: "That's funny, but I go to art school." She described herself as "not really bad at art." In spite of her age I thought we would use the squiggle technique, at any rate as an opening gambit, and she got into it very quickly. She showed herself to be a slow and careful draughts-man. She asked me to pass her bag which contained her glasses and we talked about her ring which she got for 2/6d but it was worth £5. In this way we were quickly making a contact with interplay. We used whole quarto sheets (instead of the half-quarto sheets I use with younger children) because it seemed to me that this would be more appropriate in view of the fact that she was an art student and already 18.

1. My squiggle she turned into a fish being caught in a net. There is a fish-hook in the mouth.

2. Her squiggle I turned into a plant.

3. Mine she carefully made into an abstract, gradually achieving something that was satisfactory to herself. She talked about inability to say what beauty is. She observed that in an abstract you can get away with murder. She said it would look nice in colours or on a big sheet of paper.

4. Hers she turned into a distorted face of a man, or it could be a woman. She named it Celia for some personal reason of her own.

5. Hers I started to make into a mermaid. She helped me out with this so that in the end the drawing was a combined effort. I talked about the mermaid at Copenhagen. She wondered how the mermaid legend arose. I pointed out to her that the idea of a mermaid came from me although it was from her squiggle and she said: "Oh yes I had forgotten."

There had been a danger here that we would have got bogged down in the mermaid theme introduced by myself, while the squiggle certainly did not necessarily demand that idea. Instead of that she got on to something which was more important to her which had to do with the pleasure she gets at art school.

She made the comment that schools kill, and she discussed the difficulty that she is in because although teaching kills originality, never-theless when she went to the art school she could not draw a thing and now she can. She is in a conflict here which is not resolved in her mind.

It may have been that in playing the squiggle game we were already making a contribution to an understanding of this central conflict.

6. Mine I made deliberately of a circular variety. She said: "All I can see is people; oh well, I will do a person again"—and she called the person Phil (a name that can refer to a boy or to a girl). "Daddy hates long-haired girls. I hate people with short hair. I think long hair looks nice. Definitely No. 6 is a boy." No. 6 has to do with several boys she knows. "They wear long hair and it has nothing to do with wanting to be girls. Why do they make such a fuss about boys with long hair? Look at the Stone Age. I never went out with any of them; or one I did go out with."

From here I managed to take her to the idea of dreaming. "My dreams are mostly frightening. I had one the other night. It was about mother. You will think it daft. They are all ridiculous. When I am awake I wonder why I can have dreamed such silly dreams and then when I am asleep it all comes pouring back. In this dream mother said she was going to die. Everyone knew. She said: 'Put me in my coffin before you go to school!' So there she was in the living-room in her coffin. Every time I went in I was afraid she would be dead."

7. Illustrated this dream about her mother dying.

From here she went on to talking about the two opposing trends in her relationship to her mother. She has got on better with her since going to the art school but there was a long phase when things were very bad and she mentioned the ages 13, 15, and 16. "It was all petty arguing. About things that didn't matter." An example would be: "Can't you see that the chair ought to be there and not here?" She added the general comment: "When you think that one could be angry with world affairs and then here one is just being angry about whether a chair ought to be here or there!" She added: "I am not really of the argumentative type. Nowadays we end up laughing."

About father: "Oh, he wouldn't say boo to a goose"—and she obviously despised something about him and admired something about her mother.

One got the feeling here that the argumentation had as its root a suppressed or perhaps totally unconscious homosexual bond between her and her mother which could not be brought to a satisfactory outcome. There is no intimacy as far as I could make out between herself and her older sister.

She went on about dreams: "They are not logical. They are like another life. After you die what goes on? It is as if you die while you are asleep and so you get the dreams; heaven or hell."

After a pause she said: "So I go to hell but I haven't killed anyone."

I now brought up the subject of her spina bifida, and her general condition due to congenital deformity. I pointed out to her that I felt that she was exploiting to the fullest possible extent her sense of guilt and responsibility for things, indicating how much she would like to feel that her troubles were really natural troubles arising out of the aggressive and destructive and hateful things in her own nature. The difficult thing for her, I suggested, was that the main trouble had nothing to do with her at all. It was what people call "act of God" or the operation of pure chance.

She co-operated with me to the extent of coming over for a moment on to this side of the argument and talking about the way in which it is not fair when people are born in such condition that they cannot become normal. We discussed the logic of a feeling of blaming God.

She spoke about the end of the dream. She woke herself up to see if her mother was alive. "Really she had died in the dream." I assume that this was in fact also the death of herself.

It was not possible to make notes of all the discussion that we had around this theme. What I know is that I ended up with a statement of positive feeling. I felt so easily drawn towards this nice but badly deformed person that I thought I would put my feelings into words. I had certainly not ignored the deformity which makes her short and very awkward when she walks and which of course has involved her in a long period of incontinence. I did, however, say easily and truthfully: "You have a nice face."

At the end of this consultation Hannah went away feeling, I think, that we had not been discussing a deformity but a person, herself, a student at an art college, and someone who has every intention of making a life for herself. If she got relief it was from the somewhat unusual way in which we reached to her resentment at the unfairness that belongs to her having been born with a congenital deformity of a severe kind.

I would guess that the drawing of the mother in the coffin was a significant feature in the consultation as it brought her very closely into touch with the idea of death and revenge, all within a framework which allows for love in the relationship between herself and her mother.

In my letter to the Agency I wrote:

It is uncertain how far this one visit to me has been of any value to Hannah. She came with considerable difficulty because of her troubles with the lower limbs, but somehow or other she negotiated the frozen snow and stayed with me an hour. We probably ought to have had two hours but I had not been able to allow for this in my programme.

We made quite a good contact of a certain kind, in which I made no attempt whatever to get down to the practical issues which are rather important in her case. Probably she has plenty of advice here anyway. I thought it was more important to let a relationship develop between us in which her personality could blossom in so far as it was able to do so. I found her to be surprisingly well integrated. She has a rather good face and this proves to be an accurate indication of what she is like. Perhaps what she has not been able to do is to reach to her resentment at the unfairness that there is in being born with a congenital deformity. Who is one to be angry with?

I very quickly got on to the idea of her interest in pictures through seeing that she was looking at the ones that were hanging on my wall. We therefore continued our relationship in terms of drawing and the interchange of drawings, playing a game at first as if she were much younger.

As you know, she is at an art school, and therefore she was interested in the difference between being taught to draw accurately and the freedom of using a pencil on paper with spontaneity and without anything to do with drawing well. Together we arrived at some things which had significance, including a frightening dream which I believe it was important for her to communicate to someone. She quite rightly, however, defended the drawings against being looked at to see what ideas they contained, because drawing, for her, has to do with pleasure and self-expression and not with providing material for interpretation.

I need not say any more to you about this patient at this moment because this is not what you are wanting of me. To get an indication about future procedure I think I must wait to see what kind of effect this consultation had on Hannah. We must wait a few weeks. My immediate impression is that Hannah does not need psychiatric help and that she can manage on her own. Nevertheless she might like to follow up this visit to me perhaps two or three times a year so that there is someone outside the family who is watching her progress, quite apart from her physical progress. I would like to leave it rather in the air. It was a pleasant job seeing Hannah because of something very real about her.

The Agency wrote back as follows, after receiving a letter from Hannah's mother:

The mother said she had tried to stop Hannah from coming on that very snowy evening to see you, but Hannah insisted on doing so. She had been very thrilled that your appointment letter was sent to her direct. She also suggested to Hannah that she should not go off to work that morning but should stay at home until it was time to leave for her appointment, but Hannah refused this. She also refused to consider her mother's suggestion that she should change into something more suitable than her old jumper and trousers. Hannah retorted: "Well, he wants to see me as I am doesn't he, so I'll go like this." When Hannah returned home from her interview with you her parents asked how she had got on and she replied: "He's quite nice" and then said nothing else. The mother said she had not pressed Hannah as the agency had warned her beforehand that the girl might not wish to say anything, but she was very astonished at her reply since whenever Hannah has been to see a doctor about her physical condition she has given practically a verbatim report to her mother of what she said and what the doctor said! Since seeing you Hannah has not been harping on her condition as she had done previously. However, she still insists on wearing trousers and has refused to go to a dance recently. I gathered that the mother had expected you to wave a magic wand.

In answer to the mother's questions, the social worker told her that you had enjoyed meeting Hannah and were prepared to see her again and that you thought she was very well integrated considering all that she had been through. The mother expressed some ambivalence about Hannah seeing you again, but has agreed that we should talk to Hannah herself about this when she is on holiday.

We were interested in your comments about the father and sister. Over the long time we have known the family we have had the impression that the father has been very much pushed out and on the periphery. The social worker says, too, that the sister, who is a hairdresser, is also rather out of the picture, the intense relationship being between Hannah and her mother.

In my reply I wrote:

I am quite satisfied with the way in which Hannah negatively reported what had happened between her and myself. I would hate to
think that her visit to me was just another visit to a doctor, as she
has visited so many about her physical condition. I hope that no
pressure whatever will be put on Hannah to talk about what went
on, because in fact it would be very difficult for her to report it even
if she wanted to. I have even forgotten it myself, but if Hannah and
I were sitting in the room together I should remember it.

I think the important thing was that we met as two persons and
not as a doctor and a patient with a deformity. You could quite
safely leave her relationship to me to work itself out. Sometime or
other she may very likely say she would like to see me again, in
which case I will do my best to fit in with her request. It may be that
she will not need to see me again; that would be even more satisfactory, indicating an independence which I believe she can manage
although of course in regard to her deformity there must be dependence on specialised surgical skill.

A few weeks later I had a further letter from the Social Worker:

When talking about Hannah the mother said that Hannah had now
made friends with an older girl who had been to a grammar school,
who was attending the same art school as herself. Apparently she
had begun to be friendly with this girl before she saw you but she
had refused to join in any activities with her outside the home. However, since seeing you she has started to go to a very modern church
with this girl; the vicar here is a young man who holds services in a
coffee bar and instead of the usual type of service he has a kind of
"Quiz Bee," where he encourages the youngsters to ask as many
questions as they like. Hannah goes there regularly with this girl
now and has also decided to go to evening school, which she has
already started, in order to see whether she can get G.C.E. subjects
like her friend.

After the mother had told us about this, she suddenly stopped and
said: "Well, perhaps this is the result of Hannah going to Dr Winnicott, because she would never have done this sort of thing in the
past." She then asked me whether she should ask Hannah if she
would like to come to see you again, but was told that this might be
better left to Hannah.

Six months later I was sent a follow-up report.

We thought you would like to hear how Hannah is getting on. Our
social worker saw her mother last week and she told us that she had
made a steady, slow improvement ever since she saw you last year.

She has now begun to take an interest in her clothes and has stopped wearing trousers all the time; she is now wearing dresses and a skirt. She also wears high boots, but of course these are very much in the fashion. She has also voluntarily gone to a College of Technology, in order to take G.C.E. subjects, so that she can take the full art course at her own college.

She is continuing to mix and make friends with normal teenagers and has, indeed, a very full social life, which is a great contrast to the way she used to hide herself at home and refuse to mix with other young people. She is cheerful and easy and no longer continually grumbles about her condition.

In a final follow-up (two years later) I was told:

I do know one thing that Hannah seems to have benefited considerably from her visit to you. She often talks about you and she has seemed much more confident since that time. Hannah seems to have particularly talked to mother about the drawings which you got her to do and seems to have been doing her own interpreting!

The favourable outcome need not be a direct result of the consultation, although one could reasonably claim that no harm followed the work we did and did not do together in that single professional contact.

The important inference is that whereas this young woman's physical state remained deplorable and ugly, and continued to necessitate orthopaedic interference of a remedial kind, Hannah's attitude to her disability changed, so that her personality could go forward in its developmental processes where it had been seriously held up.

An important factor was the easy co-operation of the mother, who did not need to be seen by me, nor did she need to be told what to do or what attitude to adopt.

The essential feature, it seems to me, was that this girl felt loved and accepted as she was before she was forced rather brusquely to recognise that she suffered from a physical congenital disability that was both crippling and ugly.

Mollie, Aged 8 Years

The other case is that of Mollie, a girl of 8 years. She had been adopted at the age of one year into a good family where there was already a 3-year-old girl. Since the adoption there has been born a boy who is now 3.

These adopting parents did not realise for a year or two that they had taken on a very restless child, seriously affected by the constant changes of management that characterised the first year of her life.

The whole extended family loved Mollie, and entirely accepted her, but it could not be denied that her constant persecution of the little boy was having an adverse effect on his personality development.

The mother had consulted a Child Guidance Clinic and had been told that she ought to find a place for Mollie away from her home, a boarding school or an alternative adoption. The mother felt this to be wrong, and she consulted me in order to learn my reaction to the proposal, which horrified her. The change might help her little boy, but it would end all hope of bringing the restless Mollie through to some form of social integration.

In the therapeutic consultation with me a great deal happened which must be omitted. There were difficult phases, because of Mollie's extreme restlessness.

What I wish to report is the unexpected turn of events after we had been playing the squiggle game for about an hour. Mollie evidently gained confidence, and she suddenly introduced a new theme. This had to do with the fact that she had come to see that she is dark-skinned (her real parents being ethnologically African) while the adopting family was English and fair-skinned.

It is necessary to think of Mollie as a child who had great difficulty in letting her mother go to the waiting-room, and who was constantly reasserting herself in relation to her mother, giving her a kiss or an affectionate embrace, and in general showing a genuine love of her mother though it was clinically exaggerated by anxiety.

We had reached drawing No. 19 in our game and this was of three pigs, father, mother, and baby. She was able to let me know that the school children had shouted out at her, in the way children do, "Adopted Pig!"

Suddenly she took the game into her own hands and said: "I'm going to draw my bottom." No. 20 was her drawing of her bottom which was at first clean and unmarked. Almost immediately she made aggressive pencil jabs at the buttock cheeks. Her verbalisation was: "Oh how I wish I were white" (like the boy that she persecutes).

It might have been thought that she was giving a picture of incontinence, but I knew this was not the correct interpretation. Mollie was illustrating denigration. The pig idea led on in her mind to eating and to cannibalistic fantasy, and she quickly made the buttocks unattractive. In other words she made them into bad pigs, pigs that no-one would want to eat.

I had to be very quick to make use of this unexpected communication, because Mollie seemed to have but the slenderest of hopes that she would be understood, and certainly with her conscious mind she had no idea what it was that she was telling me and illustrating.

I said: "You have drawn the cheeks of your mother's face, and at the same time the two breasts. The white babies and the white mother want to eat each other and that means they love each other. Then come fears about eating and being eaten and the good things must be spoiled if they are not to be destroyed. But first comes the eating, and the cannibalism and the destruction."

While she went on drawing she said: "Yes, I'm dark, but I like white better." Drawing No. 21 was of a mother's body and a mixture of destruction of breasts with a denigration of the body as a defence, but at the sacrifice of pristine quality. For her, because she is dark-skinned, white is an idealisation, but for white children white is an initial phase and quite natural, and she feels deprived of this phase, as if she had to start with a handicap.

She was struggling to cope with what she had only gradually come to find out about herself. Her family entirely accepted her as she was, and in fact she was quite beautiful, appropriately for her age, with perfect skin.

As if to show she knew what she had been deprived of she drew No. 22, showing herself giving her mother a vicious kick. She said: "I kicked mummy." Here she became anxious and rushed out to mother to re-establish the affectionate relationship.

There were some oblique references to sexual side-issues: father's bottom; my couch made her think of a doctor visiting herself or her father, and probably (I guessed) she had seen her father having penicillin being injected into his buttocks during an illness. Also the pencil she was using had a cap and she pulled this off the end of the pencil and said she was taking its pants off. She talked about a bare bottom. There was much that could be followed up here, either in further treatment sessions or in conversation with her mother. Nevertheless I knew that we were dealing with the same dynamic factors that make adolescent anorexia nervosa girls draw pictures of beautiful women, but with their faces covered with spots. The same theoretical considerations must be brought in to explain the acne of adolescence. The conflict is in the area of denigration as a defence, and whiteness or luminosity as an expression of idealisation, except in so far as it can be an experience that is properly worked through in the early stages of individual development, when the child lives in a subjective world, and just before the object has been made external by being kicked, bitten, torn or in some way spoiled.

Mollie was trying to account for the special effect that her discovery that she had dark skin was having on her, making her feel as if she was deprived of an essential feature of very early personality development and self-realisation.

She accepts her condition but feels cramped by having to dwell in a dark skin, not because of what she looks like now, but because of what it would mean in terms of the earliest stages of experience.

38
Individuation

A talk given to the Medical Section of the British
Psychological Society, October 1970

I have never liked this word and I never use it. My acceptance of this invitation to speak in a symposium belongs to the idea that I always carry round with me, that I might learn something.

A glance at the *Oxford Dictionary* shows me that this word has been respectable for three hundred years at least, and that it has been used in philosophical discussion. Nevertheless I cannot come to terms with it, perhaps for childish reasons—there is the root up to and including the "d" of "individ-," and then if one goes further and uses the "u" I feel it ought to go on in the ordinary way to produce "individualisation," cf. "civilation" for "civilisation." In the German language of course the Jungian term may make good sense.

What you want of me is not philosophy but a statement of the way an individual becomes an individual, if indeed he or she does reach such a stage.

We are talking about the inherited maturational processes of the baby and child, and a recognition that these processes do not carry a boy or girl forward except in so far as a facilitating environment obtains; and a statement of the facilitating environment and its essential qualities takes us into interesting but complex and difficult territory. I have written about all this in my own language and I have no doubt that some of the words I use in my writings irritate you as much as I myself feel irritated by this one that is under discussion. We are not discussing a word but a developmental process. I will say at once that I feel that Jung usefully drew our attention to the fact that human beings, except in so far as they are trapped in the rigidity of their own defences, do go on growing in all respects, right up to the moment of death. The Freudian statement may have seemed for some decades to give the impression that any development that has not occurred by 5, or at the end of puberty as the boy or girl changes from adolescence to adult status, will not happen at all. But we all know that this is absurd.

The baby (boy or girl) inherits a developmental process. To describe what happens we must know not only about the developmental process but also about the environmental provision. Any attempt to describe a developing baby sui generis and ipso facto must fail. If we are wise we do not try.

Obviously the environment must have certain basic qualities. A human being must be there somewhere and we do not believe in the Romulus and Remus myth because a wolf simply has not got the mental equipment to identify with a human baby.

I fear you may be only too familiar with what follows, whatever language we use. Here is my statement.

The baby at first lives in a subjective world. The baby exists precariously in dependence on the human mother-figure. Here, and nowhere else, is an experience of omnipotence. Elsewhere omnipotence is the name given to a feeling or a delusion, but at the theoretical start the baby lives in a dream world while awake. What is there when he or she is awake becomes material for dreams. Later the alternation of asleep and awake must become clear-cut, and the baby's world ceases to be a subjective one.

Thinking about the child on the way to objectivity (the encounter with the Reality Principle) nature allows the baby an intermediate position, as is clearly shown in cases where a baby employs a transitional object. Nature allows this but we must provide it. Such an object stands at one and the same time for the baby and for the mother. It is both, though it is neither. In this way life is an inverted pyramid and the point on which the inverted pyramid rests is a *paradox*. The paradox demands acceptance as such, and need not be resolved. This is permitted madness, madness that exists within the framework of sanity. Any other madness is a nuisance, an illness.

Thus the passage of time along with the accumulation of a personal experience goes to make for the conditions that are essential for the inherited growth process to carry the boy or girl baby through or over into a separate existence, an existence that can be free from merging and yet can allow the re-experience of being "merged-in-with" (then called regression).

We are allowing for a time span, weeks, months, years, and hoping for a second chance, so that the main experiences may be re-enacted by the child in his or her own home during adolescence. If the first has had reality the second is the more likely to have reality too.

But the precondition is clear. The precondition has to do with the mother, and with the two parents together, and the family and the extended family and the local social setting including the school, and so on.

To get to the essential feature it is necessary to look at the mother or mother-figure. From her is needed at the beginning a special state to which once again I have given my own descriptive term. I call it "primary maternal preoccupation," a state of affairs in which the woman has been able to allow herself to become temporarily orientated to the baby that she gradually recognises as a fact within her physical frame. She has been able to put aside her male self-identifications temporarily, and she has been helped by the endocrine apparatus and by her own experiences as a baby. With one baby it goes forward naturally, with another the mechanism creaks, or it breaks down. It's a matter of psychiatric health in the mother that she knows that the maternal identification is temporary and can be recovered from in time. The mother is affected by her total experience in her relationship with the man, who temporarily lent her his woman self.

The baby boy or girl who develops in an environment that this kind of mother can provide is able to live for an adequate period in a subjective world in which the world of external reality does not impinge. There develops in the baby a sense of predictability, and in this way the foundations of the very delicate early stages of personality growth are able to be laid. A line of life that is personal begins to be a feature. Prophylaxis in the context of mental health is the provision of good-enough facilitation at this early stage.

All of which sounds incredibly complex, but to a group such as this one any simplified statement must seem unsatisfactory or even an insult to the intelligence.

The main thing for the beginner to get used to is that although every boy or girl born into this world alive has, as one might say, a prime minister's baton in his or her nappie, this baton may remain something that might have been. It may become a hidden talent, with the individual boy or girl hidden in a false set-up, a false personality based on compliance and being good. It is a character disturbance to be good in this way.

No description of these matters, however much pared down to fit in with the Reality Principle that is a clock, can omit reference to the place of aggression. Let me say that we can never get far with our examination of the subject of aggression unless we can see its positive value. One way to see this is to watch the child becoming separate from the mother and from the environment generally. It is axiomatic that there is no relating to a subjective object. The world is only there for relating to in so far as it is objectively perceived and what we call external to the child. The outside world can be taken in, introjected or incorporated, that is eaten, by mental process.

What I am trying to say is that we can get nowhere with our study of aggression if in our minds we have it irrevocably linked with jealousy, envy, anger at frustration, the operation of the instincts that we name sadistic. More nearly basic is the concept of aggression as part of the exercise *that can lead to the discovery of objects that are external.* I show a child's drawing which is commonplace, but if you had been there you would have known that it represented a climax of adventure in the trust situation of a therapeutic consultation at which the little girl broke away from heavily loaded clinical dependence on the mother. There was much affectionate display that seemed genuine, and for a few seconds the girl (aged 8) put her mother *over there,* by kicking her. Naturally she was scared and needed quickly to re-establish her mother as available, accessible and responsive without vindictiveness.

You will see what I mean, and allow for over-simplification, if I refer to the way in which one of two worlds is waiting for each child, and it makes all the difference which you and I were born into.

One: a baby kicks the mother's breast. She is pleased that her baby is *alive and kicking* though perhaps it hurt and she does not let herself get hurt for fun. Two: a baby kicks the mother's breast, but this mother has a fixed idea that a blow on the breast produces cancer. She reacts because she does not approve of the kick. This overrides whatever the kick may mean for the baby. The child has met with a moralistic attitude, and kicking cannot be explored as a way to place the world where it belongs, which is outside.

It is now impossible for the boy or girl to begin to feel concerned, because the mother's moral code has become set up as a block to the natural growth in the baby of a sense of right and wrong, and of guilt and grief.

These two worlds are like chalk and cheese. Any discussion of the "paranoid position" in pure culture is futile unless the environmental provision is first assessed and allowed for.

When externality has been established in the baby's sorting out of life's potential chaos, the way is set for personal enrichment which has no limits, based on personal experience and making use of the mental mechanisms usually called projection and introjection. Along with the growth of the imaginative mental life, this starts the child off on a life of inter-relating that is done from the real base of a personal existence.

A statement like this that I have tried to make could be built up in terms of abnormality at various stages, brought about by the environmental distortions which render the personal line of life a fragmented thing.

It is easier, I admit, to concentrate on the way life goes when it goes well, when the baby, child, adolescent, adult finds life to be a personal experience, and not an organised series of reactions to environmental pathology.

When each boy or girl is living his or her own life, though imaginatively involved with other persons, with the other sex, and with society, then we can see that growth simply means life and living, and there is no end to life, except death. We are concerned here with the sense of fulfilment, but if I fulfil myself I must remember that I climbed to this over the dead bodies of my friends who died fighting, or for whom accident or illness made them only fulfil themselves in terms of their fellow creatures who happened to live long enough.

But I suppose that to some extent there always remains the task of the individual to become more and more independent, though retaining the hole for creeping back into. And therefore there could be a life-long applicability for a term like individualisation (or even individuation).

Part Two

Psycho-Analytic Psychotherapy with Children and Adolescents

39

Private Practice

A paper given at the annual conference of the British Psychological Society, Durham, 17 April 1955

It is probably true to say that physicians and psychiatrists are shy to give an account of their private work. If the work is good, this looks like advertising, and if it is bad—well, this is bad for the reputation. I approve this modesty implied in reticence. Nevertheless it seems to me that private practice is on the wane, and yet it has points in its favour. I would like to see clinic and private practice compared in the open, and I am confident that each has something to offer the other. I believe it would be a tragedy if private practice in child psychiatry were to disappear.

In this contribution I give you all the 54 cases that came to me in my private practice in 1953. (I have excluded those that came in the previous year or two, and that may have been attending for subsequent interviews.) My practice is chiefly psycho-analytic and I have not chosen to describe this which occupies the major portion of my working hours. Also I have my clinic at the Paddington Green Children's Hospital, which is based on medical out-patient practice.

These half hundred cases that squeeze themselves into my practice each year simply come along because of the law of averages.

I have chosen the year 1953 because it is near enough, so that I remember each case clearly, and also it is far enough away, so that a follow-up has value. In nearly all the cases I find I am able to get a recent report.

My contention is that private practice provides an *economical psychiatric method*. There are certain cases that need a clinic for management and for thorough investigation, and especially is this true when a report is needed for the magistrates of a Juvenile Court. A psychiatrist working in private can scarcely do without a clinic, and nothing I say or recommend annuls the value of clinics of one kind and another. Nevertheless, if results are at all comparable, then I think that, in terms of man-hours, private practice has a great deal to say for itself.

I am attempting to spread out the results of one year's work, so that you may judge by comparing results with ordinary clinic results. But first let me make the following comment: Private practice is team work, and the team consists of the psychiatrist and his secretary. It would not be possible to do this work without a secretary who is able to take part in the work, work which is intimate to a degree, and which is made safe and productive only by being kept strictly within the framework of the professional relationship.

This team is a small one, and for the sake of simple description I shall not continue to refer to it as a team. By contrast the clinic depends for its value on the work of a team, and one of the major tasks of the clinic psychiatrist is the integration of the information gathered.

These 54 cases involved about 100 man-hours of work (plus the work done by the secretary). I think this compares very favourably with the work done in a clinic, provided the results are as satisfactory.

In a few cases an I.Q. was needed, or was done as a matter of interest.

The main body of my communication is my attempt to present the 54 cases in intelligible form. It could be said that the work was done in the consulting room, and now I am merely concerned with referring to it in an orderly manner.

I have chosen to classify the cases according to the type of problem that I had to deal with, rather than by the children's personal psychiatric diagnoses. This inevitably involves much overlap and in some cases the classification must remain arbitrary.

To make myself clear in picture form I have surrounded each case number by a square if I feel that the parents got what they came for. I have used the word "fruitful" here, but success depends on the standard expected. For instance, success when I was consulted about a psychotic state simply means that I dealt with the management of the case, or explained the problem and the task to the parents. Where I was simply asked for advice I have used this square to indicate that the result was satisfactory to the parents. At the other extreme there are the children who had *amenable symptoms,* including the 13 in category H, and here I measure success only in terms of clinical cure. It is just here in Category H that private practice wins, I believe, because it is just as effective as clinic practice, and all the side issues are avoided. The child needs a highly specialised personal psychotherapeutic interview, and even in a clinic this has to be given, unless the case is to fail.

General Considerations

There are various details that can be put forward for discussion.

1. In private the psychiatrist has the whole case and takes the whole responsibility. When this can be maintained the result is good. The only drawback is that the doctor in private practice always has a stomach-ache; some case is always in a difficult phase, and it is a matter of good fortune if several cases do not blow up at the same time. I would say that in clinic practice one avoids the stomach-ache too easily; perhaps the psychiatric social worker enjoys that function.

2. In private it is easy to see the parents, the nurse, the general practitioner, the school master, anyone concerned. Also one can see the child first, or one can see the parents alone and advise them not to bring the child. A great deal is done over the telephone, and one gains from the fact that parents of private patients are in the habit of phoning, and can do more over the phone than make arrangements. Sometimes one can put patients off altogether by this means, so that they never come, and so save themselves guineas and oneself time.

3. It is often a matter of difficulty in team work *to initiate action at the right moment,* in the right direction, and from the right quarter. In private practice the one person who is fully responsible can act even on impulse, even on the doorstep as the mother and child enter the house. I suggest that it is not uncommon in clinic practice for a simple manoeuvre to be missed because of the complexity of the situation, though this would have met the case. Often psychiatric social workers have said that they have had to miss opportunities for action because they were gathering information for the case conference, and were not in a position to act, even though they knew they ought to act.

4. There is no waiting list in private practice, and this is good. The cases just roll up, and if one cannot fit a case in it goes to a colleague.

Actually in my clinic I have had no waiting list either, because the clinic worked within the framework of an ordinary medical out-patient department, and whoever wanted to see me could do so in the out-patient clinic by simply waiting a few hours on a hard bench on the appropriate morning. Waiting lists are generally acknowledged to be bad in psychiatry; the result of a waiting list is that the ordinary cases that can be helped never reach the psychiatrist or the team, and the psychotic children and the delinquents claim attention. It is the ordinary case that can be really helped, the case that drifts to the medical out-patient department.

5. Undoubtedly in private practice one gets the type of case in which the parents are able to take a responsible part in the search for the right school. In this work a great deal is done by careful placement in prep and public schools, apart altogether from the diagnosis of maladjustment. It is surprising how many schools for normal children are willing to take a few children who show abnormalities such as low I.Q., "deprived child" complex, some degree of psychosis, and neurotic disturbances (including bed-wetting). This is no new feature and I myself can remember at my two schools how we carried a certain number of what I would now call psychiatric cases.

These are ideas thrown out for discussion; but the main issue hangs round the two questions: (1) Are private practice results good enough? and, if so, (2) Is there an advantage in terms of man-hours?

If private practice is both good and economical, then I suggest that it is good for the psychiatrist, in that by being able to be self-reliant he can work better in the clinic with the team.

Particularly I suggest that the children who come off best in private practice are those who can be helped quickly and deeply by psychotherapeutic consultation.

Private practice, 1953. 54 cases, 41 male, 13 female; took 100 hours.
Case numbers in squares and circles:
41 fruitful outcomes (squares); 13 unfruitful (circles).

A. *Dominant psychiatric illness in parent(s)*

12 cases
5 fruitful
23 hours

1. *Father's illness dominates*

(3) ♂ 9 yrs 3 hrs
Writing difficulties
Father refuses psychology

(4) ♀ 5 yrs 2 hrs
Paranoid father
Discuss ex-wife's treatment of daughter

2. *Mother's illness dominates*

[1] ♀ 20 months 1 hr
Mother cannot play

(15) ♂ 10 yrs 1 hr
Mother cannot co-operate

[35] ♂ 2 yrs 1 hr
Temper tantrums
Mother schizoid

(36) ♂ 4 yrs 6 hrs
Restlessness
Mother chaotic

(41) ♂ 11 yrs 1 hr
Enuresis, etc.
Mother in conflict of loyalties

3. *Psychiatric illness in both parents*

(14) ♂ 8 yrs 1 hr
Father advised therapy

[20] ♂ 4 yrs 2 hrs
Restless parents

(22) ♂ 16 yrs 1 hr
Complex home
(Now in mental hospital)

[24] ♂ 8 yrs 2 hrs
Parental over-control
(No direct effect)

[38] ♂ 12 years 2 hrs
Home breaking up

B. Old cases, new problems
cases 2
fruitful 1
hours 2

(18) ♀ 27 yrs 1 hr
Psycho-analysis by D.W.W. at 10–13 yrs for psychosis

[34] ♂ 19 yrs 1 hr
Abscondence from army (Known homosexual)

C. Birds of passage
cases 8
fruitful 7
hours 12

[21] ♂ 8 yrs 2 hrs
Having psychotherapy

[26] ♂ 18 yrs 2 hrs
Helped out of army
Having psycho-analysis

[28] ♂ 4 yrs 3 hrs
Having psychotherapy

[30] ♂ 10 yrs 1 hr
Psycho-analysis arranged (not successful, new analysis due)

(33) ♀ 8 yrs 1 hr
Severe anorexia
Psychotherapy arranged

[40] ♀ 5 yrs 1 hr
Having psycho-analysis
Psycho-analysis interrupted

[46] ♀ 5 yrs 1 hr
Psycho-analysis arranged

[51] ♀ 14 yrs 1 hr
Having psychotherapy
Referred for diagnosis and support

D. Guidance sought
cases 7
fruitful 6
hours 13

[7] ♂ 8 yrs 2 hrs
Mother's secret

[37] ♂ 9 yrs 1 hr
Parents' ambitions

(43) ♂ 7 yrs 1 hr
Father uninformed

[45] ♂ 12 yrs 5 hrs
Father's death

[49] ♀ 3 yrs 1 hr
"Spastic" problems

[50] ♀ 3 yrs 2 hrs
Mother uninformed

[54] ♂ 6 yrs 1 hr
Eczema-asthma

E. Low I.Q. dominates

5 cases
5 fruitful
8 hours

1.

[2] ♂ 13 yrs 3 hrs
School found

[19] ♂ 6 yrs 1 hr
Neurological case
School found

[47] ♂ 7 yrs 2 hrs
Parents' attitude corrected

2. *Mentally defective*

[11] ♂ 10 yrs 1 hr
Parents' guilt allayed

[13] ♂ 4 yrs 1 hr
Neurological case

F. Childhood psychosis

5 cases
3 fruitful
13 hours

1. *Manic-depressive*

(10) ♂ 16 yrs 1 hr
Endocrine: fits

(17) ♀ 15 yrs 1 hr
Known since 3 yrs
Psycho-analysis prevented by mother

[39] ♂ 17 yrs 5 hrs
Mother responsible for accident:
M.D., fits

2. *Schizoid*

[52] ♂ 12 yrs 5 hrs
Secondary defect (placed)

[53] ♂ 7 yrs 1 hr
Secondary defect
Psychotherapy (medical cover)

G. "Deprived" complex

2 cases
1 fruitful
4 hours

[5] ♂ 16 yrs 1 hr
Psycho-analysis contra-indicated
(Mother having psycho-analysis)

(27) ♂ 12 yrs 3 hrs
Advised against psycho-analysis while at
home (but psycho-analysis has been successful)

H. *Amenable personal child problem*

13 cases
13 fruitful
24 hours

1. *Psycho-somatic*

| 6 | ♂ 8 yrs 1 hr | Colic (?appendix) |
| 42 | ♀ 8 yrs 2 hrs | Severe colitis
Psycho-analysis continues |

3. *School*

9	♂ 12 yrs 1 hr	Masochistic defence
12	♂ 15 yrs 1 hr	Father-son clash
29	♀ 11 yrs 1 hr	Envy of male
44	♂ 15 yrs 2 hrs	Father-son clash

2. *Puberty*

| 8 | ♂ 11 yrs 2 hrs | Paranoid anxieties |
| 31 | ♀ 14 yrs 1 hr | Paranoid system |

4. *Hysterical conversion*

16	♀ 14 yrs 2 hrs	Crippling paresis
23	♀ 15 yrs 2 hrs	Morning vomiting
32	♂ 9 yrs 3 hrs	Laryngeal tic, compulsions (Mother's depression)

5. *Anxiety*

| 25 | ♂ 11 yrs 1 hr | Reaction to mother's physical illness |
| 48 | ♂ 8 yrs 5 hrs | Hypersensitive twin
Paranoid anxiety
Homosexual compulsion |

40
The Squiggle Game

*An amalgamation of two papers: one, unpublished,
written in 1964, the other published in 1968*[1]

In my child psychiatry practice I have found that a special place has
to be given for a first interview. Gradually I have developed a technique for fully exploiting first interview material. To distinguish this
work from psychotherapy and from psycho-analysis I use the term
"psychotherapeutic consultation." It is a diagnostic interview, based
on the theory that no diagnosis can be made in psychiatry except over
the test of therapy.

The basis for this specialised work is the theory that a patient—
child or adult—will bring to the first interview a certain amount of
capacity to *believe* in getting help and to trust the one who offers help.
What is needed from the helper is a strictly professional setting in
which the patient is free to explore the exceptional opportunity that
the consultation provides for communication. The patient's communication with the psychiatrist will have reference to the specific emotional tendencies which have a current form and which have roots
that go back into the past or deep into the structure of the patient's
personality and of his personal inner reality.

In this work the consultant or specialist does not need to be clever
so much as to be able to provide a natural and freely moving human
relationship within the professional setting while the patient gradually *surprises* himself by the production of ideas and feelings that have
not been previously integrated into the total personality. Perhaps the
main work done is of the nature of integration, made possible by
the reliance on the human but professional relationship—a form of
"holding."

Although opportunities do occur for interpretative comment, these
can be kept to a minimum or, in fact, can be excluded deliberately. In
this way, suitably selected consultants can do this work while in process of learning how to do psychotherapy that includes verbalised

1. Published in *Voices: The Art and Science of Psychotherapy* 4, no. 1 (1968). Also
published in *Therapeutic Consultations in Child Psychiatry,* © 1971 by the Executors of
the Author's Estate; reprinted by permission of Basic Books, Inc., Publishers.

interpretation. The rewards of this work are great because the consultant is able to learn in this way from the patient, and it is necessary for the consultant to be ready to learn rather than to be eager to pounce on the material with interpretations. In selection of consultants, as in selection of psychotherapists in general, those who are eager to pounce on the material by interpreting should be reckoned to be temperamentally unsuitable for psychotherapeutic practice, and this is particularly true of suitability to carry out therapeutic consultations.

In doing this work, which I call "therapeutic consultation," with a child (or adult for that matter) it is necessary to be able to use the limited time profitably and to have techniques ready—however flexible these may be. It has to be assumed that in many of these cases what is not done during this consultation will not be done at all. The first consultation may be re-duplicated, but if the child needs to see the consultant several times, then the case already is changing over into one in which the team work of the clinic is becoming necessary and quite possibly the child will need to be handed over for treatment in long-term psychotherapy.

It is interesting that the cases that do not need to go over into casework or psychotherapy are relatively common. This is partly due to the fact that the majority of children do have good-enough homes and schooling, although they may at times present acute clinical problems. A little help given to an individual child can often lead to better relationships all around; the family and the school are waiting to do the rest of the treatment.

In regard to any technique that the consultant must be prepared to use, the basis is playing. Elsewhere[2] I have made the statement that in my opinion psychotherapy either is performed in the overlap of the two areas of playing (that of the patient and that of the therapist), or else the treatment must be directed towards enabling the child to become able to play—that is to say, to have reason to trust the environmental provision. It has to be assumed that the therapist can play, and can enjoy playing.

One useful technique has been called the Squiggle Game, which is simply one method for making contact with a child patient. It is a game any two people can play, but usually in social life the game

2. See "Playing: Creative Activity and the Search for the Self," in *Playing and Reality* (London: Tavistock; New York: Basic Books, 1971; Penguin, 1974).

quickly ceases to have meaning. The reason this game can have value for the psychotherapeutic consultation is that the consultant uses the results according to his knowledge of what the child would like to communicate. It is the way the material, produced in the act of playing, is used that keeps the child interested.

The method can easily be learned, and it has the advantage that it greatly facilitates the taking of notes. If a boy or girl communicates by talking or by recounting dreams, then note-taking is a truly formidable problem, and it must be remembered that I am not referring to those few cases that we treat by prolonged psychotherapy, but to the many that come for consultation. Each one of them hopes for more than a diagnosis—each hopes for a need to be met, even if help can only be given in regard to one detail or in one area of the vast extent of the personality.

Nevertheless I have hesitated to describe this technique, which I have used a great deal over a number of years, not only because it is a natural game that any two people might play, but also, if I begin to describe what I do, then someone will be likely to begin to rewrite what I describe as if it were a set technique with rules and regulations. Then the whole value of the procedure would be lost. If I describe what I do there is a very real danger that others will take it and form it into something that corresponds to a Thematic Apperception Test. The difference between this and a T.A.T. is firstly that it is not a test, and secondly that the consultant contributes from his own ingenuity almost as much as the child does. Naturally, the consultant's contribution drops out, because it is the child, not the consultant, who is communicating distress.

The fact that the consultant freely plays his own part in the exchange of drawings certainly has a great importance for the success of the technique; such a procedure does not make the patient feel inferior in any way as, for instance, a patient feels when being examined by a doctor in respect of physical health, or, often, when being given a psychological test (especially a personality test).

At a suitable moment after the arrival of the patient, usually after asking the parent to go to the waiting room, I say to the child: "Let's play something. I know what I would like to play and I'll show you." I have a table between the child and myself, with paper and two pencils. First I take some of the paper and tear the sheets in half, giving the impression that what we are doing is not frantically important, and then I begin to explain. I say: "This game that I like playing has no rules. I just take my pencil and go like that . . . ," and I probably screw up my eyes and do a squiggle blind. I go on with my explanation and say: "You show me if that looks like anything to you or if you can make it into anything, and afterwards you do the same for me and I will see if I can make something of yours."

This is all there is by way of technique, and it has to be emphasised that I am absolutely flexible even at this very early stage, so that if the child wishes to draw or to talk or to play with toys or to make music or to romp, I feel free to fit in with the child's wishes. Often a boy will want to play what he calls a "points game"; that is to say, something that can be won or lost. Nevertheless, in a high proportion of first-interview cases the child fits in sufficiently long with my wishes and with what I like playing for some progress to be made. Soon the rewards begin to come in, so that the game continues. Often in an hour we have done twenty to thirty drawings together, and gradually the significance of these composite drawings has become deeper and deeper, and is felt by the child to be a part of communication of significance.

It is interesting to note, regarding the squiggles themselves, that

1. I am better at them than the children are, and the children are usually better than I am at drawing.

2. They contain an impulsive movement.

3. They are mad, unless done by a sane person. For this reason some children find them frightening.

4. They are incontinent, except that they accept limitations, so some children feel them to be naughty. This is allied to the subject of *form and content*. The size and shape of the paper is a factor.

5. There is an integration in each squiggle that comes from the integration that is part of me; this is not, I believe, a typically obsessional integration, which would contain the element of *denial of chaos*.

6. Often the result of a squiggle is satisfactory in itself. It is then like a "found object," for instance a stone or piece of old wood that a sculptor may find and set up as a kind of expression, without needing work. This appeals to lazy boys and girls, and throws light on the meaning of laziness. Any work done spoils what starts off as an idealised object. It may be felt by an artist that the paper or the canvas is too beautiful, it must not be spoiled. Potentially, it *is* a masterpiece. In psycho-analytic theory we have the concept of the dream screen

(Lewin), a place into or onto which a dream might be dreamed.[3]

All this is linked to the very early stage of maximal dependence when the infant self is unformed. The ego is very weak, unless (as usually happens) the mother's ego gives ego-support. The infant starts off living with the mother's ego which she lends by her sensitive adaptation to her infant's needs.

It must be understood that no two cases are alike, and I would be highly suspicious if two cases resembled each other, because I would think then that I was planting something out of some need of my own. The description of only one case must be deceptive, and a student of this technique would certainly need to go through a score of cases in order to see that, in fact, no two cases *are* alike. For this reason I have already published a dozen or so of these cases, and propose to collect several together in a book.[4]

I have chosen one case[5] for presentation here, and I cannot say that I have chosen it for any special reason.

(Here the reader must be willing to tolerate my change of subject. I shall now, unavoidably, be describing a case, not describing the Squiggle Game. At the end I will return to the main theme, and make some comments on the game as it was used by the child and myself in the case.)

Case of L., Age 7½ Years, 1/19/66

The mother brought L. and the two waited for me in the consulting room where I had placed several copies of *Animals* magazine. This no doubt influenced the material of the consultation.

Family history:

Girl	12	years
Boy	10	years
L.		7½ years

---

3. Bertram D. Lewin, "Inferences from the Dream Screen," *International Journal of Psycho-Analysis* 29 (1948).

4. *Therapeutic Consultations in Child Psychiatry* (London: Hogarth Press; New York: Basic Books, 1971).

5. The material of this interview has also been used in a book entitled *Handbook of the Psychotherapy of Children*, ed. G. Bierman (Munich: Ernst Reinhardt, 1968), which contains a chapter by Dr Winnicott entitled "Meeting the Challenge of the Case in Child Psychiatry."—D.W.W. (Now also published as Case 3, "Eliza," in *Therapeutic Consultations in Child Psychiatry*.)

Girl   5 years
Boy   3½ years

I had a few minutes with the two together in which we talked about the animal magazine. I got L. to go with me to the waiting room which I had prepared for the mother, complete with coffee, all of which interested L. L. came back into the consulting room with me without any difficulty. We settled down quickly to the Squiggle Game, which I simply introduced and to which she acquiesced. She did not know about it as a game.

L. is a fair, slightly built girl, looking quite sweet as a child may do at 7, fairly independent and completely trusting in the context of the relationship which I had with her.

We started away with:

1. Mine.

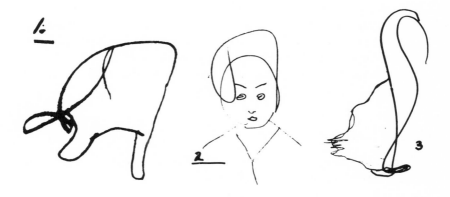

As far as I know L. had not been told previously why she was coming to see me. She was obviously much at home with a pencil. She took my squiggle and put another leg on it, leaving a space between the legs.

I said: "What is it meant to be?"

She said: "Something gone wrong."

It is not unusual in my experience for a child to plunge immediately into deep matters in the way that she did.

I made a mental note that the combination of the space where the belly might be and the words "something gone wrong" might be giving me a definite indication, even at the very beginning of the session, that L. was aware of a problem, and that this problem could have to do with the belly. *I did not say anything.* Naturally I wondered whether there might not be some problem of the "Where do babies come from?" variety.

2. Hers, which I made into a head, which she seemed to like. I did not do this for any reason, only because this is what I found myself doing.

3. Mine, which she immediately made into a bird, and in doing so showed her capacity for self-expression in drawing.

4. Hers, and I discussed with her what it might be. She was pleased with the idea of wash hanging out on a line although this does not come in the daily experience of the family. "Everything goes to the laundry" seemed to be the comment, but not as a significant contribution from her as far as I could tell. It was more that she followed up on my drawing with a reference to life at home.

5. Mine, which she turned into someone with a long hat. She seemed to think it rather fun that the hat comes off the side of the head. It could be a boy or a girl.

Interpolation

It is necessary here to refer to the fact that I had had a significant interview with the mother three months previously. This chiefly concerned the mother. Nevertheless in the course of describing L. the mother had told me of an incident that had had importance in L.'s early childhood. This concerned *hats*. If I had let what the mother

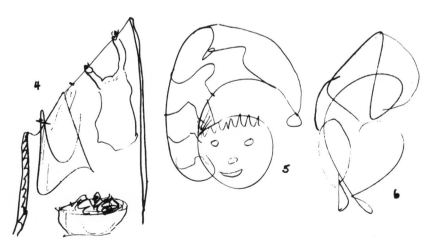

told me dominate the ideas in my mind I would have perhaps thought that drawing 5 indicated a main theme of hats; but as *I always take my cue from the child,* I had already been informed in this interview with L. that the main theme would have reference to the space between the front and back legs (drawing 1), whatever that might come to mean. However, hats undoubtedly came in as a secondary theme. I shall describe the hats complex at the end of this description of the session with the child.

The Game, Continued

6. Hers, which she quickly saw as a kangaroo with a hat on. She did something here which emphasised the kangaroo theme and linked it to the idea of a place of significance between front and back legs. She pointed out that the kangaroo had its knees bent up in the way that kangaroos do, and she illustrated this by drawing her own knees up to her chest. One can see that one of the effects of this is that it hides the belly, and, in any case, the kangaroo is an animal that children often choose on account of the pouch, and to indicate a visible instead of a hidden pregnancy.

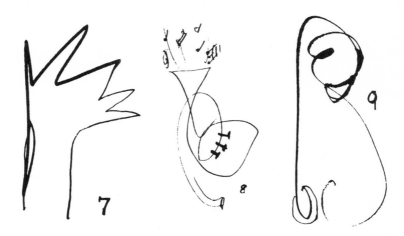

7. Mine, which she turned into a hand or glove.
8. Hers. Together we turned this into a trumpet.
9. Mine, which she turned into a "dog or something." It will be noticed that this drawing also contains a space between the tail and

the place where the limbs would be. *Evidently she felt this because she went back to drawing no. 1 and put in a line giving the tummy.*

10. Hers, which I discussed with her. I said, "That really is complete in itself; it doesn't need anything doing to it. I wonder if it isn't (and here I had to get from her the family names for products of defecation) a 'busy.' If there is no tummy to the animal this could be the sort of thing that would drop out."

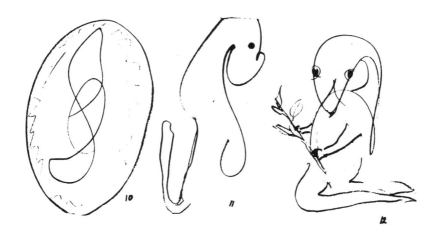

She looked at me as if it was interesting, but as if I was talking a language that was not hers, and she said it was a snake. So I put a plate round it and I suggested that we could have it for lunch.

11. Mine, which she turned into a fierce dog. It seemed to be "ready to punch somebody." This was evidence of L.'s ability to get to something in her nature which does not show in her usual behavior or in what she looks like. (Incidentally I was thinking of joining the punching with the idea of the belly which was absent, and I made a mental note that of course she had had to witness developments belonging to the two pregnancies that came after hers, especially the second when she was 3½ to 4 years old.)

12. Hers, which I turned into "an elf or something." She thought that he was going to eat the leaves off the branch. She liked this one as a drawing and as an imaginative idea.

13. Mine, which she dealt with in a highly imaginative way. "It is something going under a tunnel. It might be a mole." I felt that in this

there was the symbolism of defaecation or birth or sexual intercourse, and I left the matter at that without interpreting.

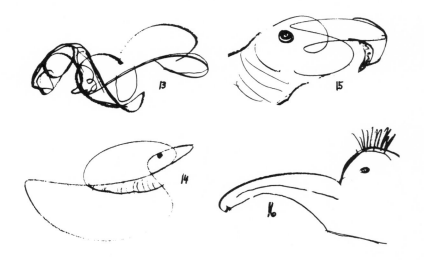

14. She made hers into a sort of duck that you see in the dark. This meant that we were near to ideas that turn up in the mind just before sleeping. We were near to real dream material.

15. Hers, which I turned into the head of some kind of a bird.

16. Mine, which she dealt with in a similar way. She gave the bird feathers on its head.

By this time there had developed quite a game which had to do with placing the pictures side by side on the floor; she was getting quite excited about taking each one as it was finished and putting it at the end of a row so that we now had pictures spreading into the other half of the room. When she went to put a picture there or see its number, which interested her also, I would say: "Goodbye," and when she came back I would say: "Hallo." She was not over-excited, but she was vitally interested in what was going on, and we were both enjoying ourselves.

17. Hers, which I made into a duck (imitating her and saying so). I gave it a fish to eat.

18. Mine, which she made into a fierce something.

By this time I had made some tentative inquiries about dreams that she might have had, but she was not finding it easy to tell me about them. She had ventured the comment that her dreams were horrid. I had pointed out that there was evidently something horrid that is part of her but which she does not know what to do with, and I reminded her of the fierce dog (no. 11). The theme was continued in this drawing (no. 18) of the "fierce something that has claws and big ears and one curious big eye so that it can see in the dark."

I said something here about the way in which things would fall out of the inside if there was no tummy; perhaps something fierce would fall out like what she had drawn.

I also said something about the claws and her ideas of getting at whatever was inside Mummy's tummy when her Mummy was going to have one of the two babies that came after L. This was a new idea to her. She was not quite sure that she remembered anything about mother being in a stage of pregnancy. (We did not, of course, use this word.)

19. Hers, which I started out doing something with, and together we turned it into an insect.

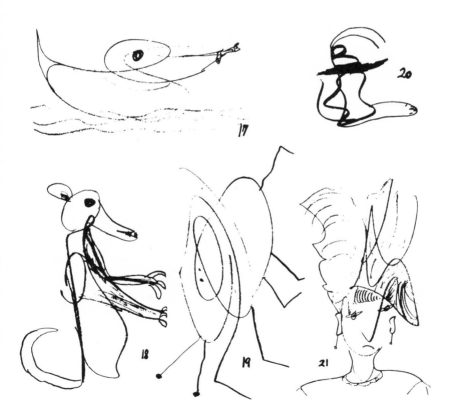

20. Mine, rather unlike the other squiggles, and more concentrated. I said: "That's a silly one, isn't it!" And she said: "No!" and she turned it quickly into "some kind of an animal with feelers." "It has a big foot and a tail. It can be nice *or* horrid."

Somewhere here I tried to get from her some information as to whether the fierce and horrid things were male or female but I got no satisfactory indication.

21. Hers, which I drew into what she called a "posh lady." While I was drawing this she was doing the next one,

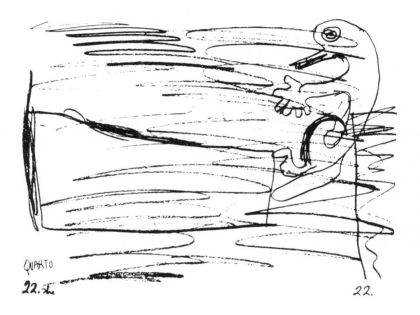

QUARTO
22.

22.

22. on a quarto sheet of paper. This was "very difficult for her to do" and she had to be "very brave." "It is a frightening dream." She started off with the dark and then put in the bed with herself lying on it. After this she got down to the details of the THING that plunges down on her. It has its knees up (in the way that she described when drawing the kangaroo and that she had also shown me with her own body). It has one big foot and one small foot and one eye. From her point of view this thing is "as horrid as possible."

I tried to get from her what it would do to her if it got at her and all she could say was: "It would be horrid to me."

I explored round with the idea here of sexual stimulation, either in the form of a seduction of some kind (which is unlikely in her family setting) or form of masturbation. I used words that she could understand. I did not force this issue at all, but let her know that I knew about it and she looked at me with wondering eyes as if this was the first time that she had self-consciously thought about masturbation and the guilt feelings related to masturbation. Obviously here I was speculating, basing my ideas on what I thought I saw going on. I went very carefully and made sure that I was in no way endangering the relationship which existed between us, which had very powerful positive features which could be relied on to cover big risks.

At this stage I gave her the choice to do something else or to draw, and she chose to do two more in the Squiggle Game. In this way I gave her every chance to get away, or to change the subject, or to play and see what might happen.

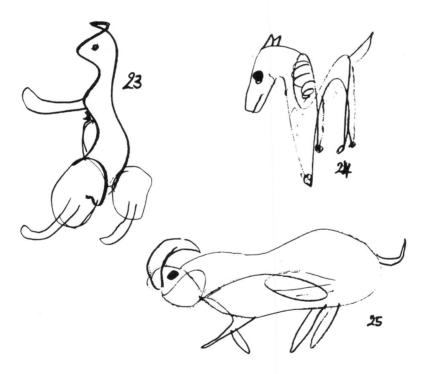

23. Mine, which she turned into another kangaroo. This time the kangaroo had a big belly or pouch with a baby kangaroo in it. The knees were not up. I talked about the use of a kangaroo for thinking

about a belly that has a baby in it without actually coming directly to the idea of mother being pregnant. She talked about the kangaroo as an animal that does things with its legs and jumps. I gave L. some more of my own idea that this very awful thing that comes at her represents something which she had never properly accepted, which is that she has feelings like that about the baby inside her mother's belly. The horrid THING would then be a return of something of her own that she could feel to be horrid.

24. Hers, which I made into an animal which she liked. She seemed to want to continue, so I let the game proceed.

25. Mine, which she made into a goat charging. I assumed (but said nothing) that for L., as for other people, a goat is a symbol of male instinct.

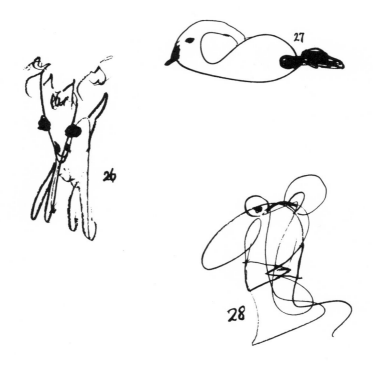

26. Hers, which I changed into another little animal, which pleased her.

27. Mine, which she said was going to be a mouse. In any case it

had a big ear. We now came to what she said would be the last of the series.

28. The final one. Hers, which she turned quite fantastically into a man's head. It started off with glasses and was fairly obviously a portrait of me. The man was reading a newspaper. "No, he is crossing his arms." She was very free at this point and she could now see whatever she liked to see into her own squiggles.

She was now quite ready to go, and I told her that we would fetch Mother, so we gathered together all the drawings which she wanted to re-examine in their right order. We went over all the significant details, including the fun and the interpretative work. She took out the big quarto (no. 22) drawing of the dream and put it aside as "different," and I think if Mother had come in she would have wanted this drawing to be kept as private to herself and me. In any case I put all the drawings in the folder and said that they were hers, which she could have any time if she wanted them, but I would keep them for her. It is my usual practice to say this at the end, and the children very seldom want to take the Squiggle Game drawings home.

Now she fetched her mother. As she went out of the front door in a very contented state I said: "Perhaps we will meet again one day." She said: "I hope."

Comment

The reader who is studying this technique, and who is also trying to use the material for making an assessment of L.'s psychiatric state, will wish to examine what has been presented without help. No doubt various opinions could be expressed, with the accent placed now on one aspect of the case and now on another.

Nevertheless a comment must be made for the reader to use after making a personal study of what transpired.

General Remarks

This intelligent girl comes within the meaning of the term "normal," or "healthy" in a psychiatric sense. That is to say, she shows a freedom from any rigid defence organisation. In a more positive way, she is able to play and to enjoy playing; she easily accepts my playing and allows our playing to overlap, and she shows a sense of humour with-out being manic.[6]

L. is able to use her imagination, and after duly testing out the situation she becomes able to give me a dream of significance, in which appears *fierceness,* the one feature that is clinically lacking in her personality as it presents itself to those who know her.

There appear certain themes which draw attention to areas in L.'s "total personality" organisation which give her some trouble because of conflict, ignorance and muddle. These themes are as follows:

A. Main Theme

Something wrong (no. 1).
Space instead of line for belly (no. 1).
Line put in later (at the time of no. 9).
Kangaroo theme introducing confusion in respect to pregnancy.
Genital pregnancy understood, but pregenital (alimentary tract) fantasy of pregnancy relatively under repression.

It is as if she had been given information about babies coming from the womb, but the information had not "taken" because L. was still struggling with babies in terms of what comes from the inside—the alimentary fantasy system. It cannot be decided whether the fault here came from the mother or from the child, or both, because it is clear that the anxiety centered on the horrid THING in the alimentary tract fantasy system, and this was related to the horrid or destructive ideas that she may have had towards the THINGS in the mother's belly that, at times, made her fat.

L.'s arrival at these matters in the relationship to me had the effect of making her much more of a relaxed person, so that the parents were well satisfied with the clinical result of the consultation. This would point to the possibility that L. was ready for a more imagina-tive and childish explanation of the origin of babies than she had in fact been given.

B. Secondary Theme

There was a recurring interest in hats, and this may well have been an aftermath of the significant episode to which the mother referred,

6. The term "manic" implies, for me, that there is a depression mood that is being denied, replaced by contra-depressive manifestations.—D.W.W.

and which I have not yet recounted. It can be given here without (I hope) interfering with the main issues of the case.

Near the end of the mother's interview with me, which was mainly about herself, she told me of something that she felt guilty about in the management of L.'s early life. She said: "It seems ridiculous, but this is what happened when L. was 10 months old. I had to go away for a few days, and I did so reluctantly, but left the children (L. was the youngest then) in the safekeeping of a nurse in the constant surroundings and routine of the home. I thought it would be quite all right, but I must have felt guilty because when I came back I rushed into wherever L. (the baby) was, without taking off my hat first. The awful thing was that L. froze up. She did not react to anything I did at all. I took her and kept her in my arms and eventually she relaxed and became just as she had been before I went away. All returned to normal, except that L. now had a phobia of hats. For a long time, many months, the baby L. would not pass ladies with hats on."

It was probably because of this phobia of hats, and the possibility of there being a residue of L.'s three-day loss of her mother at 10 months, that the mother decided to bring L. for psychiatric consultation, not the bed-wetting which really did not worry the mother at all, and the bed-wetting cleared up round about the time of the consultation.

It was important, as has already been pointed out, that I followed the child's material, and not that of the subsidiary theme of hats which I could have recognised from what the mother had told me about L.'s early years.

C. *The Third Theme*

The third theme was eventually the most important. It had to do with exactly the feature that was missing in L.'s personality, the *fierceness* that appeared first in the "fierce something" (no. 18) and then the THING in the dream (no. 22). This fierceness had to do with her fear of the things that she imagined were growing inside her mother's tummy, based on an ingestion-retention-elimination (or pre-genital) view of bodily functions. It also linked onto her own aggressive drives, anger with mother who was withdrawing from her because of the new pregnancy, and her attack in fear of the imagined horrid objects inside mother. Behind all this was the overlaid attack on the mother's contents belonging to instinct-driven object-relating, or primitive love impulse, with a pre-history of the idea of attack on the contents of the breast, or greedy appetite.

The work done in this one therapeutic consultation was enough to free the primitive love impulse from the secondary angry impulses, and the consequence clinically was that the child's personality became more free generally, and there was a greater ease in the to-and-fro of feeling between her and her mother.

The main part of this work was the child's own discoveries, or ordered sequence, culminating in her being able to use the dream which she had had but from which she had not been able to derive full benefit.

In other words, the interpretations did not produce the result, but they helped towards the child's own discovery of what was already there in herself. This is the essence of therapy.

Summary

a. An attempt has been made to describe the Squiggle Game.

b. This is a game with no rules.

c. There is nothing new in this game, and very little that is new in the use of it in psychotherapy. What is important is the use made of the material that the game may produce, especially in this type of one-session work which I call "the therapeutic (diagnostic) consultation."

d. To describe the game, therefore, it has been necessary to give an example, and this has involved a case-description. But no two cases are alike, and one example may therefore be misleading. The student is invited therefore to study this case along with other published cases.[7]

e. In many of our cases we are, so to speak, batting on a good wicket. It is these (common) cases that provide the best material for this kind of work in child psychiatry. Whatever there is of a clinical improvement following the session naturally produces a favorable response in the home or school.

f. If the work of the session does not produce a clinical result, then the case naturally passes over into being classified as one needing a different approach, such as case-work or a long phase of psychotherapy. The Squiggle Game will not be found to dominate the scene for more than one session, or at most two or three. It is convenient to

7. See *Therapeutic Consultations in Child Psychiatry*.

think in terms of re-duplicated first sessions, so that then one can say that the Squiggle Game or its equivalent is useful as a first-session technique.

g. It would be against my intention if the Squiggle Game should become standardised or too clearly depicted. The principle is that psychotherapy is done in an overlap of the area of play of the child and the area of play of the adult or therapist. The Squiggle Game is one example of the way in which such an interplay may be facilitated.

41

The Value of the Therapeutic Consultation

Written in 1965[1]

There is an aspect of applied psycho-analysis which has come to interest me more and more in the past two decades. This is the exploitation of the first interview, or the first few interviews.

First I must make it abundantly clear that what I am describing is not psycho-analysis. If starting an analysis I do not adopt the procedure described here. Nevertheless I hold the view that in order to prepare himself to do this work the therapist should make himself thoroughly familiar with the classical psycho-analytic technique, and should carry through to the bitter end a number of analyses conducted on a basis of daily sessions, continued over the years. Only in this way does the analyst learn what has to be learned from the patients, and only in this way does the analyst master the technique of withholding interpretations that have validity without immediate or urgent relevance.

I would not say that a full-scale analysis is always better for the patient than a psychotherapeutic interview. Treatment by psychoanalysis often leaves the symptomatology untouched for a period of time during which social repercussions may infinitely complicate the issue; moreover, treatment may necessitate the child's removal from a good-enough home to a strange setting and this again is a complication that were better avoided. In other words, there are cases in which a quick symptomatic change is preferable to a psycho-analytic cure even though one would prefer the latter.

Apart from this, there is a vast clinical demand for psychotherapy that is not related in any way to the supply of psycho-analysts, and therefore if there is a type of case that can be helped by one or three visits to a psycho-analyst this vastly extends the social value of the analyst and helps to justify his needing to do full-scale analyses in order to learn his craft.

1. Published in *Foundations of Child Psychiatry*, ed. Emanuel Miller (London: Pergamon Press, 1965).

It is well known that the first interview in an analysis can contain material that will come forward for analysis for months and even years. Students are advised to make careful notes of first interviews, notes which can be used at all later stages and which make possible a reconstruction of the analysis in terms of the discovery of deeper and more subtle meaning in events and free associations given in the first session.

That which I am calling the psychotherapeutic interview makes the fullest possible use of this relatively undefended material. There is real danger in this work, yet there is danger of doing nothing at all, and the risks come from the therapist's timidity or ignorance rather than from the patient's feeling of having been tricked.

The psychotherapist at this the stage of the first interview is a subjective object. Often a child will dream of the psychiatrist *the night before* the day of the interview, so that in fact the psychiatrist is fitting into the patient's preconceived notion. In another language, the patient brings to the situation a certain measure of belief or of the capacity to believe in a helping or understanding person. Also he brings a measure of suspicion. The therapist cashes in on what the patient brings and acts up to the limit of the chance that this affords. The patient goes away without having made an objective perception of the therapist, and a second visit will be needed to get the therapist objectified and shorn of magic.

There is a difference, then, between this technique and that of psycho-analysis in that whereas in the latter the transference neurosis gradually unfolds itself and is used for interpreting, in the psychotherapeutic interview there is a fore-ordained role for the therapist, based on the patient's pattern of expectation. The difficulty often is for the therapist to do as well as he could find himself allowed to do. Many patients do indeed expect to be basically understood immediately, and it might be said that we either fit in with this or else we work on the basis of "psycho-analysis or nothing." Of course we cannot understand immediately unless we are briefed, and in the first interview the patient is often willing and indeed eager to brief the therapist, giving all that is needed for the deep significant interpretation.

It often happens that we find a child has given all to the psychologist who is performing an intelligence test, and the fact that the material presented has not led to understanding (this not being included in the psychologist's aims) has proved traumatic to the child, leading to a strengthening of suspicion and an unwillingness to give the appropriate clues.[2] For this reason I have always seen my patients first, referring them to the psychologist where necessary, after I have come to grips with the case by doing something significant in the first interview or first few interviews.

I would say that it is a common thing for patients to go away from a first interview disillusioned and unwilling to make a further attempt to seek psychiatric help, because of the failure of the consultant to use the material presented. It is comparatively rare for a patient to be hurt by wrong interpretations made in a genuine attempt to use what is presented, the mistakes in omissions being due to the limits that belong to all human endeavour. I learned this from my psychotic patients (borderline schizophrenics) who are remarkably tolerant of an analyst's limitations of understanding, though they may be at the same time extremely intolerant of irregularities in the analyst's behaviour (his unreliability, an uneven performance, display through reassurance of unconscious hate, bad taste, etc.).

Technique

In order to make the most of a first interview the therapist needs to be very careful not to complicate the situation. All sorts of things need to be said and done which simply belong to the fact that the therapist is human and is not sitting on a professional high-horse and is nevertheless aware of the sacredness of the occasion. This is true regardless of the age of the patient.

> A little girl, 2½ years old, saw me five times. She demanded that she should see someone to ask about a fear which her parents could not understand, and when she got some help from me she insisted on making further use of me until she had resolved her problem. Each time she gathered herself together for the interview and after it she emerged in a relaxed state. The fifth time, for instance, she came up (by train journey) curled up on her father's lap, sucking her thumb or her father's finger. She was very tense right up to her arrival at my door, and on entry she immediately went into my room and took up her position on the floor among the toys. After this interview she (now 3 years old) was in a happy state as usual. She was interested

2. This especially applies in T.A.T. tests in which the patient has reached to unexpected ideas, fears, states.—D.W.W.

in everything she could see on the way home by train. In the afternoon she was playing constructively and with great satisfaction. In the evening she made one remark that was appropriate to the work of the session.

This was like a child's reaction to some analytic sessions but there was, in a sense, more at stake, because of the distance of the child's home from my room, which she actually talked about in the session.

A boy of 6, with a relatively low I.Q., the backwardness being secondary to an infantile psychosis, came to his first and only interview in a state of apprehension. The mother wrote: "He naturally wanted to know where we were going and we had to give him a definite answer because of his experience at 4 when he had his tonsils out. I didn't quite know what to say, so I mentioned something about learning at school and his sometimes annoying habit of finger-sucking. Anyway he mentioned after the interview with you that you hadn't asked him about this. He seemed to feel that I had misled him slightly . . . When he asked again why we had gone to visit you and not taken our other boys I replied that you were a friend and that we thought he would enjoy meeting you, and we had only taken him as he was our biggest boy. He was contented with this answer. On that morning he had been very anxious to go straight to you and not waste time on proposed shopping."

This boy made significant use of his interview, and came away "delighted," and he was jealous of his parents when they came to see me a few weeks later.

It is good to be able to prepare the parents beforehand, perhaps by phone, that it will probably be best for the child to be seen first. The fact is that the parent may have to be neglected on this first occasion. It is the patient's right to be the patient, and if the parent cannot co-operate in this arrangement then one needs to consider whether in fact the ill person may not be the parent rather than the child. If it is the parent who is the patient, then the parent should be seen first, in which case it may be best to do nothing with the child, so as to avoid raising hopes that cannot be met.

It is axiomatic that if a proper professional setting is provided the patient, that is the child (or adult) who is in distress, will bring the distress into the interview in some form or other. The motivation is very deeply determined. Perhaps it is suspicion that is shown, or too great a trust, or trust is soon established and confidences soon follow. Whatever happens it is the happening that is significant.

A boy of 8 had a very rich interview with me; we had worked hard and I had been able to give help on the basis of the clues provided. At the second interview nothing happened at all. I allowed the boy his full hour, and all I said was: "I don't know what is going on but I do know that you have reason to be in control of me. Last time you helped me to help you; this time I can do nothing." So we parted. That evening this boy casually told his mother while he was in the bath that a man had tried to assault him in the park; the mother said: "Did you tell Dr Winnicott?" and he said: "No!" in a surprised way, as if he could not have imagined this to be an important thing to do. He had in fact told me in a better way, by being suspicious of me and by having me in his control. I saw him next day as an emergency case, and he gave me another richly rewarding interview, reporting the incident and his own imaginative homosexual yearnings, based on a relative father-deprivation.

The point in all this was the boy's communication through making nothing happen, and my acceptance of this as a communication.

There is no clear-cut technical instruction to be given to the therapist, since he must be free to adopt any technique that is appropriate to the case. The main principle is that a human setting is provided and while the therapist is free to be himself he does not distort the course of events by doing things or not doing things because of his own anxiety or guilt, or his own need to have a success. It is the patient's picnic, and even the weather is the patient's weather. The end of the interview belongs to the patient too, except where there is no structure to the interview because of a lack of structure in the patient's personality or in the patient's relating to objects, in which case this lack of structuring is itself communicated.

A student attempting to study my personal technique would need to study the way that I behaved in a long series of cases, and it would be found that what I did in each example belonged to that particular case.

I hope that the only set feature that will be observed after a broad examination of my cases will be a freedom on my part to use my knowledge and experience to meet the particular patient's need as displayed in the one session that is being described.

One more observation: it is necessary to do this work in a wider setting in which there is opportunity for a case to slip over into another kind of child psychiatry category. There is no need for any case to fail (except where one lacks the necessary understanding, in which event there is no need for self-criticism). If the psychotherapeutic interview should prove inadequate even under the slogan: "How little need we do in this case?" then a more complex mechanism can be set in motion. The case can become one of those that need the full child psychiatry system of management.

It is wise, however, not to think in terms of *psycho-analysis* for the cases in which the psychotherapeutic consultation with its limited objective does not succeed; better, if psycho-analysis is likely to be a practical proposition to work from the start on the basis that psychoanalysis will be instigated. The reason for this is that a high-powered use of the first interview tends to make the initial stages of a classical analysis difficult, especially if the analysis is to be done by someone else, other than the initial consultant who went deep quickly in the first interview when attempting to make a diagnosis.

Summary

1. A diagnostic interview must of necessity be a therapeutic one, since one of the main criteria for diagnosis is the response that indicates the degree of rigidity or relative lack of rigidity of the defence organisation. The overall clinical picture may be deceptive without this additional key to the assessment of the patient's personality.

2. A human setting is provided, and into this setting the patient brings and displays the immediate strain and stress.

3. The psychiatrist is a subjective object, and the use that is made of the interview represents the patient's capacity to believe in significant persons, that is if the psychiatrist does not interfere with the pattern of the interview.

4. The psychiatrist needs to have training and experience based on long treatments, in which the work is done on the transference material as it gradually evolves, and which allows for the patient's objective perception of the analyst.

5. In this work interpretation is reserved for the significant moment, and then the analyst gives as much understanding as it is in his power to give. The fact that the patient has produced the material specifically for interpretation gives the therapist confidence that interpretation is needed and that it is more dangerous not to interpret than to interpret. The danger is that the patient will feel confirmed in the belief that no-one understands and that no-one wants to understand.

6. This is not "wild" interpreting; though even wild interpreting may convey the idea of a wish to understand.

A girl of 10 said to me: "It doesn't matter if some of the things you say are wrong because I know which are wrong and which are right." A little later on in the treatment she said to me: "I shouldn't go on guessing if I were you," implying that she could tolerate my not knowing.[3]

3. This article originally included a description of the case of "Ashton," Case 9 in *Therapeutic Consultations in Child Psychiatry* (London: Hogarth Press; New York: Basic Books, 1971).

42
Deductions Drawn from a Psychotherapeutic Interview with an Adolescent

A paper given at the Twentieth Child Guidance Inter-Clinic Conference, London School of Economics, 11 April 1964[1]

My contribution to this discussion has prescribed for itself certain rather narrow limits. A great deal can be got from an examination of adolescence as a whole phenomenon. My idea here is that eventually we get down to the individual boy or girl. If it be true that one cannot generalise from one case it is even more true that one cannot see the individual in a broad survey.

Definitions

The word "puberty" describes a stage in the physical maturational process. Adolescence is the stage of becoming adult by emotional growth. It is a common thing for boys and girls to go through pubertal development without experiencing adolescence, and without arriving at the emotional maturity which is the better part of the adult state.

Adolescence covers a period of time during which the individual is a passive agent to growth processes. I have referred elsewhere[2] to the *adolescent doldrums,* the time during which there is no immediate solution to any problem. The only cure for adolescence is the passage of time, the passage of three to six years at the end of which the adolescent becomes an adult—that is, becomes able to identify with parent figures and with society without the adoption of false solutions.

Adolescents abhor the false solution and this makes them awkward

1. The papers from this conference were published by the National Association for Mental Health.—EDS.
2. See "Adolescence: Struggling through the Doldrums," in *The Family and Individual Development* (London: Tavistock; New York: Basic Books, 1965).

to handle. But society recognises the rightness of this awkwardness. Or does it?

One other thing before I describe one case: adolescence is always with us, but we must remember that this is not a comment on the actual boys and girls who are awkward since these are all the time growing up and becoming adult. It is always a new set of boys and girls who are providing the new variety or the new phase of awkward behaviour.

Jane, aged 17 years, was referred to me by her General Practitioner, who wrote:

> I understand that Jane has always been a great problem though I must admit I find her a very charming and intelligent person. There was apparently some disturbance—about which I have not been told anything—this was the beginning of the present upset. Jane has completely contracted out of all family relationships. I don't think that there is any doubt that she has intense dislike and an unreasoning jealousy of her sister who is superficially the more graceful and accomplished of the two. There is a family history of mental disease and instability . . .

Now what would you do in these circumstances? Would you arrange to collect all the facts, see the parents, and then see the girl? I suggest that the only good way to take a history of a case is to take it as it comes from the patient; that is, once one has decided who is the ill person in the group. A history taken from the patient has a truth of its own, though the facts may be inaccurate or contradictory. Moreover, history details taken as they come can be used by the psychotherapist, whereas details gathered accurately by a fact-finding commission are valueless except for the purposes of a case-conference.

I saw Jane herself and afterwards adjusted my relationship to the parents by telephone and letter. In this case I have not seen any of the family except Jane. This may put a strain on the family, which I fully acknowledge—in case they are present!

At this point I must remind you that there is nothing more difficult than to decide whether one is seeing a healthy boy or girl who is in the throes of adolescence or a person who happens to be ill, psychiatrically speaking, in the puberty age. Is one seeing adolescence, or a hold-up or distortion of adolescence due to illness? I hope this case illustrates this difficulty.

First Consultation

Jane came in and we sat down at a table and the beginning was not difficult. She said that her father was a physics teacher in a technical college and that her mother also had a job; also that she had a sister, 14 months older than herself. I asked about her family. I said: "Is father very brainy?"—and she seemed to think he was, and that her sister, too, was intelligent. She said: "I have obviously been brought up in an educated group and I take these things rather for granted."

Let me describe Jane as she appeared in her interviews, two of which I am to report to you. In this first interview Jane herself looked the part. She had rather long straight hair like an inverted V which started from her forehead and gradually opened out to display a nose and mouth. Protruding out of this was a very sharp chin, and her mouth, certainly not sensuous, indicated an intellectual approach; possibly there was a deliberate protrusion of the lower jaw on top of the natural formation.

At the first interview one immediately got the impression of a strong personality and of intelligence and of someone who was quite able to look after herself. Jane did not seem to mind the fact that I was taking notes in a desultory fashion. (If I hadn't you wouldn't have had this.) I kept a wide open eye for this because of the natural suspicion of adolescents, but I found no trouble here. When she became suspicious she said so.

All this was a rather conscious piece of acting. The second time she came she was frankly depressed. She looked it. At the fourth interview, six months later, she had become a natural adolescent, in very tight canvas jeans, and she wore her hair any way. There was no act and no mood. When she came a fifth time just recently she had on a coat and skirt and already one could see the adult state creeping up on her.

I want you, unless you do these things yourselves (and most of you do), to watch out for the way the interview develops. A good interview in child psychiatry develops momentum of its own accord, or holds itself back if it must. I must be myself, alive and awake, but if I jog things along I am a bad interviewer. I can be natural. I can hum, or do doodles or scratch my head, but if I try to make the interview follow a pattern I am interfering with a natural process. For it may be taken as *axiomatic* that if a child or adolescent or a grown-up is suffering, some of this will appear in an interview if conditions are provided which might possibly lead to understanding.

To continue:

> Jane described the household arrangements, and this involved her in telling me about her parents, their not getting on well together and living apart from each other.
>
> She said about her mother: "She is intelligent and much deeper than I myself; mother is the deepest of the lot of us. (Pause.) (Of course, I can't give the pauses. This would make it into a two hours' talk, but the pauses are important.) I myself am now, I hope, out of my sister's influence, but this has been a real struggle. Everybody admits that my sister is inordinately jealous. Now she has gone away to another town. She is really in trouble and liable to marry someone who is not really suitable."

Later she gave me a different version of this, but what is true for the patient NOW is the truth that I am after.

> Here I asked her: "If you were coming here of your own accord, what would it be like?—what would you be asking me or using me for?"

I wanted to make sure she was not just being compliant, coming because of her mother.

> She said: "I *am* coming of my own accord. For three or four years I really ought to have seen a psychiatrist. It's not really that I'm a disturbed person, but mother gets worried. We have rows, usually when my sister is at home. Recently my sister got fed up with mother and I refused to get mixed up in it all; so I withdrew, and this meant that I got cut off."

Here she was referring in her own way to the withdrawal described by the G.P.

> Jane continued: "Of course you know I always add melodrama and lying to everything. Mother gets troubles on all sides; you know, I am very fond of my sister really but really she's only 14 months older than me and that's a lot of the trouble, because we've always competed as if we were level. But now she and I are separate. Thank goodness I have separated myself off from my sister. She is a demonstrative person, whereas I am not. She doesn't like secrets. People think that I am eccentric and that I've no contact with convention; father's rather conventional."

Here then is a general layout of the home situation and a specific reference to trouble arising out of the fact that only 14 months separated these two sisters. This theme eventually developed in an unexpected way, towards the end of the second interview. I will remind you of this theme from time to time.

I asked about father and mother and she said: "They don't get on well together. My parents were never happy together; there's father away being a teacher, shut up in his own little world. There was a phase when I was 14 and my sister 15 when we were jealous of each other relative to *mother*. I was surprised when this turned up, but apart from this short phase I have not had the sort of feelings about mother or any-one that would make me jealous. My sister, on the other hand, has always been of a jealous nature. In a way I gave my sister to father; she can confide in him about sexual matters in a way I would never do. When we were children we did not know that father and mother were at loggerheads, although there is an early remark of mine which indicates that I may have known; it was when I was 9: my sister asked mother about her and father, and I remember I said: 'No don't!'—I didn't want mother to answer. I felt desperate because I knew that she would have to say that things were not good between her and father. I am glad always to be alive, and especially glad at times. On the other hand I am rather cynical in my way of dealing with life. I and my sister have always known the facts of life. I went to school satisfactorily till six, and then I went to a school where I was *really* happy and this school I still have an affection for, but I got fed up with it. I became unhappy *but I was basically happy, as I always am*. Eventually school became a nuisance and I went to a crammers. Here I found a relaxed atmosphere. The great thing is that its co-education and 50 per cent of the students are foreign. You are responsible for yourself at this school. Some girls don't know how to use this emancipation, but it suits me. I didn't get on at all with A levels because I don't believe in the stuff. The work is futile. Or perhaps I'm lazy, I don't like working hard. I like the *idea* of work, and in phases I can work hard. I have girl friends and several boys and am liked *in a way*. My sister, on the other hand, was never popular. This is something which has always distinguished us from each other. My sister had to go straight to emotional relationships because of having no *friendships,* and when she discovered heterosexuality she plugged herself as attractive, and let rip. Now she is engaged, and will probably get married quite soon, as I said before. Perhaps the man isn't unsuitable but he's foreign."

(By her tone she seemed to indicate that she linked foreign with beyond the pale. You'd agree, wouldn't you, that in the unconscious "foreign" signifies incest, and at the same time the opposite extreme to incest, exogamy.)

> "I have always been popular. What really worries me is that I've no real moral standards. I can't feel that this or that is wrong. I'll tell you what I mean. I've got a friend who is very happy at home, unlike me, and she got involved with a foreigner who is quite sweet but who works rather fast, and she fended him off; she said about this: 'Well I don't know; it would break mother's heart.' It must be wonderful to have something like that that you can say which tells you where you are . . . you see I really love my mother very deeply but I don't want any intimacy and I don't want any emotional entanglement. That's why I wanted an older brother who could be a mother to me without being a mother; he could have offered me a shoulder to cry on; but I would never cry on my mother's shoulder. You see I get really fond of people like mother but I don't get emotionally churned up. There's my sister feeling terribly guilty. I don't feel guilty about anything. My sister says: 'Mother doesn't understand.' My mother doesn't get my hostility because she fits in with what I need." Jane went on talking about herself, saying that she couldn't be demonstrative, that she really loved her mother deeply: "You see I am trying to be an individual, yes, to establish my own identity; and while I am doing that I can't afford to take on mother's worries. You see, mother's nearly all the time in tears, although she's really a very controlled person. She would never try to make me take on her worries; but I easily could, and *then I wouldn't make it* . . . Nowadays I seem to be a bit tired all the time."

The full significance of this conflict in relation to the mother became more evident as this interview and the next interview progressed.

> We talked a little about dreams and the imagination and she then eagerly told me about her early childhood games with her sister. She said: "My sister and I were catalysts for each other. In all kinds of mediums we played together and had worlds of our own which we shared, and there really was a marvelous imaginative experience in all this. The awful thing was when all this stopped. It stopped when I was 13; really because of moving from the house where we all lived and where father lives now. All these games were so intimately

mixed up with the house that they could not be re-established any-where else."

Jane then went on to talk about "the glorious irresponsibility of childhood." She said about childhood: "You see a cat and you are with it; it's a subject, not an object."

I said: "It's as if you were living in a world of subjective objects."

And she said: "That's a good way of putting it. That's why I write poetry. That's the sort of thing that's the foundation of poetry. Of course (she added) it's only an idle theory of mine, but that's how it seems, and this explains why it's men who write poetry more than girls. With girls so much gets caught up in looking after children or having babies and then the imaginative life and the irresponsibility goes over to the children. I kept a diary but now I only write down things that I feel in poems; in poetry something crystallises out."

We compared this with autobiography which she said she felt be-longed to a later age. She said: "There is an affinity between old age and childhood." (Here she looked at me rather pointedly whilst speaking.) "I don't show my poems to anybody because although I am fond of each poem for a little while I soon lose interest in it. I am not interested in the question: are the poems really good or not?—that is to say, would other people think them good?"

I asked her about dreams and this led on to the subject of day-dreaming and abstracting herself from the world. Obviously there had been a great deal of this, which she now did alone instead of in the games with her sister. She said: "After O levels I went to an art school but I fiddled it. I have an ability to draw and I could do better than I have done, but I won't. Sometimes I might draw a figure which you can see by its position is the figure of a *depressed person*. That may be done as a picture of someone but it really is *myself*. But the funny thing is that there's a joie de vivre always present in me, however depressed I am. There seem to be some inner resources so that I never *have to do* things; others seem to be always *having* to do something or other; but that's not me. On the other hand I have some things that make people think I am eccentric; I seem to have to say things out, like having to be natural. I'm not really an eccentric but people think I'm odd."

I asked her about the subject of a façade and she took this up. She said: "I'm really very introspective. I live on a sub-level. When I'm with people it's only as I feel they exist. I've met about five or six people in my life who have an effect on me that I know when I'm in the same room with them that they are slightly off. One was an aunt who became schizophrenic and suicidal, which showed me that I am very sensitive to something in people which has to do with madness. The thing is I feel what's underneath the surface more than I do what is on the surface. You see I can't play with a facade. The result is that with boys I find myself leaping in and out of bed with them because I can't play about with a barrier or façade. I can't feel that it's cheap to leap in and out of bed with boys. *I simply can't get a sense of low degradation.* There's no deceit possible, or hypocrisy. On the other hand I tell lies and I don't know why."

Here she said: "By the way, it's quite safe, isn't it?—you won't tell of this to mother?"

And I said: "Yes, I suppose I'm a subjective object; it's no more dangerous than talking to yourself."

She accepted this very easily. I went on taking notes, she not seeming to mind this at all.

You will see that Jane was giving a picture of an affinity with each psychiatric abnormality in turn. She knew about melancholia, she was at one with schizophrenia, and she played about with all the schizoid defences such as depersonalisation, derealisation, splitting; she accepted a division into a true self and a false self, and she had thought-disorders. There was trouble in the intermediate area of transitional phenomena, the place where sparks fly in moments of intimacy between persons. She had a more than nodding acquaintance with suspicion and the paranoid trends. In the psycho-neurotic area she was in touch with homosexuality (as would appear later), and she now went on to show her antisocial tendency related to deprivation.

I asked her about stealing, and she said: "Well, only once when I was 7, I had a period in which I was constantly taking pennies or 3d, anything of that nature that was lying about the house. I have always felt extremely guilty about this and I've never told anyone at all. It's really very silly because it's so slight."

Here I made an interpretation. I spoke to her about the difficulty that she really does not know why she stole these pennies; in other words she was *under a compulsion,* and she was very interested in this. She said:

"I know that children steal when they have been deprived of something or other but I've never thought of this before, that of course the trouble is that I *had* to steal and I didn't know why, and it's just like that with lying."

(You see she's read all the literature and she knows all the things that belong to this age, but intellectually).

"You see it's pathetically easy to deceive people and I'm a wonderful actress: I don't mean that I could act on the stage, but once I get caught up in a deceit I can carry it through so well that no one can know. The thing is, it's so often compulsive and meaningless. For instance somebody asked me what I was going to London for, and it was quite unnecessary for me to tell a lie, but I quickly found myself saying that as my friend has had (giving the name of a rare and exotic illness) I had to go and see a doctor to know if I was all right in this respect. Of course I can see that if I had said I was to see a psychiatrist then this would bring the whole thing into discussion and it would be a public affair. There was a compulsion to tell a lie and I did it quickly and easily."

There was a pause of the stock-taking variety.

"What really worries me about myself is that I've got no soul-mate. I can't pretend that there's more than there is in anyone or in anything or in any situation. I am as fond of sex as the next girl, but it's different with me because I have to look for a boy who will take on the sexual relationship with no strings attached. It must be absolutely understood that it's going to end in a few days. This of course eliminates any boy who would be suitable for marrying. There seems to be no way of being certain of *one* boy or of knowing that you want to *marry* anyone."

This led on to a conversation on the subject of difficulties between parents. She said: "Father is himself a deprived person."

(She followed this up in detail which I'm not giving because I wish to keep the case unrecognisable. All along I think you can see evidence of the insight that belongs to this age of development.)

I then spoke to her about her very great need for a father-figure or even for an older brother. She said that she hadn't even got a cousin that she could use. "I have an uncle, but he is not really happy with *his* wife."

It turned out that she feels she has absolutely no responsible older male person to whom she can turn.

I said "You are therefore a father-deprived person," and we ended the first interview with as clear as possible a statement on this matter.

Jane went away in a very relaxed state and seeming to be friendly with her mother whom she collected from the waiting-room.

She wrote asking to see me again after two months had lapsed.

Most of us find, I think, that it suits the adolescent if we are willing to work on an "on demand" basis.

Second Consultation

This time Jane came on her own and I found her in the waiting-room reading. She was looking less spruced up and less of a set-piece; in fact, rather untidy. The "act" had been dropped, and instead Jane was plainly in a depressed mood. She was very easy throughout the interview, which lasted an hour and a quarter. I can only give a part of this interview.

I started by asking "How's mother?"

There was really no special need for me to do anything, but at the same time no special reason why I should not.

She said: "She's very tired; really I am her main worry. My sister is married now and so I suppose mother feels that I am the only thing left to make something of. I am all the time worried about mother. You see, she's the only one of the family that I am close with. At the same time whatever she does irritates me. She's about the most tolerant and understanding mother that you could think of having and she's very intelligent. *But I have to do everything to keep her at a distance.* I quarrel with her rather than let us get near to each other. Mother tries to help. She comes and sits in my room; she doesn't mind if nobody talks; but all the time I am tense. I absolutely trust her. I know she won't push for anything. I absolutely hate to hurt mother but I am wounding her the whole time."

How many mothers have been in this position, and puzzled! Later she and I returned to this theme and made an attempt to undo some of the rigidity of this defence.

I asked her about her own life and she said: "Oh yes, it's all right superficially. I have crowds of friends. I can say that life is both good and lousy."

I said: "Are you working?" and she replied: "I do absolutely nothing. Our flat's not a home. *No one lives anywhere.* The trouble for mother is that she can't make a home. We are not a family. This distresses mother all the time. I suppose she sees herself as going on being lonely all the time—for ever. The trouble is, mother always has ideas that she *may* be able to bring father out of himself and back to a life with the family but it's absolutely hopeless and I don't know why she can't see it."

Another long pause.

"I don't talk to my sister now; after she got married she snubbed me and that was the end of it. My sister says she loves me but she has always been jealous of me and she hates me."

It was evident, however, from the way she said this, that something was retained of a positive relationship to the sister. At a later interview she reported her great fondness for her brother-in-law, and a complete rapprochement.

I said: "Why is your sister jealous of you?"

Jane replied: "Well, because I have always had an easy-going nature and she has always been difficult."

(This was a first effort to explain. Soon this develops into the main theme.)

"Mother said I was to be sure and ask you why I am tired all the time." (In other words, to report depression.)

After a talk about her doctor which I must omit, although it contained significant details, I made a further comment in the form of a question: "Are you perhaps defending yourself against a sexual element in your relationship with your mother?"

You will see that I was attempting to deal with Jane's rigid defences in her relationship to her mother, and her conflicting feelings towards her sister. This idea of a defence against homosexuality made sense to her, and she discussed this so easily that I quickly realised that the main difficulty did *not* lie *here* where I had expected to find it. She said that she realised that her "repulsion of all contact with her mother was the negative of the sexual element in the relationship." This took her back to the age of 7, a time of particular difficulty in her relationship with her mother and a time therefore of special defence against the sexual element.

She said: "I don't know whether mother told you what I was like as a small child. My sister of course was always screaming and active, but I was withdrawn and quiet and made no noise. I did a great deal of sulking and hiding in cupboards. The trouble always is this, that if mother has only me I may get caught up in something, so that although my sister and I hate each other it is a great relief if my sister is around. At any rate there are then two of us."

Here she implied the tremendous need which might arise out of the mother's unhappiness and loneliness. There was an element here, however, that I did not understand, and the explanation only came after the further development of the theme of her relationship with her sister. In other words, we wanted new light on the defence against intimacy with the mother.

> After discussing her relationship with her mother in some detail Jane said: "Mother has a vision of loneliness and I don't want to be involved in it. Mother feels real and sees people as individuals and of course there is always a sexual element where there are feelings."
>
> Jane said how she herself hated to be close to anyone in her family. She had to sleep in the room next to her mother and she could hear her mother breathing and this was hateful because it was too close. And she then went on to repeat how really lucky she was in the fact that her mother was an exceptionally intelligent and understanding person, and emphasising also her distress at having to wound her mother all the time.
>
> She said: "Mother tries to help but I can't let her. I come home at 4 A.M. and she knows perfectly well I've been sleeping with a man but she never interferes in any way at all."
>
> Jane put in a word here to suggest that she slept with a man and came home late to wound her mother as much as to have a man. The general trend of the conversation here had to do with Jane's ability to manage her own affairs.
>
> She said: "The thing is I can't stand social or political pressures and I hate competition. If really left to myself I can manage *because of something that goes on inside myself.*"

She was describing her own ego-organisation and her capacity to believe in something in herself, and therefore in the world too. It was this which gave me confidence in my relationship to her and enabled me to lean back on her own processes and overcome her reticence. Some people are too ill and one knows one can't do that with them.

> We went on to talk about Jane's own position in regard to homosexuality; for instance, a girl of 14 took to her, so she fostered her. Obviously the girl had a pash on Jane. They did not meet for a bit and then she bumped into the girl at a party. They talked and she found herself talking in a horrid way, implying that the girl had no significance. Jane said: "I kicked myself while talking in this way. Afterwards I felt certain that the girl was now antagonistic to me and I translated something that happened in these terms. Apparently the girl seemed to cross the road to avoid meeting me. Nevertheless I found that this was a *delusion,* because the girl still continued with

her passion." She added: "Younger girls are always having crushes on me, and small boys too."

Here was Jane's acquaintance with the paranoiac's ideas of reference, and with the association of all this with homosexuality.

She then gave me a picture of life in a girls' school. She said: "Automatically the girls separate off into boys and girls, and I quickly became a boy in this grouping process." She then described the relationships between the girls, how futile things go on at the point of contact, things which neither of the two girls would approve of, things that are said and things done. Together we worked out that this had to do with *keeping the two girls essentially separate.* I got a picture here of techniques for indefinite postponement rather than for coming to grips in a relationship. Jane went on to describe actual boys who were mad to get into bed with girls, not because they wanted sex or because they liked the girls. For them it was a technique for dealing with the relationship; the boy and the girl each really wanting to remain intact and isolated. In this way, which was Jane's own way, we approached the main theme, the conflict underlying Jane's ambivalence towards her sister and her defence against intimacy with her mother.

There was a special importance to her of this merging and defence against merging. We did not get to this immediately. In other words, the physical sexual act kept the two personalities free from merging and other mechanisms that might threaten the intactness of the individual. She was looking out for and finding the kind of boy who gets into bed; they have a sexual relationship and then they part. They've met and separated and neither has affected the other, and each time a danger has been averted. Each one has retained his and her own individuality. So here again is a subject which is specially important to Jane but also belongs to every adolescent. Here followed an account of the origin of Jane's present depression in a failed attempt to get into contact with father. I must leave this out, but in the course of this she said: "Mother was all the time trying to help, but it was impossible for her to do anything at all except irritate me. I said to mother: '*Don't trust me*'; *but really, you know, I am trustworthy.* I know what is happening. I know I won't go off the rails, and of course I also know that there is always this histrionics on top of everything else, like exaggerating to spite someone, or compete with my sister."

So then followed for me what was the surprising piece of insight which concerned Jane's relationship with her sister, whom she loves and hates. I shall end with the report of this detail, which cleared up some of the mystery in her relationship with her mother. (It was difficult for me to take notes as it always is at the significant moments of an interview. I guess most people in this room know this).

I think I said: "So it turns out that the withdrawn states and the sulkiness are your insurance policy." She agreed to this, but there was obviously something more complicated that had to be stated. We talked about the relationship to her sister and how something persisted from the early years in the relationship to her sister and how it was at present in a negative phase. I spoke about the very rich relationship she had had with her sister in the childhood games and she took up this matter.

(You will see that I was still trying to get at the *homosexuality in the relationship*—a false line of research as it turned out.)

Jane was not unwilling to see homosexuality, and she had already dealt quite freely with the homosexual idea in relation to her mother. But she said that this was not what happened between her and her sister. The relationship with her sister in these games was that *their personalities merged*. They were two aspects of the same person, she said. She then went over to the history of the development of the relationship. Here was her sister, a screaming active child who absolutely hated Jane's birth when she was 14 months old. The reaction of the two sisters was not identical, of course.

(At that time of growing up they were, of course, always at different ages, but here we are dealing with a specific thing—14 months is not usually old enough for a total reaction of a child to the birth of a new baby. There's a lot of difference between 14 months and 16 or 17 months, isn't there? Identification with the mother and other mechanisms are not fully developed.)

"My sister hated me, and also took me over as an aspect of herself. In response to this I allowed myself to be taken over as an aspect of her and alternatively developed a technique for withdrawal. The games therefore were between two aspects of one person, and these two aspects were composed of the halves of each of us. My sister's half was the dominating one."

In spite of the pathology of all this the extreme richness of the mutual play could never be lost, although for the time being it is wasted because these two sisters are now separate; each is trying to establish a total unit self. Possibly one day there will be a re-uniting in some way or other which will be acceptable.

The way the patient gave it to me was clear enough, but I haven't given it to you clearly. There was herself and half of herself was involved in her sister. That was her sister's way because of her inability to have a mature relationship to this idea of a new baby coming. So herself and her sister were like one whole person; but Jane was left with a half which is the most important part of her which was to spend most of its life in cupboards and withdrawn. Being withdrawn was what she came to me for. And her sister had her other half which repudiated the idea of a sister and was very extrovert in temperament and led a life that had to be separate from the sister's and had to deny the importance of Jane. The sisters had to separate from each other to establish themselves as unit selves.

> Following on from this piece of insight Jane was able to describe a further very important detail of her trouble. She enumerated all the schizophrenia that existed on both sides of the family. She said that what bothered her in her illness was that there were two of herself; one was outside and looking at the other one that was withdrawn and being looked at. This seemed to be the important thing that Jane came to tell me although she did not know at all when she came what it was that she was coming to tell me.

Here I made another interpretation, taking up what I had been told. I was able to go over the relationship to her sister as she had described it. Outside the merging there existed both the withdrawn half of Jane and the extrovert half of the sister.

> I said that I could see that the trouble between herself and her mother was not only this defence against homosexuality and against getting involved in mother's essential distress and loneliness. I could see that there was a worse danger felt by Jane that if she made use of her mother then there would be from Jane's end a repetition of the merged relationship of the type that had had so much danger and so much positive in it in relation to the sister. In other words she feared lest the mother would take over the sister's place in this merging for this would start up again the abnormal state of affairs which was really, historically, based on the sister's hate and Jane's adaptation to her sister's hate. Jane's hope lay in an evolution out of the withdrawn state but this meant that she would have to tolerate feeling split and have to tolerate holding on to the idea that both the observer and the observed in this split added up to her unit self.

Before relating to the mother she must achieve a unit self or identity.

All this made sense to Jane because it was complex and it was true: any simplification couldn't have made sense at all: and we then went on to a businesslike discussion of the way to deal with Mother.

So a year has passed now since these first two of the five "on demand" interviews, and I can report good progress, neither forced forward nor held back. I am still being used as a brother-mother.

Conclusion

I hope you will have got from this case description something of what I got in the actual experience. I felt very close to this adolescent girl's sensitivity and her live contact with her primitive mechanisms and near-illness states. There is practically no psychiatric disorder that is not touched upon, and yet I think this girl is healthy. I doubt whether she will be so interesting, or so painfully near the raw truth when she is 25. At 17 she is a remarkable and awkward young person.

Incidentally, the process of the psychotherapeutic consultation carried Jane and me on to this unexpected insight into the aetiology of her painful split in her relationship to her sister, and this gave an explanation of the girl's fear of involvement with her beloved and lonely mother. The momentum of the girl's reaction to the psychotherapeutic situation took us through to an aetiologically significant factor, and it is this that I especially wish to stress in presenting this clinical detail, just the picture of one girl.

43

A Child Psychiatry Case Illustrating Delayed Reaction to Loss

Written for a collection of essays in memory of Marie Bonaparte, 1965[1]

On his eleventh birthday Patrick suffered the loss of his father by drowning. The way in which he and his mother needed and used professional help illustrates the function of the psycho-analyst in child psychiatry.

In the course of one year Patrick was given ten interviews and his mother four, and during the four years since the tragedy occurred I have kept in touch, by telephone conversations with the mother, with the boy's clinical state as well as with the mother's management of her son and of herself. The mother started with very little understanding of psychology and with considerable hostility to psychiatrists, and she gradually developed the qualities and insight that were needed. The part she was to play was, in effect, the mental nursing of Patrick during his breakdown. She was very much encouraged by being able to undertake this heavy task and by succeeding in it.

Family

The father had a practice in one of the professions. He had achieved considerable success and had very good prospects. Together they had a large circle of friends.

There were two children of the marriage, a boy at university and Patrick, who was a boarder at a well-known preparatory school. The family had a town house in London and a holiday cottage on an island off the coast. It was in the sea near the holiday cottage that the father was drowned when sailing with Patrick on the day after his eleventh birthday.

1. *Drives, Affects, Behavior: Essays in Memory of Marie Bonaparte*, vol. 2, ed. Max Schur (New York: International Universities Press, 1965).

The Evolution of the Psychiatrist's Contact with the Case

The evolution of the case is given in detail and as accurately as possible because this case illustrates certain features of child psychiatry casework which I consider to be vitally important.

Whenever possible I get at the history of a case by means of psycho-therapeutic interviews *with the child*. The history gathered in this way contains the vital elements, and it is of no matter if in certain aspects the history taken in this way proves to be incorrect. The history taken in this way evolves itself, according to the child's capacity to tolerate the facts. There is a minimum of questioning for the sake of tidiness or for the sake of filling in gaps. Incidentally, the diagnosis reveals itself at the same time. By this method one is able to assess the degree of integration of the child's personality, the child's capacity for holding conflicts and strain, the child's defences both in their strength and in their kind, and one can make an assessment of the family and general environmental reliability or unreliability; and, in certain cases, one may discover or pinpoint continuous or continuing environmental insults.

The principles enunciated here are the same as those that characterise a psycho-analytic treatment. The difference between psycho-analysis and child psychiatry is chiefly that in the former one tries to get the chance to do as much as possible (and the psycho-analyst likes to have five or more sessions a week), whereas in the latter one asks: how little need one do? What is lost by doing as little as possible is balanced by an immense gain, since in child psychiatry one has access to a vast number of cases for which (as in the present case) psycho-analysis is not a practical proposition. To my surprise, I find that the child psychiatry case has much to teach the psycho-analyst, though the debt is chiefly in the other direction.

First Contact

A woman (who turned out to be Patrick's mother) telephoned out of the blue to say she had reluctantly decided to take the risk of consulting someone about her son, who was at a prep school, and she had been told by a friend that I was probably not as dangerous as most of my kind. I certainly could not have foretold at this initial stage that she would prove capable of seeing her son through a serious illness.

I was told that the father had been drowned in a sailing accident, that Patrick had been to some extent responsible for the tragedy, and that she, the mother, and the older son, were still very disturbed and that the effect on Patrick had been complex. The clinical evidence of disturbance in Patrick had been delayed and it now seemed desirable that someone should investigate. Patrick had always been devoted to his mother, and since the accident had become (what she called) emotional.

In this brief account of a long telephone conversation I have not attempted to reproduce the mother's rush of words or her skepticism in regard to psychiatric services.

First Interview with Patrick (two months after this telephone conversation)

Patrick was brought by his mother. I found him to be of slight build, with a large head. He was obviously intelligent and alert and likable. I gave him the whole time of the interview (two hours). There was no point in the interview at which the relationship between him and me was difficult. Only during the most tense part of the consultation was it impossible for me to take notes. The following account was written after the interview.

Patrick said he was not doing very well at school, but he "liked intellectual effort." We were seated at a low round table with paper and pencils provided, and we started with the Squiggle Game. (In this I make a squiggle for him to turn into something, and then he makes one for me to do something with.)

1. He made mine into an elephant.
2. He made his own into "a Henry Moore abstract." Here he showed that he was in contact with modern art and later it became clear that this is something which belongs to his relationship to his mother. She takes an active part in keeping him well informed in the art world, which has been important to him since the age of five years. It also shows his sense of humour, which is important prognostically. It shows his toleration of madness and of mutilation and of the macabre. It might be said that it also shows that he has talent as an artist, but this comes out more clearly in a later drawing. His choosing to turn his squiggle into an abstract was related to the danger, very real in his case, that because of his very good intellectual capacity he would escape from emotional tensions into compulsive intellectualis-

ation; and because of paranoid fears, which later became evident, there could be a basis here for an organised system of thought.

3. I turned his squiggle into two figures which he called "mother holding a baby." I did not know at the time that here was already an indication of his main therapeutic need.

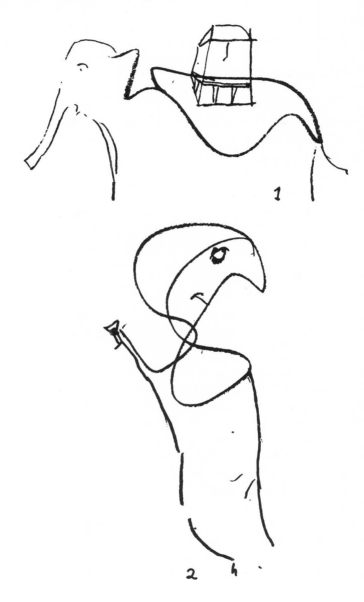

4. He turned mine into an artistic production. It was done quickly and he knew exactly what he was doing. He said it was a tree at F. I did not know at that time that F. was the site of the tragedy, but in this drawing there was already incorporated his drive to cope with the problem surrounding his father's death.

5. This is his drawing, done at my request, of the holiday island, with F. shown.

6. He turned his own into "a mother scolding a child," and here one might see something of his wish to be punished by the mother.

7. He turned mine into Droopy.

8. I made his into some kind of a comical girl figure.

9. This was important. He made my squiggle into a sculpture of a rattlesnake. "It might have been by a modern artist," he said. In this case he took hold of a squiggle with all its madness and incontinence

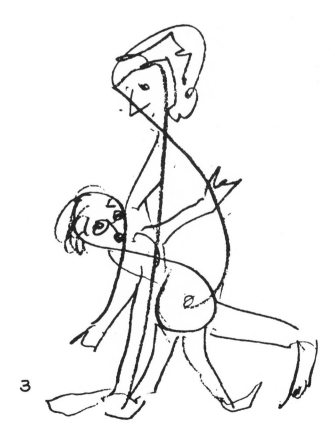

3

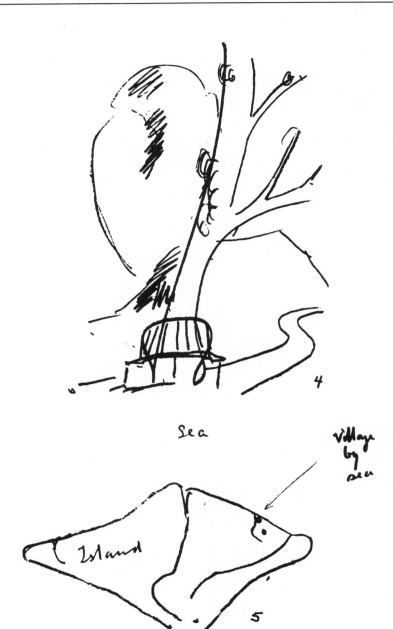

4

Sea

Village
by
sea

Island

5

and turned it into a work of art, in this way gaining control of impulse that threatens to get out of control.

10. In the next I turned his into some kind of a weird hand, and he said it might be by Picasso. This led to a discussion of Picasso in which he displayed his knowledge of Picasso in a way that sounded a little precocious. We agreed that the recent Picasso exhibition at the Tate Gallery was very interesting. He had been twice to it. He said he liked Picasso best in the "pink" and "blue" period and seemed to know what this meant, but I was aware that he was talking language which belonged to his discussion of these matters with his mother.

11. This was rather a surprising picture. He made my squiggle into

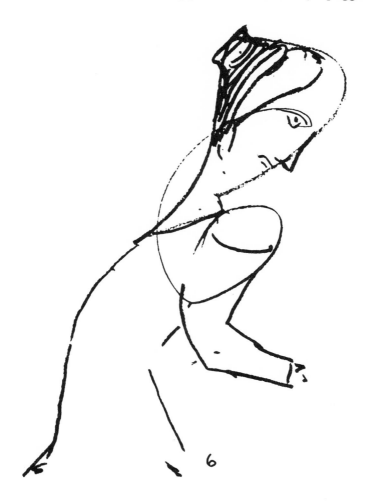

a person who slipped into some dog's food. There is a lot of life in the picture, but I was not able to find out why this idea had turned up. I would think he was mocking me or perhaps all men.

He then started talking, and drawing became less important. What we talked about included the following:

In the first term at school he had had a dream. He had been ill with some kind of epidemic two nights before half-term, which he said is "an exciting time for a new bug." In the dream the Matron told him to get up and go to the hall where the tramps are fed. The Matron

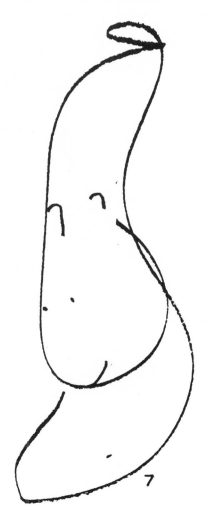

shouted: "Is everyone here?" There were fifteen *but one was missing;* nobody knew that one was missing. It was weird in some way because there was no extra person. And then there was a church with no altar, and a shadow where the altar had been.

The rest had to do with a baby jumping up and down, of which he drew a picture (no. 12). The baby was screaming, going up and down on the mattress. He said that the baby was about 18 months old. I asked him whether he had known babies and he said: "About three." It seemed, however, that he was referring in the dream to his own infancy. This dream remained obscure, but its meaning became elucidated in the fourth interview, four weeks later. It was thought that

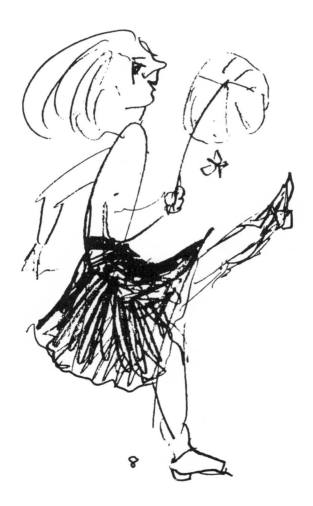

there was a reference to the dead father in the one person missing.

At this stage I did not know that he had not been told at once about his father's death.

13. Here is his drawing of the church with a shadow instead of an altar.

I asked: "What would be a nice dream?" He said quickly: "Bliss, being cared for. I know I want this."

When I put the question he said he knew what depression was like, especially since father's death. He had a love of his father, but he did

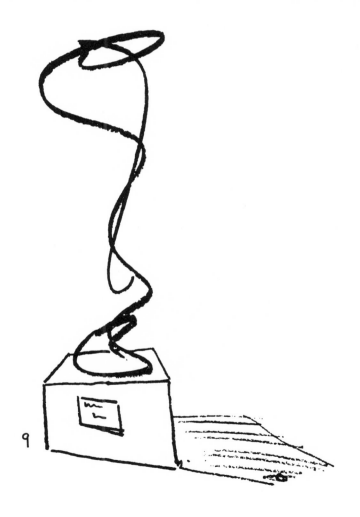

not see him very much. "My father was very kind. But the fact is that mother and father were constantly under tension." He went on to talk about what he had observed: "I was the link that joined them; I tried to help. To father it was outrageous to prearrange anything. This was one of his faults. Mother would therefore complain. They were really very suited to each other, but over little things they would begin to get across each other, and the tension would built up over and over again, and the only solution to this was for me to bring them together. Father was very much overworked. He may not have been very happy. It was a great strain to him to come home tired and then for his wife

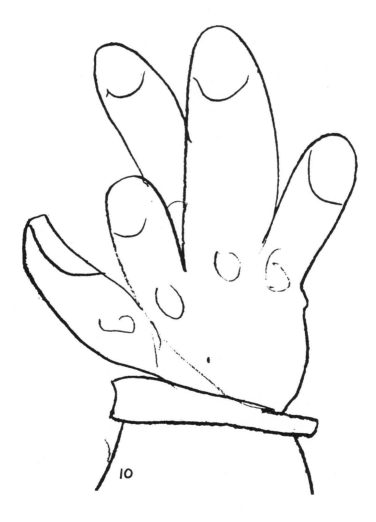

10

to fail him." In all this he showed an unusual degree of insight.[2]

The rest of this long and astonishing interview consisted in our going over in great detail the episode in which his father died. He said that his father "may have committed suicide"[3] or perhaps it was his own (Patrick's) fault; it was impossible to know. "After a long time in the water one began to fight for oneself." Patrick had a life belt and

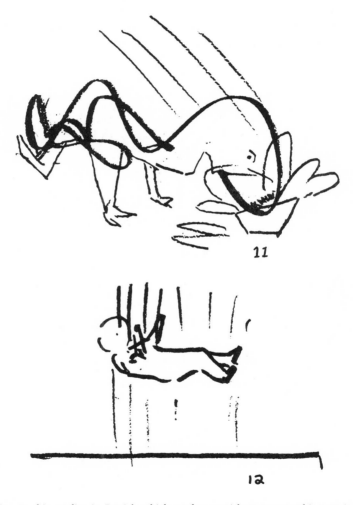

11

12

2. It was this quality in Patrick which made me wish to present this case in Marie Bonaparte's book, because we have clear evidence of the deep insight that was Marie Bonaparte's when she was at the latency stage; see *Five Copy-Books* (London: Imago, 1950).—D.W.W.

3. There is good evidence that neither parent was in fact suicidal.—D.W.W.

the father had none. They were nearly both drowned, but sometime after the father had sunk, just near dark, Patrick was rescued by chance. For some time he did not realise that his father was dead, and at first he was told that he was in the hospital. Then Patrick said that if his father had lived, he thinks his mother would have committed suicide. "The tension between the two was so great that it was not possible to think of them going on without one of them dying." There was therefore a feeling of relief, and he indicated that he felt very guilty about this. (It will be understood that this is not to be taken as an objective and final picture of the parental relationship. It was true, however, for Patrick.)

At the end he dealt with the very great fears he had had from early childhood. He described his great fear associated with hallucinations both visual and auditory, and *he insisted that his illness, if he was ill, antedated the tragedy.*

14. This is a drawing of Patrick's home with the various places marked in which persecutory male figures appear. The principal danger area was in the lavatory, and there was only one spot for him to use when urinating if he would avoid persecutory hallucinations.

There was a quality about this phobic system that seemed to be-

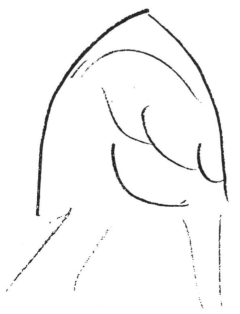

13

long more naturally to an emotional age of 4 rather than to 11 years, with phobias closely linked with hallucinations. The whole matter was discussed in terms of dream life spilling over into the waking life, and along with this the idea of the tragedy as a hallucination and yet real. Patrick described panic as being in a nightmare when awake. The hallucinations he feels are ghosts of a returning vengeful man, but they antedate the tragedy.

It will be noted that a drawing that came with a powerful drive from the unconscious (no. 12) had no meaning for him. I did nothing about it, though it seemed to me to convey a manic defence quality. This proved to be the most significant of the drawings, but I had to wait till the fourth interview (about a month later) to gain a precise understanding of it.

The accent in this interview was on the drowning incident, remembered and described in a rather detached way. After two hours we both had had enough. Probably we both knew there was much more to be done, but we did not say so to each other. The effect on Patrick was that he gained confidence in me, and the effect on myself was that I now knew a good deal about him from inside him.

From this first interview I got a glimpse of the personality and character of the patient. In addition, I learned:

1. Patrick was beginning to feel guilty about the father's death.

2. He did not yet feel sad.

3. He felt threatened by the arrival of feelings that had been so long delayed.

4. He had a fear of illness, and there was a basis for this in the hidden illness dating from early years with a liability to hallucinosis.

5. There was an indication of an important unknown factor represented by the unexplained bouncing baby drawing.

6. At school he had had undefined illnesses for which he had

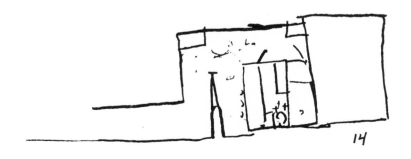

14

sought the Matron's care. Later I found that he had produced his symptoms deliberately, not knowing how else to get the special and personal care that he needed. This had taken place in the autumn when he was supposedly quite happy and well, and "unaffected by his father's death."

7. There was a strong indication that Patrick had a belief in the existence of reliable persons, and I noted that this faith of his could be used, if necessary, for therapeutic purposes: in the breaking down of his defences and a regressive re-living of his experiences. In such a case he would need a high degree of dependence on someone. In fact I was able to use the mother, who in spite of giving a neurotic impression proved herself to be able to act as Patrick's mental nurse. The good dream: "Bliss, to be cared for; I know I want this" was the indication which I later used as a pointer for management. I had nothing to tell me at this stage whether the mother could or could not meet his need (to be cared for); in fact, it seemed that she might be the worst person rather than the best.

Patrick returned to boarding school.

The next event was an emergency call from the mother and from Patrick: Would I see him immediately? Patrick had run away from school, and had taken the train home laden with Latin books. He said he had to get home to work at Latin, since he was not able to work at school and he was letting the school down. He had made a terrific effort to learn Latin all the way in the train, and at home he retired to bed to continue the intellectual effort. It will be noted that he was completely unable to ask for help on account of the threat of mental breakdown.

Second Interview with Patrick (two weeks after the first)

This was a comparatively uneventful interview. Patrick said that he had thought of running away in the autumn term. The thing was that a boy had made an elementary mistake and a master had said of this boy that he was fit to be caned and that he was not fit to be in the school. Patrick had reacted strongly to this minor incident. He had made himself sick, and had gone to the sickroom. Generally he displayed a paranoid disposition with hypersensitivity to any idea of punishment or censure. His housemaster, ordinarily a benign figure in his life, had become a threat.

Clinically Patrick had become a psychiatrically ill person, with no insight, and with paranoid-type anxieties.

After a quarter of an hour he dropped the rationalisation that it was fear of failure in Latin that had brought him, and he said openly that it was the first interview and what he got from it that had brought him back, *though he had not known this till he actually came to see me.* He described how the faint word of disapproval on the part of the schoolmaster linked up with hallucinated voices. He did not fear being actually punished, because being punished was kept separate in his mind from the hallucinated voices.

I advised that he should stay at home over the week-end, and arranged this with the school. The staff told me they considered Patrick's mother was *too disturbed to be good for him,* but I insisted that he should stay at home.

Third Interview with Patrick (four days later)

On a Sunday Patrick was due to go back to school. He locked himself in the bathroom and would not come out, and would not see me. He was coaxed out and brought to see me as an emergency. I had to lure him out of his brother's sports car.

This third interview was a very intense one, and I was not able to take notes. It was a communication in a deeper layer, in which Patrick told me a great deal about himself and his family, and at the end I said: "You are not going back to school, but you are going to your cottage on the island. *You are ill.* As long as you are ill you can stay with your mother, and I will tell your mother what to do. And I will deal with the school for you." The important thing was that I told him he was ill.

He made a last effort to protest, remembering all he had looked forward to in the summer term at school, especially painting, and then with a sigh of relief he accepted what I said.

Comment: He was now *officially ill.* This was the crucial moment in the management of the case. It could be said from this moment he started on a slow process of recovery. But the first jump forward clinically came after the next interview in which the unknown factor of the first interview became elucidated.

The school was helpful though skeptical. The headmaster came to London and visited Patrick, and it was arranged that Patrick could go back to the school when well again, and without being hurried or harried.

Fourth Interview with Patrick (three days later)

Patrick came alone. He said that he had come for a specific reason, which was that he now understood the bouncing baby drawing (no. 12).

Trying to get at the meaning of this unexpected drawing, he had been talking things over with his mother and she had told him the story of his behaviour at one and a half years when she had had to go away for "six weeks" for an operation. While his mother was away he had stayed with friends who were supposed to be suitable, but they got him more and more excited. His father visited every day. In this period Patrick had become overexcitable, seeming happy, and always laughing and jumping up and down. He said: "It was like the drawing, and when mother told me about it all I remembered the bars of the cot." When his mother came back from the hospital (he went on to tell me) he saw her in her car, and suddenly all the bounce went, and he got on to her lap and went straight to sleep. It is said that he slept for twenty-four hours, and that his mother had kept him with her all that time. (This was the mother's first experience of the mental nursing of Patrick, and she was just about to have a second.)

Patrick had been describing to me a real incident, the feeling of which he had remembered. It was a period of danger at one and a half years, of a crescendo of manic defence, which quickly turned into a depression at the mother's return. Evidently there had been a real danger at this time of a snapping of the thread of the continuity of his being. The mother had come back only just in time, and she knew she must let him sleep on her lap till he should wake.

Patrick told me all this with deep feeling, and went on to say: "You see, I have never been able to be quite sure of mother since, and this had made me stick to her; and this meant I kept her from father; and I had not much use for father myself."

In all this Patrick was describing the illness which *antedated* the tragedy in which the father died. Patrick felt at this stage that he had manoeuvered the whole episode, which of course might have ended happily, but which in fact ended in disaster. He said he really had expected his mother to be pleased when his father died, and the mother's unexpected grief had simply made him confused. He had not been able to react to the actual drowning episode (except for the psychosomatic disorders at school) until the first interview with me, that is, eight months after the tragedy.

Patrick went away from this interview *immensely relieved,* and his mother reported a marked clinical improvement which persisted and gradually led on to his recovery.

Patrick now became able to criticise his mother without losing his love for her. In his words: "Two days of her, fine! Two plus, ghastly!"

Incidentally, describing an art exhibition that he went to with a friend, he said: "Pictures and painting, that's why I'm alive." He could now tell me: "Depression means that the world comes to an end."

Regression as a Feature in the Clinical State

There now started up an indefinite period of regression. He turned into a boy of 4, going everywhere with his mother and holding her hand. Nobody knew how long this would last. Much of the time Patrick spent in the holiday cottage. There a stray cat conveniently had four kittens. Patrick seemed to be completely identified with this mother cat. Eventually he brought the kittens to London for me to see them and opened the zip-fastener of his bag in my room, whereupon four kittens jumped out and went all over the house.

The mother telephoned (three weeks later) to let me know she had had a letter handed to her, written by Patrick in a very childish hand, it said:

1. Do you love me?
2. Thank you very much.
3. Can I see Dr D.W.W. soon?

So a new visit was arranged for the next day.

Fifth Interview with Patrick

Patrick had had a dream, and he had been frightened the whole day. This dream was dreamed for the interview, and it is interesting that he knew he was liable to have this dream, so that he asked for the interview several days before he dreamed it. It was a long dream (no. 15), some of which I was able to take down.

The Dream

There was a church and the church had an altar (cf. previous dream of church with no altar). There were three boxes and it was generally understood that there were corpses in them. It was thought that the far one on the left was most likely to turn into a ghost, but actually it was the near one that became a ghost. It showed some signs of life and sat up. It had a waxy face and looked as if it had been drowned. Curiously enough this ghost was female. It was a girl, and in describing the girl he used the word "pristine." (It is rather characteristic of him to use a word like that.) He said it was ominous.

Some of the analysis of this dream was done in the course of the analysis of other dreams. In the end it turned out that he felt that this ghost was the ghost of his father, but of the female aspect of his father. He now said that the quarrels between his father and mother were between his mother's masculine self and his father's female self. In fact, as he said, he has not entirely lost a father because a father is still present in the mother.

The dream went on in rather a long-winded way. Roughly speaking, this concerned a woman and a school in the island. They arrived there with a school friend. There was something about the tradition in the service in the chapel. This is why the boxes were in front of the altar. The seniors knew what was in the boxes. Patrick was told

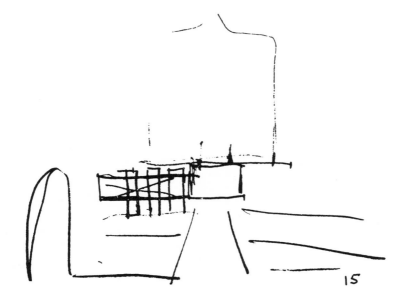

15

to go up to the altar and he suddenly knew that there were dead people in the boxes. After this there were two other episodes, each of which involved water. They went to watch a cricket match. There was something grey about it. He saw the school was going to collapse because of erosion by water, so 300 boys were drowned. Then his mother and the woman were with two boys. Water was rising higher and higher and lapping at the houses which started to crumble. The water covered his brother's sports car. The school friend seemed to get lost in the course of this, but he and his mother got away in the sports car, which by this time had reappeared.

From the associations spontaneously given it was clear about this dream that the fear of water was joined up with the general crumbling away of morale during the drowning episode. *In the telling of this dream Patrick reached very close to the actual agony of the drowning situation,* although in the first session when he told me about the drowning episode he had not been able to reach to deep affect.

He asked me two other things. The first had to do with his grandmother, who has had a stroke. He said: "Will you please tell me how either to alter her so that she is not so difficult with mother or else to make it possible for me to stand it when she is really quite impossible?" I told him that I had no way of altering either of these two things at all. There was nothing to do but to survive the awfulness of the relationship, particularly that existing between his mother and the grandmother, a relationship which had a history going right back to mother's early days and which, as Patrick said, very much accounted for mother's personal difficulties.

The other question had to do with Patrick's experiences during the last week of holiday. A boy with whom he had been camping provokingly pulled down the guy ropes: Patrick said: "All right, I'm going off" and the boy said: "I never did want you, *and my father never did want you either.*" This was very disturbing. He said he felt that other boys would be able to deal with this sort of thing in a friend, but for him his friend's behaviour produced a crisis. When his mother collected him in the car he broke down into crying. He emphasised that he felt that he ought not to be as upset as all this about such an incident. He gave all this as an example of the way he becomes upset and this joins up with the reaction to the criticism of another boy by the Latin master before he ran away from school. (If people are not friendly, then they quickly become associated in his mind with the latent paranoid potential.)

Comment: Patrick had now had time to get into touch with his guilt feelings and with the full agony of the crumbling morale, when he watched his father drown and when he himself nearly drowned too, but was rescued.

In dreaming this dream he showed that he had gained control over the episode, and in remembering and reporting it he had further displayed the strength of his ego-organisation; also in arranging to see me he had shown his capacity to believe in his mother, and in me as a father substitute, and in our working together as parent figures acting in unison.

Sixth Interview with Patrick (nine days later)

Patrick used this interview to go into details about his depression that was related to his mother's absences. This was related in a complex way to the demands made on his mother by her own mother. He also told me that the threat of depression had always been with him, at least since the episode at the age of one and a half.

First Interview with the Mother (a month later, five months after the initial telephone conversation)

This was the first personal interview I had with the mother. The main reason why I had not seen her was that the case had come my way when I had no vacancy whatever, and I had to be economical in my use of my own time. The following account is built up from notes made during the interview. At this time Patrick had regressed to a state of dependence and immaturity, in the care of herself and the people in the locality. Here the mother's basic reliability had shown up.

The mother first of all talked about her relationship with her own mother, whose old age exaggerated her usual demanding nature. She went on to speak about Patrick and his anxieties about work and school. It appears that during his period of regression he got permission to go to a local school when he felt like it. Then Patrick found a blind man teacher.

I insisted, and in doing so supported the mother in her own ideas, that whatever was done in the way of education at this stage had to be done only if Patrick really wanted it, and no tests whatever were to be allowed. The mother described how sensitive Patrick could be:

"One sarcastic word annihilates him. He easily feels the ground cut from under his feet." I explained that her job was to wait for spontaneous forward movement and in no way to expect anything of Patrick at this stage. The mother said that Patrick already understood that he was getting better, and he had said it in these words: "If I were still ill Dr W. would see me immediately, wouldn't he!" This was in reaction to my having to make him wait for an appointment, the first time that I made him wait since he had come under my care. I took great trouble during this consultation to support the mother's intuition, or what she called her "instincts," especially as she felt the lack of the support that she used to get from her husband in her management of the children. Already Patrick had begun to think about his position in the school on his return and to worry about the possibility of having to stay down in a lower class for a year while his friends would move up. (A great deal was said during this consultation which was important from the point of view of the mother but which could not be noted at the time.)

Seventh Interview with Patrick (a few days later)

Soon after this consultation a complication arose due to the school's failure to believe in Patrick's illness: examination papers arrived from the school and the result was almost a disaster. Patrick painfully gathered himself together out of his withdrawn state and attempted to meet the challenge. At the same time he lost all his capacity for relaxation and became seriously anxious and "persecuted." For the time being he emerged from his regressed and dependent state.

I arranged to see Patrick immediately and told him that I *absolutely prohibited* all tests and examinations, and that he should throw the papers away. Actually I said: "Put them in the lavatory and pull the plug," which was suitable in the circumstances, but when reported to the mother these words seemed to her to be dangerous. The mother had a parent's anxieties about school authorities, and she was afraid lest I had put these words in my letter to the headmaster. My perhaps clumsy interference in regard to the examination papers caused consternation in the school, and in any case it was not understandable to the headmaster and the housemaster, or to the school doctor, that this boy should be away from school leading a carefree life in the charge of his "neurotic" mother, without any father figure in his life, and completely neglecting his education. Yet this was exactly what he needed.

The immediate result of this consultation and of my making the decision about the test papers in a firm way was that Patrick regained his relaxed manner and returned quickly to a withdrawn and regressed state and became once more completely happy in the country cottage. In this way he did quite a lot of work with the examination papers without anxiety, and he called this "playing with them."

The First Anniversary of the Drowning Episode

It was important that the mother asked me to discuss with her by telephone the arrangements for the first anniversary. There had been a tendency to arrange for a sort of party, with a lot of people coming in, and the sort of feverish activity which would cover up the wound. This would have been a new version of the bouncing baby episode. With my help the mother and Patrick arranged to be alone together on the afternoon of this the first anniversary of the tragedy, which was also, of course, Patrick's birthday.

Afterward the mother described what happened. She said that Patrick looked excessively tired, and indeed they were both worn out. They sat together all the afternoon and heard the clock tick by. Thus the time passed. Then Patrick said: "Oh thank goodness that's over, it wasn't half as bad as I thought it was going to be." Immediately he seemed a much more healthy boy. His face "came undone." It could be said that the regression and withdrawn state changed at this point into a progression, a movement forward towards independence and participation.

Eighth Interview with Patrick (six months after the initial contact)

Patrick came and reported a dream he had had. He was talking with Sir X (a well-known writer and art critic and a friend of the family). There was emphasis on the word Sir. He was very nice. The "Sir" probably related this father figure to the idea of his housemaster. In this way Patrick was reporting to me the return of live father figures in his inner psychic reality. There was a good deal more in what Patrick talked about which had to do with men, and also about his older brother.

Ninth Interview with Patrick (two months later, a year and a half after the drowning episode)

This was more or less a social event in which we talked about a wide range of matters and Patrick drew a skyscraper which he called "Sunset over Rio" (no. 16).

Letter to School

Before this ninth interview I wrote to the school recommending Patrick's return, and I included in the letter the following paragraph:

> I want to emphasise that I do feel that Patrick has had quite a serious breakdown. I would say that he has now recovered and that probably he is in a better state than he was in before his father's death. Certain symptoms of early childhood have disappeared. There is a residual symptom which may give a little trouble and that has to do with his extreme sensitivity in regard to praise and blame. It may help those who are working with him to know that it is not the big things that worry Patrick; he is not really disturbed if somebody is very angry with him, because this is real and is related to the actual situation objectively perceived. What so easily upsets Patrick is just a very little blame or praise and the effect of these two can be quite

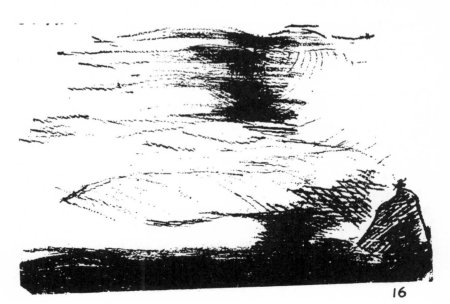

16

out of proportion to anything real. I think he knows about this and will try to stop himself from excessive reactions. If you have to be openly angry with Patrick, then this is not the sort of thing that I believe will cause trouble.

From the point of view of the school Patrick was in a satisfactory state. The staff soon forgot that he had been ill and probably found it difficult to believe that Patrick had in fact had a serious breakdown.

Second Interview with the Mother (after the last interview with Patrick)

This second interview with the mother was important, and was necessary because of the mother's anger with me, which needed to find expression. In the course of the interview it emerged that I had put a very big strain on her, and indeed I knew I had done this. I had in fact asked her *to postpone her own reaction to her husband's death* in order to nurse Patrick, and I had relied on her to take responsibility for him during his breakdown. Moreover, there were many ways, some undoubtedly reasonable, in which Patrick's mother found herself annoyed with me. I had left her "out on a limb." After thoroughly expressing her dissatisfaction with me and letting me know that the school was also angry with me she became very friendly and grateful. She then told me how helping Patrick had helped her herself.

Third Interview with the Mother (a week later)

I was able to check up with the mother on the details of her leaving Patrick when he was one and a half years old. It was *after* my first long interview with Patrick that she told Patrick about this. While she was telling him he became intensely interested and said: "I remember hitting a cot." The reason why the mother told him this story was that after the first consultation with me, when Patrick was very much changed by his contact with me, she began to think back.

She talked to a woman friend who told her that the place where Patrick had been sent when she went away from him at one and a half years was not a good place, and that she had known this at the time. She added: "It was a family in which everyone is pepped up, and children are trained vigorously." Recounting these details made the mother think of a still earlier incident. At five days Patrick was hospitalised for six weeks on account of vomiting, and his weight went down from 9 pounds to 6 pounds. At six weeks the mother took him home, whereupon "he put on weight like a bomb."

Fourth Interview with the Mother (six months later, two years after the husband's death)

The mother reported that Patrick had made good progress. He was top of his form at school (not a high form) and he was enjoying work; the school report was good. She said he was happier and sleeping well and his phobias, which he had had at home since he was a little boy, had dwindled to nothing. He had enjoyed his holidays, being always occupied in his own way, and he had stayed with a school friend in the cottage, which he got ready for his mother.

His insight is shown by the plans that he was making for the second anniversary of the tragedy. He found that he had arranged to go with friends to another island! When he realised the date for which this expedition had been planned, he said: "Not that day. No. It would not be good to be by the sea then." So he cancelled this holiday to which he had been looking forward. There was no wish to bypass the tragic moment. He was still not quite at ease when near the sea and he made the comment: "Fancy it's nearly two years," implying that he was still very near to the feeling belonging to the tragedy. The mother was helping him to plan a very simple day for the second anniversary.

Reconstruction of Patrick's Illness

1. Unknown effect of the hospitalisation at five days to six weeks with sudden clinical improvement dating from the moment of the baby's return home.

2. The dangerous separation from the mother at one and a half years. The family in which he was placed encouraged a manic defence, but on the return of the mother there was sudden recovery in the form of depression, which was clinically hidden in the twenty-four-hour sleep on her lap.

3. Following this there was a bond between the boy and the mother which had behind it not only love but also his uncertainty about her reliability. *Here was a relative deprivation.* This made Patrick some-

what mother-bound and it interfered with the development of his relationship to his father.

4. The development of Patrick's personality during the latency period was distorted and, as the mother put it, it seemed as if he was destined to become mother-fixated.

5. Then came the tragedy which, though partly accidental, was felt by Patrick to be engineered by his unconscious processes.

6. Next followed the delay in the development of Patrick's reaction to the tragedy. He seemed unaffected and went back to boarding school. Here, however, he tended to go to the sickroom for obscure disorders. He engineered these, but without knowing why.

7. The first interview with me. This was brought about by the mother, who began to sense that Patrick was becoming oversensitive and liable to psycho-somatic disorder. Here was a paranoid clinical state of increasing severity. The mother also knew that Patrick had not reacted to the tragedy. In this interview Patrick took the trouble to make me understand that *his difficulties started a long time before the tragedy*. He drew a picture which in a later interview gave the clue to the original trauma.

8. Truancy from school for a subsidiary reason. In the second interview Patrick knew that he had come to me for help, and that he was threatened with a mental breakdown. A regressive withdrawal state could appear instead of the paranoid illness because of the fact of his belief in me, which had been engendered in the first interview.

9. *My decision that he was ill,* and that he must not go back to school for an indefinite period. This quickly led to his reaching a deep level of regression to dependence and to his becoming withdrawn. The mother met this dependence more than adequately. To do this she had to postpone her own reaction to the loss of her husband.

10. The arrival of feelings appropriate to the tragedy (fifth interview). At the depth of his breakdown Patrick brought the dream, which led to his experiencing the affect that had been experienced neither at the time of the traumatic episode nor subsequently. After the experiencing of these feelings Patrick began to lose his need to be ill. He began to recover.

11. Return to boarding school. He was now nearly well and had not lost much ground in schoolwork. He entered his old form for another year and accepted the situation. He quickly resumed emotional growth appropriate to his age.

Final Comment

Patrick had a delayed reaction to a tragedy in which he was involved at the age of 11 years. The delay belonged partly to the fact that he was already ill at the time of the tragedy, and the tragic episode could be said to be a part of the boy's total illness. This illness had as an aetiological factor a dangerous period of separation from the mother at one and a half years. (Possibly, a pattern for his reaction to this illness was set up by his earliest illness and separation from five days to six weeks at the beginning of his life.) The acute illness, for the management of which I was responsible, started with the tragedy and the delayed reaction, and this illness can now be said to be at an end.[4] The total result is that Patrick has lost the major part of the illness from which he suffered *before* the tragedy, which was of the nature of a deprivation reaction, and which was characterised by a degree of mother-fixation, by a schizoid distortion in his reality testing (phobic system), by a tendency to deny depression, and a personality disturbance leading towards homosexuality with a paranoid coloring.

The main therapeutic provision was the way in which the boy's mother met his regression to dependence, and along with this there was specific help given by myself on demand.

4. Follow-up: Four years after the tragedy the boy's development can be said to be natural and healthy.—D.W.W.

44

Physical and Emotional Disturbances in an Adolescent Girl

Written in January 1968[1]

My contribution to this collection of studies must be a clinical one. I propose to describe a case. One case proves nothing, but it may illustrate much, and may illustrate phenomena that, though significant, do not show up in conventional scientific investigations.

Case of G.

I was consulted by the parents of a girl who was 14 yours old. G. had always been a healthy energetic child, and she had certainly been much wanted by her parents. The family was a stable unit and a going concern. There was a great deal of feeling experienced in the home situation, and G. had displayed affection and aggressiveness and what the father described as a big range of feeling. G. had a sister four years older than herself and she had always felt challenged and had made a very big attempt to compete with her sister. There was a boy three years younger, and towards him she had had phases of open jealousy.

Briefly a description of G. would be a description of a child living it up. She could be described as developing in an extrovert manner. There was an incident in this girl's life, as in the life of so many, which I knew about because of the confidence that the parents had in me. This was an encounter with a man who had a perversion in the form of a compulsion to seduce children. In fact he tried to get her to micturate in front of him in an exposed way. The incident was closed but it left G. with a certain amount of increased frequency of micturition. At 11 years G. began to menstruate; she had been prepared for this. Clinically she became awkward at about this time, clumsy and walking in a waddling manner, and repudiation of the feminine role be-

1. This is a draft of a chapter for a textbook of obstetrics and gynaecology; it was not, in fact, published.—EDS.

came a feature. Along with this was a growing interest in boys and an identification with her mother, who looked after the house. From the age of 12 she became rather heavy, languid, and quiet, and developed a leucorrhoeaic vaginal discharge. This was considerable in amount and necessitated much extra washing of clothes.

A competent physician was consulted, and after physical examination the doctor told the parents that the girl was physically ill and recommended tonsillectomy with appendicectomy later. This was all based on physical findings, and further investigations were made which seemed to confirm the doctor's diagnosis. It is possible that the doctor did not impress the parents as having properly assessed the girl's personality and the history in terms of the development of this adolescent girl from a little girl and from a baby, taking into account her place in the family. The parents were puzzled because they had watched these things develop and they felt that something was being ignored.

At this point I was consulted, and I was able to see all the reports and to take my time in allowing the mother to give me the history of the child's development.

In the interview with the mother I was able to become informed in regard to the way that all the symptoms started up and how they interwove with the girl's moods and actual experiences and with a group of symptoms such as nail-biting which could not possibly be part of the physical illness which had been diagnosed by my medical colleague.

In close confidence the mother was able to tell me that the incident with the man took place when the girl was 4 and that he manipulated her genitals. It could be noted here that these kind of details are often omitted when parents give a history because they have no idea what kind of attitude towards parents and children the doctor will have. Alternatively they give these details in some sort of way that is disproportionate, so that the doctor's reaction is to say that they are putting too much stress on one event. In this case there is no doubt that the incident was to some extent brought about by the child and the state that she was in at the time, developing as she was in an extrovert way and always somewhat excited.

I had an interview with G. herself, and as a result of this and a general survey of the whole problem I decided to come down heavily on the side of a diagnosis of *health* complicated by emotional and physical disturbances that belong to a certain kind of development. I knew of course that there was no half-measure in this matter. I must either support my medical colleague or else make a very definite statement of an opposite kind to his and take the risks involved. The risk could only be to my own reputation since it was possible to keep the case in review and a modification of diagnosis would not have presented difficulties.

I therefore told the girl on the spot that I considered her to be quite healthy. Moreover I told her that the leucorrhoea was regularly a feature accompanying fantasies and dreams of a sexual kind such as she at her age would be having, and I found that she understood what I was talking about. I had to assume that the tenderness which made my colleague think of appendicitis was ovarian tenderness associated with activity of the whole genital apparatus.

I did not make a physical examination, and naturally I was more inclined to avoid examination of the genital region when I learned of the incident with the pervert. As far as I could tell G. had not remembered this incident, or at any rate had not been obsessed with the memory of it.

The girl went out of my room, therefore, diagnosed as healthy and normal, and I followed this up with a very definite statement to the parents quite simply stating that we were looking here not at an illness but at a girl developing in a certain way.

As a result of this consultation and of my attitude the girl was very much relieved and the parents responded to the immediate improvement in her general health. The father wrote me that the consultation had a very marked effect on G., who started to feel bright and to be what he called "her usual self" from the time of the consultation. The vaginal discharge quickly lessened in quantity and ceased to be a nuisance. No more was thought about the physical troubles and neither did G. have her tonsils removed nor did she have appendicectomy.

The conflict about identification with boys or with girls continued and gradually worked itself into a solution as G. grew on into puberty.

Four years later I was again consulted by the parents and I followed up the work with four further personal interviews with G.

At that time G's complaints were more definitely psychiatric. They included fear of dying, "sense of heart-beat," fear of cancer and appendicitis, etc. She had told the father that she knew what it was that worried her but she would rather not tell him, and for this reason she came to see me.

By this time she was 18 years old and very much involved in heterosexual relationships. The father was able to see what came out very clearly in the consultation, that there was still a conflict of sex roles. He felt sad about this because of the fact that she was very much a young woman from the point of view of observers, and very much loved as such.

In the interview I found that G. was gradually solving her conflict of sex roles by very careful choice of a man to whom she could hand over the rather strongly developed male self which was part of her fantasy life. This had not affected her clinical state, so that no-one in contact with her would think of her as masculine. It was fairly obvious that G. was coming quickly up to the idea of a marriage and of the care of children of her own. In this context it would not be valuable for me to describe the content of these psycho-therapeutic interviews, but it is worth mentioning that G's fantasy and dream life was very strongly coloured by lions and tigers and other symbols of ruthless appetite just as it had been when she was a little girl. It was fairly clear that the breast feeding of her babies would be a matter of great significance to her.

The psychiatric disturbance proved to be temporary, and G. went ahead with her personal development without further consultation with me and without psychiatric help.

Sixteen years later I was consulted by G. on account of her 8-year-old daughter. She also had another child. I saw this 8-year-old girl three times in therapeutic consultation and was given very rich material illustrating her personal problem. The detail which is important from the point of view of what is being stated in this chapter is that this healthy little girl, also living in a good family, was able within the limits of the specialised technique of the interview to let me know about her reaction to the masculine element in the mother of whom, by the way, she was very fond.

In short, the mother's very copious breast feeding had acted for her rather more than it does usually for a woman as an expression of a masculine activity. This girl, like her mother, had a very great conflict in regard to sex roles and spoke about it at length, drawing pictures to illustrate her remarks, as children like to do during what I call a therapeutic consultation. She gave a dream and her illustration depicted a bag of poison. "It looks like a pig." Later she developed this idea in terms of her mother, reassuring me that really her mother is very nice but this is what she dreams about her mother. At one point she became dramatic in describing what she would do to her mother's breasts. She shouted out: "I don't want any of her horrid milk." And then she spat. She then drew a woman whose breasts hung down in the front like the cords of her father's dressing-gown which she had drawn in another picture, and then she said: "I think there would be holes instead of breasts."

It is not to be expected that the reader of this chapter will find this material convincing, because of the following circumstances. Firstly, the reader is not necessarily in touch with the extremely complex special subject of the emotional development of the human being including the fantasy content of the child's mind. Secondly, it is not possible in this context to give the complete account of the four interviews, which could in fact be given, because accurate notes were taken and the child's drawings illustrate every step.

What can be stated is that from the point of view of myself conducting the interview this child was able to show me without any lead from myself that she was reacting to a powerful expression of the masculine identification which she detected in her mother and which disturbed her. She would of course have liked to have found all this in her father who perhaps is more maternal than masculine.

It is to be understood that in terms of psychiatry these people, adults and children, are not to be described as ill. It is more that they have certain patterns which if exaggerated and fixed could then be diagnosed as illness patterns. The important thing that is being emphasised is that to my surprise the child had picked out for description the very element in her mother which had turned up in the mother's presentation of herself to me two decades previously and which had been a feature of her (the mother's) childhood life.

Looking back then on the whole complex one can see that the leucorrhoea which provided the reason for the original consultation with the physician and which could so easily have led to an unnecessary series of operations was one very small part of a total personality problem which was not even outside the wide area of the concept of health which one has to employ in the practice of child psychiatry.

Comment

It is likely that this kind of clinical contribution may come as a shock to the reader of a book which has as its title "The Scientific Foundations of Obstetrics and Gynaecology." Nevertheless it is necessary for those who make very carefully controlled observations and who draw conclusions from their work that they shall be reminded that in the practice of medicine it is not possible to ignore the total personality and family pattern, without the danger of more harm being done than good.

The clinician is the one who provides the material for scientific work, not the pathologist or the specialist in mechanical tests. Perhaps then there is a place in this book for this thumbnail sketch of a vastly complex clinical situation.

45

Mother's Madness Appearing in the Clinical Material as an Ego-Alien Factor

Written for a book on psycho-analytical psychotherapy, 1969[1]

In a recent case of mine the sudden intrusion of "foreign" material needed to be noticed, understood, and interpreted. The patient was a boy of 6 years who was referred to me on account of his being unable to make use of his good intelligence; instead, he would bite holes in his gloves, coat, tie, and jersey, and he would only defecate in a chamber pot near one of the parents. Further, he demanded routine that was strict in many details, and he was restricted in the foods he could eat.

There is no need for a detailed description of the case here, where I have the limited aim to describe the psychotherapeutic interview that he had with me on the only occasion that I saw him. The interview had a good effect because I was able to sort out the muddle in the boy's mind from the muddle introduced into his life by certain characteristics of the mother. It can be taken for granted by the reader that this only child was loved by his parents and that the family was in no danger of breaking up. The father was of professional class, and the mother had had her own training as a teacher.

In order to give a useful picture of the session I must ask the reader to follow many details which need to be reported simply because they give continuity to the material.

He and I played the Squiggle Game together, and it was easy for me to find his capacity to enjoy playing and to play along with him. This is what happened alongside the drawings: after a desultory discussion of his home and his family situation, we prepared the paper and two pencils, and I started with the first squiggle.

1. Mine, which he made into a donkey, giving alternatives: pig,

---

1. Published in *Tactics and Techniques in Psychoanalytic Therapy*, ed. Peter L. Giovacchini (London: Hogarth Press; New York: Jason Aronson, 1972).

cow, horse, dog. "It has a funny eye." Here in the "funny eye," we already had a reference to the unpredictable.

2. His, which he said was a head, and I gave it a girl's body.

3. Mine, which he turned into a funny head. Note the recurrence of the theme of "funny," indicating its significance. He made a reference to me which belonged to the mother's assessment of me. Apparently she possesses a book by me and he had seen this, and he said: "You do good head writing." I think the elaborate scribble on the forehead referred to brains, as if it were a portrait of me seen through the mother's eyes. "The man has a funny nose with three nostrils. His ears are behind so that you do not see them."

He told me about other things he could draw, including a bus, and he was very keen to get coloured crayons. He had already used me to talk to about the idea of something funny about the mind. I, of course, made no interpretations. The three nostrils could be thought of as mad, but within the area of the boy's play activities.

4. Here the paper got torn in the process of vigorous drawing. He did not manage to draw anything at first.

5. This has some sort of mystery to it. It was his and up in the corner he made a mark. This mark was also part of an M. There is a pun on his name here. He said, "It's a nothing." He had reached an extreme defence, for if he is a nothing then he cannot be killed or hurt by the worst trauma imaginable.

I followed up the theme in talking to him here of drawing as a way of getting something out of his head onto the paper. He talked about the way in which the train sometimes has to stop to allow an express train to come through. He said, "Our train gets blocked because they have to change the points and then we can come back again."

Here he just saved the pencil from falling onto the floor, and these and other small things seemed significant, indicating that there was chaos rather than order in his immediate experiences. Now the pencil slipped off onto the floor. Nevertheless he was not in a frightened state, and it could be said that he had found a position from which to look at the express train coming through.

We had an interlude here. I used the pause to ask him about dreams. He said, "I don't know." Now he was back doing no. 4. "It is an engine. That is a good window. It is like a real engine's window, a steam train."

He was getting towards the traumatic express train, which evidently reminded him of Mother. "In Battersea Park there is a train

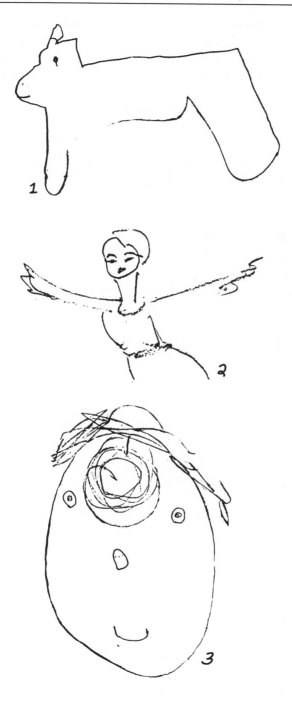

that looks like a steam train but really it is a diesel. Mummy thinks it is a steam train!" He went on about steam trains that he sees on the underground. He watches real shunting and he has seen one lots of times on various trips to Victoria Station; backwards and forwards. "I have seen in the paper something on the other side of the world that was on fire. People weren't killed; well, not while it was a little fire."

The immense potentialities for danger are indicated—a comment on the fire in the steam engine. "Oh we forgot the coal tender." And he started to try to add it onto the back of the engine; many other

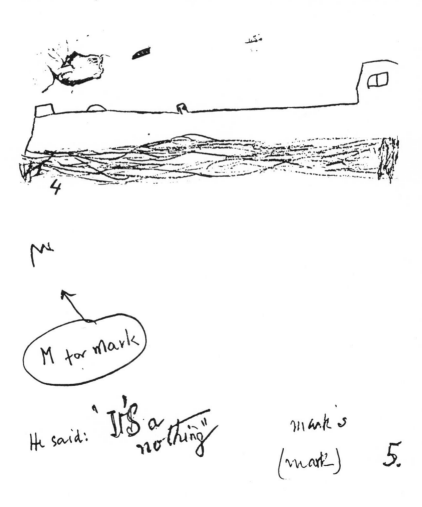

small details got lost at this point, and then he suddenly manifested something quite new and out of the general trend of the material.

The Traumatic Agent Arrives

At this point he started to behave quite out of character. I could hardly recognise him as the same boy. A new thing had come and had taken hold of him. This that was new had to do with hearing a funny noise; it was a booming sound. It might come from the gasfire, a sort of sound when it is leaking. He went over to examine the gasfire, but there was no smell to it, so it wasn't leaking.

It was not possible to be sure whether he was hallucinating or remembering in auditory terms. I fished around by making an interpretation about hearing the parents in the other room, to which he gave a strong No, and he said: "It was very high up on the hills or perhaps right away at the source of the Thames."

I continued with my theme, saying, "Like it might be the beginning of Mark, something happening between mother and father."

He followed up my theme in an effort to comply by saying, "I started inside Mummy and I ended up out of Mummy at the hospital. There was no noise, babies crying."

I said, "I wonder if there was a noise inside Mummy," and he said he had his eyes closed so that he could not hear. I, myself, was bewildered and I seem to have persevered with this primal scene interpretation as if at a loss.

It was difficult to take notes of the chaotic way in which material was appearing. He made noises illustrative of the sort of noises that he was hearing or remembering, and they seemed to include the word "no," and this sort of thing repeated itself many times. It was all frenzied or hectic. He interrupted this by saying, "What are you doing— writing more books?" referring to the notes that I was taking. So I wrote "Mark" very big and in several different ways. He said, "It's not good writing; it's scribbling."

I think it was here that no. 4 got torn by Mark making his mark more and more vigorously. Here he found he had completely lost his pencil. This seemed significant, although for a time he went over to an interest in an old penknife in the pencil box. Together we explored this and he said, "I am allowed a knife." With the knife he jabbed the paper and sometimes jabbed the table, and it was at this point that most of the damage to no. 4. was done. Several times the sheet got new damage, and I think he was showing why he had to be nothing if he was to let the traumatic "thing" arrive. Here, too, was the penetration theme that we had already obtained of the origin of Mark.

He was then exploring the tin containing pencils and crayons. Have I got a "rubber"? (I haven't.) "My goodness!" And so on. The game was now at an end and he began walking around starting some new theme. He took something from his right and left pockets and stuffed them in his right and left ears, and it seemed legitimate to suppose that he was dealing with the hallucinated sounds and moreover that he had come prepared to deal with them, and had brought right and left bits of paper for use in this respect.

He was manifesting a confused state, but he quickly changed the subject and referred to my roof garden which he could see from the window. He referred to a story in a comic and he wondered where the comic might be. Probably Mother had it in the waiting room, he thought. In this way the actual Mother came back into his mind, and I was able to see that *the express train had been a mad Mother.* I was still unsure of my ground, however, and postponed making the main interpretation.

Anxiety showed still further by his saying, "I might be going home soon, or now." He referred to fear of the noises, and there was some fun about the chair walking away and behaving as if it would kick Mother or get knocked over.

I made a reference to the madness that this represented. Either he or I said, "Everything's gone mad," and there was some laughing. I said, about the head, "It's got eyes but no ears," and he said, "Yes it has, but if fell over and now it's upside down."

There was a moment of a mad world and some kind of sound like "Woof, woof" inside the mad chair, and then this noise went out on the other side of the chair. I made a remark about a mad place inside his head or possibly inside his mother, and I began to have a conviction that this boy was bringing me a picture of his mother as an ill person.

Continuing the primal scene theme, I said, "And then Mummy did a big noise and it was called Mark." Eventually I definitely stated. "*Mummy sometimes goes mad when you are there. This is what you are showing me.*"

He was distracting himself by talking about the care that you have to take with electric gadgets. He said, "I was born a boy."

I said, "You were born a big noise!" And he said, "I didn't!"

He was now wanting to go but saying that he was not scared, simply that he wanted to see his mother, so we went together to collect her.

Comment

When I had a new look at the mother, I realised that she does carry with her a severe personal problem, and when I spoke to her about this she was very willing to admit that she was often an ill person.

Later the mother said she was so very glad that I had seen in the way the boy behaved that she does go mad in front of the child, and she knew that it was this that was disturbing him. She is herself having treatment for her mental condition.

In this example of a therapeutic consultation, it is possible to watch a boy of six years communicating a complex and dynamic personality pattern, not a profile but a representation in depth, integrated in a space-time continuum.

He quickly senses the special conditions of the professional situation and develops the necessary trust in myself. On this premise he plays around with personal madness, testing out whether I can stand the "funny" eyes and the triple nostrils. Then he shows the way he has learned to adopt the extreme defences of nothingness or invulnerability. He is no more than a mark, a mark that can be easily unnoticed. He happens to have the name Mark and he uses this in a playful way.

Now the stage is set. He is there playing with me, and all is well. He warns me of the trains that have to go into a sideline to let through the express. In terms of the details of the steam train, he tells me about an immense potentiality for destruction: fire on the other side of the world.

Then suddenly he goes mad, but it is more true to say that he is *possessed by madness*. It is no longer him, but it is a mad person that I watch—one who is completely unpredictable. The express train is rushing through the station while the local train is standing still in a siding. "Nothing" is not being destroyed by the mad "something."

Then the mother's madness passes and the boy begins to want to use his mother as a mother who cares for him and whom he needs in order to get home. The boy leaves my house in a happy state. He is confident in this mother whose going mad has now been shown to me, whose going mad has become objectified and limited by its own boundaries. Mark has now become something instead of nothing, and he can play again, even play at absurdities which, being part of his own madness, are not traumatic so much as comical and laughable.

I think that I was needed in my special role as someone who could see him, think about him (clever brains in head), experience contact with him (communication through playing), recognise and respect his defence organisations (and the extreme defence of his being "nothing"), and then witness his states of being possessed by a mother's madness when his own mother goes mad in front of him. He also needed my other contact with his mother by which I could know that when not insane she is a good and responsible parent and wife to the boy's father.

Where is he when he is nothing? I think that in the consultation he relied on my having a mental image of him in my head which he could recall after the express train had gone through and the local train could come out of the siding.

Added Note

Although this is not the purpose of this paper, I wish to add that there was considerable clinical improvement following this one psychotherapeutic consultation. This showed in a clearing up of the scholastic block of which the boy's teachers complained; it also showed in the boy's general attitude at home, in his progress toward independence, and in his new ability to function normally in regard to excretions.

Part Three

On the Work of
Other Analysts

46
Susan Isaacs

I. Obituary[1]

1948

Susan Isaacs died on October 12 at the age of 63. Few can have had a greater influence in our time on the upbringing and education of children; indeed, the modern trend towards full recognition of the human aspect of nursery school and subsequent education owes much to her work.

Dr Isaacs was the daughter of William Fairhurst, of Bolton, Lancashire, and of Miriam Sutherland. Educated at Bolton Secondary School and at the Universities of Manchester and Cambridge, she became a research student at Cambridge in the Psychological Laboratory in 1912, and then lecturer in psychology at Darlington Training College. In 1924 she was invited to become principal of the Malting House School at Cambridge. It was during the following three years that she gathered the comprehensive data of children's behaviour, thoughts and feelings which she presented brilliantly in her two books *Intellectual Growth in Young Children* (1930) and *Social Development in Young Children* (1933).

In 1933 she was made head of the new Department of Child Development of the University of London, at the Institute of Education. She held this post with outstanding success for ten years. In the course of that time a large number of experienced teachers and educationists were enriched by the wide and deep new knowledge which she was able to impart, and above all by her vivid sense of every child as a full, living personality, needing to be imaginatively realised and understood in his own right.

Dr Isaacs turned to the new insight offered by Freudian psychoanalysis as soon as this work became generally known in England, and joined the British Psycho-Analytical Society in 1921. She was

1. Published in *Nature,* 4 December 1948.

385

appointed a psychologist on the staff of the London Clinic of Psycho-Analysis in the year 1931. She remained on the staff of the Clinic until her death, and contributed signally in a great number of ways to the scientific work of the Society and to the practical work of the Institute. She was a valued member of the Training Committee and of the Council.

Dr Isaacs was a clear writer as well as teacher and lecturer; her books and scientific papers are well known to students of psychology to-day. Her small handbook for mothers and teachers, *The Nursery Years,* written in 1929, is known all over the world; it was awarded the *Parents' Magazine* Medal in the United States. *The Children We Teach* is another little book which is widely popular. One of the two books published just before her death is *Childhood and After,* containing essays and clinical psychological studies which belong to the later period of her life. A chapter in it called "Children in Institutions," originally a memorandum presented to the Home Office Care of Children Committee, known as the Curtis Committee, in 1945, was probably the most important single document consulted by that Committee.

Dr Isaacs' gifts were based on a combination of intellectual and emotional factors. Her passionate interest in the conditions, first, of young children's education, and, secondly, of their general upbringing in the home, arose out of her own experiences. Her mother's death when she was just 6, terminating a fatal and incapacitating illness which started when Susan was barely 4, led her to find in her first elementary school in a Lancashire town in the 1880s a refuge and solace from the tragedy at home, but also to become very quickly a rebel against its manifold constraints and inadequacies. This disappointed eagerness and keen sense of what "school" might have been like, but in fact was not, remained in the background of her mind throughout her growth and did much to shape her later life-work.

It became clear to her at an early stage in her development that mere criticism and mere abandonment of existing methods could bring no constructive results. She quickly assimilated and adopted the most advanced educational ideas current at the time, and her immediate response to the new teaching of psycho-analysis showed that no conventional opposition or resistances could stand in the way of her unhesitating acceptance of anything that offered her wider horizons and deeper understanding. In the same way, at a later stage, when Melanie Klein's ideas were first put forward in Great Britain, she was among the earliest to sense the further sources of knowledge which were now opening up. She saw how these new ideas could be developed to the general benefit of every child's upbringing, and from that moment she pursued that knowledge, and applied it untiringly up to the very last.

Her outstanding intellectual characteristic was an extremely rapid and comprehensive grasp of the matter in view and an ability to classify and summarize it, to present it with remarkable clarity, and to discuss it from various angles. Her exceptional capacity for instantly translating her thoughts and impressions into verbal expression served as a powerful instrument for all her other gifts.

It was characteristic of Susan Isaacs that when she found that there was a great deal which she had not yet encompassed, especially in the work of Melanie Klein, she decided (although she was already a member of the British Psycho-Analytical Society) to start again as a trainee and to go through the whole course. Thus she developed further, undergoing a second long personal analysis, and greatly enriched her own work and the contribution which she was eventually able to make to general psycho-analytic research. In her last years, she devoted herself almost entirely to actual analytic practice, and felt this to be the most satisfying of the various kinds of work she had done.

In her husband, Nathan Isaacs, she had a constant friend and supporter, and a constructive critic.

II. Foreword to *Susan Isaacs,* by D. E. M. Gardner

Dated 9 September 1968[2]

When Susan rang me up and told me that she was ill and was going to die I was very angry. She reminded me of my angry reaction a year later when I saw her for the last time.

It seemed such a waste, that this very real and active person should cease to be, simply because of a cancer.

2. London: Methuen, 1969.

Susan and I got to know each other when we were both students at the Institute of Psycho-Analysis, in the mid-thirties. She had already done her basic work at the Malting House School, and it was about at that time that the Child Development Department of the Institute of Education was created for her. As a psycho-analyst she was having a second training, having become dissatisfied with her first, and this meant a second analysis and a new personal upheaval.

It was of great importance to me that Susan invited me to give a series of lectures each year to her students in the Child Development Course. I was more than surprised. She simply let me loose, in spite of my immaturities, and for some years I lectured to her students out of my paediatric experience. Gradually these lectures developed into a series, ten each year, attempting to cover the subject of the emotional development of the individual. Not only was it kind of Susan to invite me and to leave me to evolve my own method and viewpoint, but also it may have been quite brilliant of her to see that such a use of a colleague could possibly lead to anything at all. But this was typical of her. She was quite outstandingly superior, generous, and at the same time human, vulnerable, modest, and humorously tolerant. When I heard Nathan ruthlessly criticise her ideas and formulations I felt maddened, but I found that she valued exactly this from him and that she made positive use of his ruthlessness, as of his terrific intellect.

It fell to my lot to supply child cases for Susan's child analysis training, and I watched with interest her sensitive management of the total family situation, a difficult thing when one is engaged in learning while carrying out a psycho-analytic treatment involving daily sessions over years. I never had qualms about the course of these treatments, although in those days we worked in a potentially hostile environment.

Of course, if I had known that illness would come and cut short our friendship I would have forged ahead, making much more use than I did of all that she had to offer; but there seemed to be plenty of time; and in any case we all needed to recover from the war.

Then the life of this sturdy soul came to an end, and we who survived were left angry. This memoir compiled by Dorothy Gardner gives me a moment of happiness in that it recaptures some of the reality of a truly great person, one who has had a tremendous influence for good on the attitude of parents and of teachers to the children in their care. This attempt at a reconstruction will serve its purpose if it brings Susan alive to those who never knew her, so that some may feel inclined to read her books by being introduced to her as a struggling, striving, and radiant human being, one who seemed destined to achieve something significant that we cannot now define because her death stopped the process. There is still room for the study of what she actually achieved.

47
Marion Milner

Critical Notice of *On Not Being Able to Paint*[1]

1951

Let no one think that this book is just about painting or not painting. Yet it had to have its title because in that way the writing of the book started. The real purpose of the book only becomes clear to the author in the course of her experience of writing, in fact the book is itself an example of its main theme. This theme, which gradually becomes clear to the reader, is foreshadowed in an early quotation: "Concepts can never be presented to me merely, they must be knitted into the structure of my being, and this can only be done through my own activity" (M. P. Follett, *Creative Experience*).

The central concept which is presented to the reader and apprehended by the writer through the writing of the book has to do with the subjective way of experiencing and the role of this in creative process. Thus the book is in one sense a plea for the recognition of subjectivity as having its own place and way of functioning, just as legitimate and as necessary as objectivity, but different. As applied to education, it is pointed out that subjectivity must be understood by teachers, otherwise the objectivity aimed at must be in danger of fatal distortion. Painting comes in as a jumping-off place; it was the surprise of discovering the power to make "free" drawings that concentrated the writer's attention on this problem of subjectivity or subjective action.

The concept of the role of subjectivity which emerges has two main aspects, one to do with illusion, the other with spontaneity. Both are connected with what the writer calls the interplay of differences, out of which creativity proceeds, but if interplay is to be allowed in oneself one must be prepared for mental pain. Such an interplay needs

---

1. This book was written under the name Joanna Field; London: Heinemann, 1950. Winnicott's review appeared in the *British Journal of Medical Psychology* (1951).—EDS.

various descriptions according to the level being considered. At a comparatively late stage of emotional development, what is familiar in psycho-analytic literature about unconscious conflict between love and hate in interpersonal relationships is relevant, and indeed this paved the way for all other statements. Such conflict involves the problem of the preservation of the loved object from hate and from erotic attacks (whether in fact or in fantasy) and creation is seen in this setting as an act of reparation. If one considers earlier stages in emotional development of the individual, one must use other language, such as the statement that magical creativity is an alternative to magical annihilation.

If I understand the author aright she wishes to make a yet more fundamental statement about creativity. She wishes to say that it results from what is for her (and perhaps for everyone) the primary human predicament. This predicament arises out of the non-identity of what is conceived of and what is to be perceived. To the objective mind of another person seeing from outside, that which is outside an individual is never identical with what is inside that individual. But there can be, and must be, for health (so the writer implies), a meeting place, an overlap, a stage of illusion, intoxication, transfiguration. In the arts this meeting place is pre-eminently found through the medium, that bit of the external world which takes the form of the inner conception. In painting, writing, music, etc., an individual may find islands of peace and so get momentary relief from the primary predicament of healthy human beings.

Psycho-analysts are accustomed to thinking of the arts as wish-fulfilling escapes from the knowledge of this discrepancy between inner and outer, wish and reality. It may come as a bit of a shock to some of them to find a psycho-analyst drawing the conclusion, after careful study, that this wish-fulfilling illusion may be the essential basis for all true objectivity. If these moments of fusion of subject and object, inner and outer, are indeed more than islands of peace, then this fact has very great importance for education. For what is illusion when seen from outside is not best described as illusion when seen from inside; for that fusion which occurs when the object is felt to be one with the dream, as in falling in love with someone or something, is, when seen from inside, a psychic reality for which the word illusion is inappropriate. For this is the process by which the inner becomes actualised in external form and as such becomes the basis, not only of internal perception, but also of all true perception of environment. Thus perception itself is seen as a creative process. In practice psycho-analysts, just like other people, love the arts and value the work of those who traffic in illusion. This book is showing psycho-analysts a way in which they may bring their theory into line not only with their psychotherapy but also with their daily lives.

Moreover the author is reminding psycho-analysts and all teachers that teaching is not enough; each student must create what is there to be taught, and so arrive at each stage of learning in his own way. If he temporarily forgets to acknowledge debts this is easily forgiven, since in place of paying debts he re-discovers with freshness and orig-inality and also with pleasure, and both the student and the subject grow in the experience.

The second thread of the book, the role of spontaneity in creative-ness, is also something that analysts tend to allow for more in their practice than in their theory. They are well used to theorising about the effects of too rigid control of spontaneity, imposed in the interests of social living and propriety. What they, and also other teachers, are less used to considering is the stultifying effect on the creative spirit of too great insistence not just on propriety but on objectivity. This insistence on objectivity concerns not only perception but also action, and creativity can be destroyed by too great insistence that in acting one must know beforehand what one is doing.

48
Ernest Jones

I. Obituary[1]

1958

The death of Ernest Jones has prime significance for the whole of the psycho-analytic world. For the British Psycho-Analytical Society this significance is naturally intensified, since Jones created the Society and for many years dominated it by his personality and devotion. For some individual members, especially those whose analytic roots reach down to the decade following the First World War, Jones's death means a great personal loss.

Jones was born in South Wales. He was educated at Swansea Grammar School and at University College, Cardiff, and it was at University College Hospital, London, that he received his medical training. From the early stages of Jones's professional life there were unmistakable signs of his exceptional ability. He had one of the finest of intellects, and at the same time a fierce drive to work hard and to concentrate on the job in hand. His interests at this early stage included clinical medicine, surgery, neurology, pathology, and also clinical psychiatry, although the latter as we know it now was then almost non-existent. Undoubtedly the friendship of Wilfred Trotter was important to him at this stage. Trotter and Jones were associated in their "discovery" of Freud. Here was a colleague destined to be in the front rank of surgery who contributed positively in later years to the theory of group behaviour and cohesion. Such a friendship was indeed valuable during the stage described in his autobiography[2] when Jones was starting painfully to learn that physicians, surgeons, and psychiatrists did not want their terrain invaded by the discipline of a new science.

1. Published in the *International Journal of Psycho-Analysis* (1958). Copyright © Institute of Psycho-Analysis.
2. *Free Association: Memories of a Psycho-Analyst* (London: Hogarth Press, 1959).

In 1910 Trotter married Jones's sister. The development and evolution of this friendship is well described in the autobiography.

Jones qualified in 1900, with Gold Medal both in medicine and in obstetrics. In 1903 he again was awarded Gold Medal in the London M.D. examination. He took the Membership of the Royal College of Physicians in 1904 and the Diploma of Public Health (Cambridge) in 1905. After qualification he held various hospital appointments at University College Hospital, London; at the National Hospital, Queen Square, London; at the Hospital for Sick Children, Great Ormond Street, London; and at the Royal Ophthalmic Hospital, London. He held the post of pathologist at the West End Hospital for Nervous Diseases and was lecturer in practical neurology at the London School of Clinical Medicine. He quickly became active among students and colleagues and at scientific meetings, and having qualified at a young age himself he coached many others for the M.D., working through a University Correspondence College in Red Lion Square, London, W.C., run by a Mr. E. S. Weymouth. He continued this for about twenty years, even continuing when he was in Canada, although the work was exacting. Eventually it was his wife Katherine who persuaded him to conserve his energies in this direction.

Jones started to publish early, and the quantity of his output was always large, as evidenced by the list of his published works (see Grinstein's bibliography).[3]

It is perhaps of interest to look at his writings at this early stage where there already appears evidence of his immense powers of application and of the wide reading which was associated with all his written work. In 1907 in an article on "Alcoholic Cirrhosis of the Liver in Children,"[4] Jones gives 185 references! As another example illustrating the amount of work Jones was prepared to do in the preparation of an article, the paper on "The Question of the Side Affected in Hemiplegia in Arterial Lesions of the Brain"[5] may be mentioned. The aim of this paper was to expose a fallacy in the teaching of that time that the lesion of hemiplegia is apt to be found more frequently on one side than on the other. Jones quotes 5,281 published cases, and the article ends with seven closely printed pages of references, about one thousand in all!

3. Alexander Grinstein, *The Index of Psychoanalytic Writings*, preface by Ernest Jones, vol. 2 (New York: International Universities Press, 1957).

4. *British Journal of Children's Diseases* (1907).

5. *Quarterly Journal of Medicine* 3, no. 11 (1910).

This same attitude towards published work appears at a later date in the book *On the Nightmare,*[6] and also in the paper "The Symbolic Significance of Salt,"[7] as well as in very many other books and articles.

One wonders what would have happened if Jones had not met Freud's work. Is it possible that he would have exploited his intellectual capacity and lost touch with the ordinary matters of feeling? While speculating in this way it is interesting to look at his paper "The Significance of the Phrictopathic Sensation."[8] This paper ends:

Conclusion. Sensations showing the six features here grouped together under the designation phrictopathic are due to a cleavage between the esthesic sensibilities and the autosomatognostic memory-feelings of a part of the body, which results from hysterical disaggregation implicating the latter group of mental processes; the degree to which the features are marked is an accurate measure of the extent of this cleavage.

In subsequent writings Jones seemed to avoid precisely the kind of specialized cleverness which is illustrated here.

It was just at this time that Jones was assimilating Freud's contribution. He had acquired a mastery of the German language and as a post-graduate student in Munich he had become acquainted with German neurology and psychiatry. In the following year, 1909, he contributed an account of psycho-analysis to the *Journal of Abnormal Psychology.* Evidently psycho-analysis and the new interest in the emotional life of the individual brought about a deep change in him.

Incidentally, the word "phrictopathic" appears to have been his own invention. It should be emphasised that Jones was not prone to institute new terms and he was critical of those who too easily did so. His word "rationalization," however, is now part of the English language, and the value of his term "aphanisis" has not yet been fully explored.

A series of severe blows fell which broke the line of his career in London, and it is fortunate that we have an accurate description of these in the autobiography, since they produced a distorted view of Jones which persisted until the main actors in the drama died. In an attempt to rehabilitate himself Jones worked in Canada in the period

6. London: Hogarth Press, 1931.
7. *Essays in Applied Psycho-Analysis,* vol. 2 (London: Hogarth Press, 1951), p. 22.
8. *Journal of Nervous and Mental Diseases* 35, no. 7 (1908).

1908–1912, with support from Osler. There he became Associate Professor of Psychiatry at Toronto University. At the same time he kept in touch with Freud and with the group that was becoming associated with Freud and his work in Vienna. Jones's own story of his relation to Freud at this time can be found in the pages of the Freud biography, also his love of Europe and his determination eventually to return to practice in London.

While in Canada, Jones was in touch with neurologists and psychiatrists in the U.S.A. He became assistant editor of Morton Prince's newly founded *Journal of Abnormal Psychology*, a journal which (because of Morton Prince) "accepted psychoanalytic papers when other periodicals fought shy of them" (autobiography).

Jones met and accompanied Freud when the latter made his U.S.A. visit to lecture to Clark University.

In the U.S.A. Jones was partly responsible for the founding of the American Psychopathological Association (1910), and while Brill started the New York Psychoanalytic Society, Jones organised the American Psychoanalytic Association which was intended for psycho-analysts scattered over the States (autobiography).

The First World War separated Jones from the other analysts. At this time he made an important contribution to the subject of shell-shock. When contacts were renewed Freud was able to report similar findings to those of Jones; the former had been published in the German language[9] by Ferenczi and others. It was largely due to Jones that scientific exchange between psycho-analysts of enemy countries was renewed at the earliest possible moment after the cessation of hostilities.

During the war Jones was practising privately in London and was in process of integrating the British Group. He had formed the London Society of Psycho-Analysts in 1913, but he eventually dissolved this, because one of its important members favoured Jung. The reconstituted Society was called the British Psycho-Analytical Society, and came into being in 1919 with Jones as president, Dr Douglas Bryan as secretary, and Dr W. H. B. Stoddart as treasurer. The other founding members were Dr H. Devine, Mr Eric Hiller, Dr David Forsyth, Mr J. C. Flugel, Miss Barbara Low, Mrs Joan Riviere, and Major Stanford Read. In the years following the war a number of other people became interested and took part in the organisation. These

9. Freud, Ferenczi, Abraham, Simmel, and Jones, *Zur Psychoanalyse der Kriegsneurosen. Diskussion am 5. Internationalent Psychoanalytischen Kongress, Budapest, 1910* (Vienna: Deuticke).

included Dr R. M. Riggall, Dr James Glover, Dr John Rickman, Miss Ella Sharpe, Mr James and Mrs Alix Strachey, Dr Edward Glover, and Dr Sylvia Payne. In conjunction with Dr Rickman, Dr Jones established the International Psycho-Analytical Press in collaboration with the Hogarth Press, and founded the *International Journal* which he edited from 1920 until 1939, at first with Joan Riviere's assistance as translation editor responsible for translation from the German.

At about this same time the British Psychological Society was undergoing an extensive transformation. In Jones's words:

> Flugel was Secretary and I was Chairman of the Council that was carrying it out. One outcome was the founding of a special Medical Section, which proved an invaluable forum for the discussion of our ideas with other medical psychologists. To heighten its prestige we got W. H. R. Rivers, the distinguished anthropologist, to act as its first president, but the next seven were all psycho-analysts, as have been many since.[10]

During this time Jones was developing a private practice, setting the pace for psycho-analysts who since that time have combined consultation work of a rather specialised kind with their analytic practice. Jones played the principal part in the establishment of a training scheme which could be officially adopted as the training for psychoanalysis in this country. At this stage there was necessarily a good deal of ill feeling resulting from the fact that certain important and obviously skilled workers in psychiatry who applied for membership of the Society could not be accepted unless they were willing to undergo a training analysis, which is not different in any significant way from a therapeutic analysis. Some of the effects of this can be discerned today. We see now how necessary it was that the principle should be established that the main feature in training is the personal analysis. This is but one example of the way in which Jones used all his powers to support Freud and psycho-analysis, and at a time when psychoanalysis was in process of establishing itself, and by no means certain of the main principles that should underlie the programmes for the training of future analysts.

It could be said that Jones admired Freud and found it possible to believe in his work as much as Freud believed in it himself. Jones's evaluation of it seems to have been steadily positive, with the result

10. *Sigmund Freud: Life and Work*, vol. 3 (London: Hogarth Press, 1957), p. 12.

that he was able to contribute in an important way in these early stages, and we are not sure that without him we should have had an agreed training policy.

Students who were prepared to undergo analysis and to learn by apprenticeship found Jones to be a keen teacher and one who was ready to understand their anxieties and to give practical help and advice.

During the two decades between the wars, while the Society was establishing itself and developing what might be called a personality, and while the Institute was becoming organised, Jones was always there with a finger on the controls. There was seldom a Scientific Meeting or a Committee Meeting with Jones absent.

In 1940 Jones decided to live near Midhurst on account of the war, but he kept in touch with the Society and analysts who were working at the Clinic. He resigned the presidency in 1944, as he decided not to return to London but to concentrate mainly on writing, while continuing with a certain number of private patients who could live in the country. In this way he was able to make full use of his literary gifts. Executive work could now be left to others. It may indeed have been difficult for Jones to leave his central position, because the history of the development of the Society was one that he alone knew, since it was part of the history of himself. How was he to know that the Society would continue to fight for the things which he personally had devised and the main principles which he had established?

Jones now moved over into the position of elder statesman, throwing the responsibility for the affairs of the Society on the shoulders of those who were willing to take it. There followed a democratisation of the Society's affairs which was, as it turned out, good for the health of the British Society.

Into these two decades between the wars was crammed a very full scientific and private life. His first wife, Morfydd Owen, a talented Welsh musician, died in 1918, and there were no children of this marriage.[11] Jones married Katherine Jokl in 1919, and there were four children of this marriage: Gwenith,[12] Mervyn, Nesta, and Lewis.

It is difficult to understand how Jones could have done so much as

11. See biographical notes to Morfydd Owen Memorial Edition of Musical Works.
12. Gwenith died when she was 7½ years old, and this death caused Jones deep grief which matched his grief at the death of his first wife (autobiography).—D.W.W.

he did in these twenty years, developing his own home life with the children, keeping control of the rapidly expanding British Society, while constantly maintaining contact with Freud and the Continental groups, and at the same time remaining closely associated with the rapid developments in the U.S.A.

One of Jones's most important practical achievements was the establishment of the word *"psycho-analysis"* as something accepted in this country as referring to the work of Freud and to Freud's method. To gain this end Jones and Edward Glover attended many meetings under the auspices of the British Medical Association, and the result was an acceptance by the medical profession in Britain of the essential linkage between the term "psycho-analysis" and the name Freud. When the British Psycho-Analytical Society in 1928 asked Jones what he would like as a present commemorating this achievement, he asked for a chair to be used by the president at Scientific Meetings. Accepting the chair at a small ceremony he said that he could not have gained his end without the help of two persons: Edward Glover and his own wife Katherine. It was on this occasion that he made a slip of the tongue which caused considerable amusement. He said that he was sure that the gift would be greatly appreciated not only by himself but also by his predecessors in the chair!

This ceremony was referred to by Dr Sylvia Payne in her address on the occasion of the presentation of his portrait to Ernest Jones in July 1946. This portrait, which is by Rodrigo Moynihan, now hangs in the house of the British Psycho-Analytical Society.

On accepting his portrait Jones delivered a Valedictory Address to the British Psycho-Analytical Society. This will be remembered as an essentially unemotional occasion, and although it was a time for sadness it was not one when those who were present felt sad. He ended the address with a statement of his belief in the ultimate power of truth, something which enabled him "to advocate with some confidence a greater tolerance towards diversities or even divergences than is sometimes exhibited."[13]

Jones's scientific work is well known, and is in every respect as fresh and valuable for students today as at the time of delivery or writing. An idea can be gained of the influence Jones must have had during this period by a study of the list of the very many "outside"

13. "A Valedictory Address," *International Journal of Psycho-Analysis* 27 (1946).

societies and organisations which he addressed, although most of his papers were written either for the *Journal* or to be delivered to various psycho-analytic societies in England or U.S.A., or to the British Psychological Society and its Medical Section. Going out to address groups in this way involves much sacrifice of leisure hours, and one wonders how Jones can have found time as he did for his many other activities, including figure-skating, which his wife Katherine enjoyed with him, and chess, and especially reading. He was always a wide reader, and he had an accurate memory of what he had read. Whatever he had been doing he would always read for half an hour before actually going to bed, choosing to read mostly in history and allied subjects. He seldom read fiction. He was a good sleeper, and he did not therefore use reading as a sedative.

In the late thirties, as is well known, Jones interested himself in getting Freud and his family, as well as many other analysts (about fifty in all), to this country, away from Nazi persecution. These activities illustrate the comment made by Joan Riviere, who wrote that one feature of Jones's personality which formed the main instrument by which his success was achieved was his outstanding capacity to take action: "Undismayed by obstacles, he would apply every energy and every available means to further the ultimate aim . . . Whatever was needed must be done and would be done." [14]

The story of Jones in retirement at The Plat, Elsted, his very beautiful Sussex home overlooking the South Downs, is a story of enviable richness, and many analysts visited him there. In retirement he was not only free to lead a much closer family life and to grow roses, but he was also free to read more, to write and to edit his papers for publication, while all the time continuing some private psycho-analytic practice. He continued the editorship of the *International Psycho-Analytical Library* right up to and including the publication of the fiftieth volume.

About the year 1947, Jones was invited to undertake the biography of Freud. This involved no easy decision, and he and his wife Katherine talked the matter over for some time before he eventually accepted. Incidentally this meant a postponement of the writing of his own autobiography, which he longed to do and which he was never able to complete. It should go down to history that his wife typed out 1,500 personal letters of Freud all written in German script! This was

14. Obituary, *British Medical Journal, 22 February 1958.*

done because Jones had said that he had a visual memory, and that he could not properly use the letters if he had to work at each one in order to understand it. The biography, a final act of devotion to Freud and psycho-analysis, and to the psycho-analysts of the future, was done in spite of failing health. In 1947 Jones had had a severe coronary thrombosis, but from this he made a good recovery. He had a second in 1957. From the time of this second coronary thrombosis he was never well, though sometimes better and sometimes not so well. He used to say how lucky he had been in the matter of physical health, but in fact he could scarcely have known health as some know it. He suffered from an inherited blood disorder, Gaucher's disease, but this did not inconvenience him much. He did suffer, however, from chronic rheumatism, on account of which he was never free of pain. Eventually he developed cancer of the bladder (about January 1956). From the cancer he recovered, through local treatment, just enough to be able to make his American trip (April 1956) when he delivered three Freud Centenary Lectures.[15] These were: "The Nature of Genius" (New York); "Our Attitude towards Greatness" (Chicago); and "Psychiatry before and after Freud" (Chicago). He suffered very greatly, however, from the cancerous growth, which eventually killed him. The degree of pain which he suffered is evident to anyone who reads his brief comment on pain in the *Journal* of May-August 1957.[16]

On his return from the U.S.A. he conducted the Freud Centenary Celebrations in London, unveiling the plaque at Freud's house, 20 Maresfield Gardens, repeating the two lectures "The Nature of Genius" and "Our Attitude towards Greatness," and also delivering a radio talk (British Broadcasting Corporation) on "Sigmund Freud: The Man and His Achievements." A gramophone recording of this talk is available, which illustrates admirably Jones's ability to rise to an occasion.

Those who did not meet Ernest Jones will wish to know what he was like. Physically he was of small stature like many of the Welsh race; he had a rather big head, a pale complexion, and piercing brown eyes. He was vibrant with a sensitive awareness of the environment, and of the matter that was of interest at the moment. Watching

---

15. *Sigmund Freud: Four Centenary Addresses* (New York: Basic Books, 1956).
16. *International Journal of Psycho-Analysis* 38 (1957).

his eyes and mouth during the reading of a paper one could divine his feelings about it, and especially his quick detection of a new idea. He was not one to stand about with, as one might with a fisherman on the quay, with no exchange of ideas. He had but little small talk. In his home he was restful and able to be mentally in repose; what one encountered in ordinary contact with him was his lively interest in anything to which he applied himself and his quick grasp of what was good and what was bad or false. He liked to be associated with anything that would probably turn out to be valuable, and this gave him a keen nose for originality and a wish to support new ideas. His interest in what was new was reflected in one of the outstanding contributions which he made in this country, namely, his invitation to Melanie Klein to work in London, and his encouragement of her in her work, especially during the first decade after her arrival here in 1926.

Ideas were perhaps more important to Jones than anything else, and they had to stand the test. Joan Riviere writes that a most important feature in his character consisted in

> an acute faculty of perception, of insight—a propensity to recognize evidences of intrinsic worth and value when and where they appear, and to respond with a sure instinct of affirmation to that recognition. The strength and persistence of this trait in him were the mainspring of his work; it dominated him and outweighed those inhibitions which cause most of us to overlook or lose touch with various good things that are accessible. This capacity to recognize value was by no means limited to his appreciation of the work of Freud; it played an important part in his rôle as a leader, enabling him to utilize elements in different people of many different, even conflicting, kinds, in order to serve the main purpose in view. It was also evidently the source of another characteristic—the wide range of his interests.[17]

Some reference must be made to the fact that those who came in contact with Ernest Jones were often stung by something in his way of making contact. It is not easy to know exactly what it was that people experienced, but whatever it was it had to be accepted. His mother told him he had a sharp tongue. His own Celtic quickness was not always to be matched by a similar quickness in the other person, and this could easily lead to a moment of awkwardness in which there was a sense of something having gone wrong, when in

---

17. Obituary, *British Medical Journal*.

fact all was well. Jones had a keen grip on every subject that he interested himself in, and it would seem that he expected a similar preparedness on the part of those to whom he was talking; when the others were, in fact, not at grips with their subject in a way comparable to his own they were apt to feel a sense of intellectual inferiority, often only too well founded in fact.

The question must be asked: How deep did this characteristic of sharpness go in the structure of his personality? An understanding of Jones can best be made by a reading of his autobiography, which shows the amazing growth of his world from local Gower to world psycho-analysis. Apart from such a study, however, it would seem that some answer can already be given by a general survey of his writings, because it can be definitely said that in the Jones essays and lectures there are very few signs of bitterness or of a clever scoring of points, and this must surely indicate that the acerbity was a relatively superficial phenomenon. Perhaps it is only in the paper "The God Complex"[18] that one can perceive some of this, which did undoubtedly affect Jones's social contacts outside his home, and which one may suppose was related to the characteristics that he freely admits having displayed in the early years of his professional life. As he grew old he seemed more able to shed this characteristic.

The fact must be remembered that Jones not only bore the brunt of the early public resistance to the theory of infantile sexuality, but also it was he who had to discover this resistance, at least as it became a reality in England. He it was who had to be taken by surprise, and to find himself professionally ostracised. Few would have recovered from experiences such as he encountered. This isolation may have somewhat determined the way of making contact which seemed to some who met him like an attack in defence when it was probably an attack made to stimulate a significant response.

In this connection it is instructive to re-read the paragraph Jones offered to Freud as suitable for *Moses and Monotheism*, which was to be published in England. This paragraph contains no mention of the English reaction to the idea of sexuality in childhood, but refers only to the religious tolerance which characterises this country.

In no other European country has so much tolerance been shown towards the discoveries of psycho-analysis as in England. This is in

18. *Essays in Applied Psycho-Analysis*, vol. 2, p. 244.

accord with her profound trust in the importance of freedom of thought. And for some centuries now it has also been the English tradition that frank and sincere discussion of theological and religious problems is to be included in this freedom; indeed, historically it was the origin of it.[19]

From one who had suffered professional ostracism it could be claimed that this statement is generous.

It is impossible to overstress the generosity and the kindness that lay behind an attitude that often was sharp. The amount of loving care that Jones would spend on manuscripts sent him by colleagues from all over the world was amazing; also he was ready to praise when he felt he could honestly do so. Enthusiasm for the establishment of psycho-analysis as a science was constant, and with this there was a dislike of the mediocre, especially in a scientific paper.

By the time most analysts who are now alive came to know him, Jones had become free to relax from defence of psycho-analysis and from the need to establish his own personal position in the world. It was now easy for anyone with serious intentions to reach quickly through to Jones's warm appreciation and eagerness to support and help. He continued of course to feel and to show intolerance of analysts who tried to avoid the implications of the unconscious, and also to criticise those who, by their propagandist activities, betrayed their own unconscious doubts.

In looking at such a man and considering the continued contribution which he made over the span of half a century, it is natural to think of the setting in which he worked. His wife Katherine played a very important part in his life both in giving him peace and happiness and by her active participation in his interests.

19. Ibid., preface.

II. Funeral Address

Given at Golders Green Crematorium,
14 February 1958[20]

It falls on me as today's president of the British Psycho-Analytical Society to represent the Society at this solemn moment.

At the end of his long life we are here to pay tribute to a man of exceptional calibre. At the age of 79 he died, but too early. He was in full possession of his powers and had even more to contribute had it not been that illness overtook the slow but inevitable progress of age. This is our only regret. For the rest, you will want me to say that we acknowledge a very full life, fully lived.

Ernest Jones was a Welshman, born in Wales. It is not uncommon for Wales to produce men and women with big personalities and fine minds. Scattered over the Welsh villages are philosophers and scholars who reach fame only in their own locality. Every now and again for some reason or other there is a reaching out to the wider community, and then, as in the case of Jones, it may be not Great Britain but the world that forms the natural arena in which the drama of the man's life is acted.

It has been suggested by Jones himself that the fact that he was a Welshman in the British community made him understand better than others might have understood the special position of the Jewish race of which Freud was so distinguished a member.

It must have been evident that Jones was exceptionally brilliant from the beginning. I have no record of his school years. By the time he had become medically qualified at University College Hospital, where he eventually died, he had established himself as a gold medallist in several subjects, and he could evidently reach eminence in any field that he might choose to make his own. Jones was certainly one of the world's workers. His capacity for working, always in top gear, was phenomenal, and he loved to round off a job, as witness the

20. Published in the *International Journal of Psycho-Analysis* (1958). Copyright © Institute of Psycho-Analysis.

eighty contributions collected in the five editions of his essays, each essay being a small masterpiece.

His capacity for reading and for remembering what he read was huge, and persisted to the end of his life. It was not in his work alone that Jones was in the top rank. He had many personal interests, and it seems that he never failed to impress his mark on whatever he did. One of the disadvantages of his living long is that inevitably those who were associated with him in the early stages of his career are now mostly dead. Jones was engaged on writing his autobiography, and it is to be hoped that he had time to write down many details which will help us as students of this great man in our attempt to understand one more example of genius. By the time Jones himself appears in his biography of Freud he has already been through a great deal. In 1908 when he first appeared as a guest of the Psychological Wednesday Society Jones was 29.

I can only guess at the life of the brilliant young clinician who seemed to have the world of neurology at his feet, but who chose to work with Freud, thereby making himself unpopular among his medical colleagues. It is important for us in remembering Jones to remind ourselves that it was necessary for him to weather the storm of abuse. In the early 1920s, when I myself came on the scene, I found a medical profession hostile to Jones, and this hostility found direct expression in the almost indefinite delay in his election to Fellowship of the Royal College of Physicians. Unless we recognise the antagonisms to Jones and to psycho-analysis in the medical profession of the day we cannot properly assess his contribution to psycho-analysis in this country.

Gradually there has come about a change of climate, and that one is a psycho-analyst is now no longer something to hide. Jones had support from friends, but it must be assumed that the general hostility of his professional colleagues was a matter of great grief to him. He, as much as anyone, would have liked early recognition of his value. He was indeed no saint. Undoubtedly he wanted to be liked and to be known in his time, but it was necessary for him to remain relatively obscure for several decades. This was the price he paid for his quick recognition of the importance of Freud and for his unwavering loyalty to his chosen master. Surely when we consider the fact of personal ambition we must admire Ernest Jones not least in that he was not only contented but proud to work with another man whom he felt to be in all respects greater than himself.

It is difficult to imagine a more fruitful relationship between two men than that of Jones and Freud. I would say that they were not at all like each other. There was a sharp edge to Jones's wit that seems to have no counterpart in the Freud that Jones describes to us. Jones did not idealise Freud. He perceived the value and originality of his contribution. He helped in the provision of a setting in which the new ideas could be discussed and developed, and to this psycho-analytic pool he himself contributed most richly.

To Ernest Jones we owe the introduction of Freud's work into this country, and the establishment of our Scientific Society. Jones founded our Journal, and fifty books were published under his editorship in the International Psycho-Analytic Library. At this moment, however, we are not so much concerned with listing his contributions as with remembering the man.

It was characteristic of Ernest Jones that he should make a sensible retirement to the country while he was still able to enjoy his family life and his garden. In retirement he worked, of course, as hard as ever, treating patients, reading, and writing. At The Plat, Elsted, his family grew around him, and those who visited his home never failed to feel enriched by the experience. Surely nothing more could be expected, but when he was already 70 it became his great privilege and immense task to write the biography of Freud, and the story of the development of Freud's ideas. In order to write this he and Mrs Jones soaked themselves thoroughly in Freud so that, as I am told, they could play games in which they would ask each other what Freud would have been doing at such and such a date at four o'clock in the afternoon. The result of this final act of devotion to Freud is a biography which has achieved world fame.

Now we have come to the end of this man's life. The Society, its Members, Associate Members, Students, and future Students wish to offer his widow our sympathy and our love. We love her because of our affection for Jones, and also for herself as one who was obviously happy to be his wife and the mother of his children and his partner in the study of Freud. We also think of his three children and his daughter-in-law and his grandchildren, and we like them to know that something of Ernest Jones continues in the hearts of those of us who knew him. Ernest Jones will continue to be important to all those in future generations who will benefit directly from the stand that he took on behalf of Freud's claim that human nature can be studied scientifically; the whole of human nature without exception.

49
Dorothy Burlingham

Review of *A Study of Three Pairs of Identical Twins*[1]

1953

For those who are thinking of trying the experiment next time of being born twins, my advice is to choose parents who live near a library. Few parents would be able to afford to buy Mrs Burlingham's book, yet they could enjoy following the fortunes of the three pairs of identical twins the details of whose development are faithfully and clearly set out in charts. Such charts are expensive to print but they are indispensable here, and Imago Publishing Co. is to be congratulated on a beautiful as well as a valuable production.

The study is a record of work done, and the comment, which is only half the book, is presumably intended for workers in the field, since certain terms are used in Mrs Burlingham's personal conclusions, at the ends of chapters, that would be correctly understood only by those who know current psycho-analytic usage. I will return to this point later when I offer some criticisms.

Mrs Burlingham has long been known to have a special interest in twins, not only in the three sets of identicals that are reported here. A companion book on non-identical twins will be eagerly awaited. In this volume by careful planning the masses of facts are laid out for our benefit, facts which were recorded at a time of maximum air-raids, largely by persons whose own relation to home and country had been so rudely disturbed that paralysis might have been excused. This is not mentioned in the book, except that there are inevitable references to bombs, air-raid shelters and separations attendant upon war.

Details in the daily lives of the children are presented in such a way,

1. London: Imago, 1953. Winnicott's review appeared in *New Era in Home and School* (March 1953).

helped by three-colour printing, that one can follow the development of each child or of each pair without difficulty, and one soon gets to know the children quite well. It is perhaps best for the reader to start with the charts of the set of twins presented last, because these were already 3 years 7 months when they came under observation and one is on familiar ground right away, watching the development of positive and negative inter-personal relationships, and of the instinct life, and of the organisation of defences against anxiety and intolerable internal conflict.

As an example, it is easy, from the charts, to pick out, following the appropriate colour and column, that Mary, at 3 years 11 months, took over a male role. At 4 she said "I am Daddy." At about this time, being confronted with her daddy she hesitated, while Madge ran to meet him, and kissed him. This state of affairs was related to a subdued role that was being played by Madge. After Madge had been away ill, however, roles became reversed, to some extent. It was then Madge who said, "Daddy must not be killed." This is only one of very many types of theme that could be studied from the charts by anyone who has limited opportunity for the study of actual twins in development, and in a controlled yet human environment. Many of the observations of these children remind one of those of Susan Isaacs, Piaget, Gesell; they are interesting but nowadays largely supplanted by direct observations made by students in practical work. Example: Madge (5 years 2 months), "Will to-day be yesterday to-morrow?" as an example of the child's conception of time. This and other comparable observations have increased value because they are related to the emotional climate and the environmental setting (in this instance, the absence of Mary, the twin, because of illness).

Both the other sets of twins came to the Hampstead Nurseries at 4 months. Bill and Bert and also Bessie and Jessie had been evacuated with their mothers soon after birth. Both sets were fatherless. The observations of these, extending back to the early months, provide data that can only be excelled by complementary psycho-analytic studies for the development of the theory of the emotional growth of human beings.

The first question that will be asked is: When did the twins become aware of each other? Bill and Bert began to take notice of each other at 7 months and Jessie and Bessie at 8 months. In each case there was a time-lag between the first recognition and mutual recognition. The onset of response to the mother was much earlier, but was difficult to sort out from a general response to being handled by the nurses who were also known to the infants. With this important qualifying comment, it could be said that both infants (Bill and Bert) took notice of the mother's visit from 4 months, the earliest time of observation. With Jessie and Bessie the response to the mother began several months before they responded to each other. At 4 months Jessie smiled at her mother, and at 7 months both she and Bessie had contact with her, by which I think is meant had formed a human relationship with her.

These details show up the lateness of the observable mutual response between the twins of these two sets, and also have an interest apart altogether from the study of twinship. It is clear that those who were observing had no axe to grind, but were day by day making notes of what was to be seen and heard.

I give this sample to try to whet the appetite of the reader, so that the book will get properly read and used.

Mrs Burlingham gradually shows that with twins there is not only the inborn alikeness. Soon the twins begin to copy each other. They copy each other for various distinct reasons, for instance: to please themselves and to please their mother; to distract each other; because of a dependence of one on the other; because of identification, with one incorporating the other and so compulsively imitating; to strike a balance between having all or renouncing all, through fairness and the demand for fair treatment; and so on.

There is a unique opportunity in the twin relationship for team work, and Mrs. Burlingham has a comment to make on the light that a study of twinship may possibly throw on the origins of the gang, as for instance that of delinquents.

At 2 years 5 months Jessie and Bessie were separated through illness. Bessie, when told to lie down, said, "Me not Bessie, me Jessie" and lay down ordinarily when called Jessie. Mrs Burlingham points out the identification with the lost love-object illustrated here and elsewhere in the material. My comment is that with twins the magical side of identification is facilitated, which means that the imaginative side can be by-passed, so that there is less of the depressive quality to the reaction, this latter depending on (imaginative) incorporation rather than on (magical) introjection. The result of the one is anxiety due to the destructive elements in the incorporation idea, and that of the other is simple possession by the unaltered love-object.

By way of criticism I would say that some of Mrs Burlingham's conclusions are marred by the use of terms that have a limited public. For instance (p. 16); "On the basis of the pleasure principle all babies respond to whatever gives them sensations of pleasure . . ." The term "pleasure principle" belongs to a theoretical construct of Freud, and those who are familiar with the growth of psycho-analytic theory will understand what is meant. But the term adds nothing and makes Mrs Burlingham's meaning liable to misunderstanding, especially as the paragraph ends with the phrase "the desire to please *à deux*," in which pleasure is used in the ordinary way and not as a technical term with specific connotation. As a technical term it belongs to a period of theorising in which the object-seeking element in early erotic experience was being neglected in psycho-analytic writings, though (I believe) not in practice.

I could drag in other criticism of this sort but the fact remains that the book has real value, and it can be used as a source for the student, and an example for those who have detailed observations to present.

Mrs Burlingham pays due respect to the idea of twins and the contrast that exists between being a twin and imagining being a twin. I think there is more to be said about the actual twin situation. For instance, by the time twins start to show they notice each other there has already been plenty of room for good or unsatisfactory emotional development. Mrs Burlingham fully expounds the theory of the twin relationship in terms of inter-personal relationship and indeed as something profoundly affected by the satisfaction and the frustrating aspects of the ordinary triangular situation (parents and child), that is to say, the Oedipus complex. But twins are twins before they get as far as being whole human beings related to whole human beings. There is plenty of material in this book for a study of these very early matters.

It is right to make a start by studying twins as persons who have developed through these early stages (in which failure denotes a predisposition to insanity) to the stage of the Oedipus complex, in which failure spells neurosis.

But the early tasks of the infant seem to me to be understressed in this book, and yet they are probably relevant. By early tasks I refer to the following: the development of the sense of self as a unit, integration of the personality; the development of a sense of existing in the body, of occupying it all, no more, no less; also the gradual acceptance of the illusory nature of all emotional contact between persons, from which it follows that objective perception is only a relative term, referring to something that loses meaning as soon as it is out of step with the corresponding process of subjective apperception, or of creativity.

I know this is a very personal phrasing, but through it I can perhaps convey the idea that there are important things to be learned from twins that can help with the study of the roots of sanity and insanity. Probably it is once again psycho-analysis rather than direct observation that can give what is needed here. I have had two patients in long analysis who were twins, and in each case it was for a disturbance that was established prior to the stage of the Oedipus complex that my help was sought.

Mrs Burlingham will easily support me when I stress the value of psycho-analytic study that must go with and elucidate direct observation. I know she has had a great deal of experience of twins that is not referred to in this book.

This, which I have written by stretching my neck while standing on the platform that is her book, in no way modifies my opinion of the book, which is that it has no twin.

50
W. R. D. Fairbairn

Review (written with M. Masud R. Khan)
of *Psychoanalytic Studies of the Personality*[1]

1953

Fairbairn has made a sincere and bold attempt to revise psycho-
analytic metapsychology in the light of his own clinical experience
and through the private thinking that he has done while applying
himself to the therapeutic task. The reader will be able to enrich himself by sharing the gradual evolution of a personal theory which is
clearly presented by the method of a chronological order in the arrangement of the papers. Whether one agrees or disagrees with Fairbairn's theory, there is very much to be gained from a study of his way
of looking at things.

A reviewer is in a less fortunate position than an ordinary reader,
since Fairbairn makes a definite claim, and it must be this claim that
gets the appraisal and the criticism. The claim is that Fairbairn's
theory supplants that of Freud. If Fairbairn is right, then we teach
Fairbairn and not Freud to our students. If one could escape from this
claim one could enjoy the writings of an analyst who challenges
everything, and who puts clinical evidence before accepted theory,
and who is no worshipper at a shrine. But the claim is there. Incidentally, Fairbairn writes as if there were practically no other psycho-
analytic theoreticians except Freud, Abraham, and Klein, so that a
review to be complete should include the quotations from other authors that Fairbairn seems to have left out of count. This will not,
however, be attempted.

The first paper, "Schizoid Factors in the Personality" (1940), is perhaps the most stimulating and rewarding contribution in the whole

1. London: Tavistock, 1952. This review appeared in the *International Journal of Psycho-Analysis* (1953). Copyright © Institute of Psycho-Analysis. For later comments made
by Winnicott about Fairbairn, see the Postscript to this volume.—EDS.

book. Here Fairbairn suggests that the understanding of schizoid states, processes, and syndromes, and nothing else, can yield the deepest understanding of the origins and the true basis of human personality. The term "schizoid" naturally undergoes a vast enlargement in his hands, and he is aware that it covers almost every facet of human living if looked at in the way that he suggests. And that is how it should be, according to the author, because (p. 8), "The fundamental schizoid phenomenon is the presence of splits in the ego . . ." and ". . . some measure of splitting of the ego is invariably present at the deepest mental level—or (to express the same thing in terms borrowed from Melanie Klein) *the basic position in the psyche is invariably a schizoid position.*" The author adds: "This would not hold true, of course, in the case of a theoretically perfect person whose development had been optimum; but then there is really nobody who enjoys such a happy lot." Evidence that everyone without exception is schizoid at the deepest levels comes partly from the study of dreams, because all figures in the dream "represent either (1) some part of the dreamer's personality, or (2) an object with whom some part of his personality has a relationship, commonly on a basis of identification, in inner reality."

The author makes the comment (pp. 8–9, 1940): "the fact that the dreamer is characteristically represented in the dream by more than one figure is capable of no other interpretation except that, at the level of dreaming consciousness, the ego of the dreamer is split. The dream thus represents a universal schizoid phenomenon." It is important for the student of Fairbairn's theory to grasp this, since the author's concepts of psychic structure evolve from the analysis of a dream (reported pp. 95 ff., 1944); it is here that he finally arrives at the conclusion that "dreams are essentially, not wish-fulfilments, but dramatizations or shorts (in the cinematographic sense) of situations existing in inner reality," and the "figures represent either parts of the 'ego' or internalized objects." Hence (p. 99) "the situations depicted in dreams represent relationships existing between endopsychic structures; and the same applies to situations depicted in waking phantasies." In a much earlier paper (1931: "The Analysis of a Patient with a Genital Abnormality") studying the phenomenon of personification in the patient's dreams he had concluded (p. 221) "The appearance of stable personifications in the patient's dreams seems to indicate the manner in which the phenomena of multiple personality originate. It suggests that these phenomena result from the invasion of the conscious field by functioning structural constellations which become differentiated in the unconscious under pressure of economic necessity. It also suggests that Freud's tripartite division of the mind should be regarded as representing a description of characteristic structural constellations of a similar nature rather than as representing an analysis of the mind into component entities." The reduction of this "tripartite division of mind" to rigid entities on the one hand and to anthropomorphic agencies on the other is the result of analytic theoreticians other than Freud. In Freud's metapsychology the emphasis is on the functional properties of these hypothetical mental structures. The methodological route Dr Fairbairn pursues is very direct and simple: from personifications to internal objects and thence to endopsychic structures.

In passing it should also be noted that though Fairbairn is offering a total theory he offers no hypothesis to explain the dream work in dream formation. In the same way, in his psychic structure theory he does not even consider the fact that a metapsychology should be able to postulate some hypothesis about mental functioning, e.g. memory, hallucination. Freud has offered a very definite theory of mental functioning in *The Interpretation of Dreams* (last chapter), and his hypothesis that libido and primary processes are regulated by the pleasure-pain principle derives as much from this area of observation as from the study of emotional disorders.

It is possible to get something out of Fairbairn's work on dreams by considering the relationship of his concept of introjection of the bad object to the work of Freud on repetition-compulsion. If the bad object introjected (in order to be coerced or controlled) is a painful experience, i.e. something perceived but not tolerated, then the introjected experience repeatedly claims attention and gives rise to a specific dream type. The concept of repetition-compulsion carries us over the period which we need for the understanding that to get behind the repetition-compulsion the patient must rediscover the external painful situation as it was originally perceived, though at the time it could not be tolerated as a phenomenon outside omnipotent control.

But this is going ahead. It is necessary to go back to examine what the author considers to be the state of affairs in infancy, just there where the schizoid process is in operation, where the schizoid states that appear later on are created. There is a great deal of valuable material in the part of the book in which this is considered.

Our main concern must be with the author's theory of endopsychic

416 On the Work of Other Analysts

structures. Drawing on the researches into schizoid phenomena of Freud, Bleuler, Abraham, the author comes to the conclusion that if the clinical manifestations of a schizoid order have a fixation point in the early oral phase, then surely there must be a very close connection between splitting of the ego and a libidinal attitude of oral incorporation; in fact, that a fixation in the early oral phase plays a prominent part in the determination of the pattern of the schizoid attitude.

In infancy the "first social relationship established by the individual is that between himself and his mother; and the focus of this relationship is the suckling situation, in which the mother's breast provides the focal point of his libidinal object and his mouth the focal point of his own libidinal attitude." In this quotation (1940) we already meet with all the characteristics of Fairbairn's way of looking at an infant (that is to say, if he really is looking at an infant) that paves the way to his final theoretical construction. Here should be noted the designation of the mother-child relationship as a "social relationship," the equation of the infant with the adult individual he is going to be, the characterisation of the breast as "his (the infant's) *libidinal object*," and the attribution of a "libidinal attitude" to the infant's mouth.

It might be claimed for the author that he is verbalising a pre-verbal primary state, but examination of the developed hypothesis will show the reader that this cannot be called into account for what follows. Fairbairn does start off with an infant that is a whole human being, one experiencing the relation to the breast as a separate object, an object that he has experienced and about which he has complicated ideas (p. 11). It is this way of working that makes the author theorise categorically that "libido is object-seeking," etc. But the author, as we shall see later, finds it very difficult consistently to maintain this view by which the infant is always a separate entity, seeking objects from within his own entity-existence.

To return to the text, Fairbairn elaborates by giving four main features of this early oral attitude (pp. 11–12):

1. Although the emotional relationship involved is essentially one between the child and his mother as a person, and although it must be recognized that his libidinal object is really his mother as a whole, nevertheless his libidinal interest is essentially focused upon her breast; and the result is that, in proportion as disturbances in the relationship occur, the breast itself tends to assume the role of libidinal object; i.e. the libidinal object tends to assume the form of a bodily organ or *partial object* (in contrast to that of a person or whole object).

2. The libidinal attitude is essentially one in which the aspect of "*taking*" predominates over that of "*giving*."

3. The libidinal attitude is one characterized, not only by taking, but also by *incorporating*, and *internalizing*.

4. The libidinal situation is one which confers tremendous significance upon the states of *fullness and emptiness* . . .

Fairbairn does not make it quite clear what is the nature, what are the causes of the disturbances in the mother-infant relationship (§1 above). However, from remarks in other places, one can piece together his opinion. He suggests (p. 13) that "the orientation towards partial objects found in individuals displaying schizoid features is largely a regressive phenomenon determined by unsatisfactory emotional relationships with their parents, and particularly their mothers, at a stage in childhood subsequent to the early oral phase in which this orientation originates. The type of mother who is specially prone to provoke such a regression is the mother who fails to convince her child by spontaneous and genuine expressions of affection that she herself loves him as a person."

In this quotation and context it is not clear whether the mother only "provokes the regression" to this early state, or is the creator of it.

In §4 (not fully quoted) Fairbairn mentions "circumstances of deprivation," but without making it clear whether they are the result of a deficiency in mother's care or inevitable in child care. If these two are held to be the same on account of the imperfect maturity of all persons (including mothers), then it must be said that Fairbairn has not found a language that covers both the normal and the abnormal.

On page 23 the author scrutinises "the sources of that sense of difference from others which characterizes individuals with a schizoid element in their personality." He writes that the following feature stands out prominently: "In early life they gained the conviction, whether through apparent indifference or through apparent possessiveness on the part of their mother, that their mother did not really love and value them as persons in their own right." This, like many others in this book, is a valuable and penetrating observation; unfortunately the author's theoretical structure, which must be our main concern, spoils our appreciation of the flashes of clinical insight. Fairbairn's most valuable contribution is the idea that at the root of the schizoid personality is this failure on the part of the mother to be felt by the infant as loving him in his own right as a person.

It is very difficult to work out whether Fairbairn considers this maternal failure to be truly the mother's failure or the child's projection on to her of his own hate. There is much in the book to suggest that the latter is the view mainly held. For instance (pp. 110–111)

> It is the experience of libidinal frustration that calls forth the infant's aggression in relation to his libidinal object and thus gives rise to a state of ambivalence . . . From the subjective point of view of the infant it is his mother becoming an ambivalent object . . . Since it proves intolerable to him to have a good object which is also bad, he seeks to alleviate the situation by splitting the figure of his mother into two objects . . . since outer reality seems unyielding, he does his best to transfer the traumatic factor in the situation to the field of inner reality, within which he feels situations to be more under his own control . . . It is always the "bad" object that is internalized in the first instance, for I find it difficult to attach any meaning to the primary internalization of a good object which is both satisfying and amenable from the infant's point of view . . . internalization of objects is essentially a measure of coercion, and it is not the satisfying object but the unsatisfying object that the infant seeks to coerce.

(In passing, it seems hopeless to try to correlate these statements with the work of Melanie Klein, since Klein's work has been set down with great clarity, and Fairbairn's discoveries seem to run criss-cross with those of Klein. It would be easy to ask Fairbairn to make a more close study of Klein's work before quoting her, but on the other hand we must concede to a colleague the right to express his opinions in his own way, even when his work runs parallel with work being done elsewhere. It is a pity, however, that terms are used which suggest familiarity with work such as that of Klein in respect of what she named the "positions" in emotional development, the "depressive," "paranoid," and "schizoid" respectively.)

This internalising to coerce is surely a defence mechanism, one that has been well described and accepted in analytic literature. Fairbairn is thus considering introjection as a specific defence mechanism, and not as a primary process as such, nor as a kind of object-relationship. It is difficult to see how the human being could build up inner sources of strength, or the basic stuff of the inner world that is personal and indeed the self, simply on the taking in of "bad" objects through the operation of a defence mechanism. Certainly this is but a caricature of Klein's theory, if it is related to that theory at all, which seems doubtful except that the terms overlap.

This is the author's position of 1944. It is important to note that in an addendum to this paper, written in 1951, he himself has found this state of affairs unsatisfactory. He seeks to correct himself by harking back to the 1941 paper, and by writing: "The object which is originally internalized is not an object embodying the exclusively "bad" and unsatisfying aspect of the external object, but the pre-ambivalent object ... The internalization of the pre-ambivalent object would then be explained on the ground that it presented itself as unsatisfying in some measure as well as in some measure satisfying. On this assumption ambivalence will be a state first arising in the original unsplit ego in relation, not to the external object, but to an internalized pre-ambivalent object."

But this lands the author in other and possibly worse contradictions, and in any case it would seem that if this new turn to his theory be true, then his main point (which is that libido is object-seeking) is no longer a good one. This could be stated by the method of putting the argument into reverse.

In his "synopsis" (1951, p. 163) the author gives a theory of ego development. Its first tenet is: "Ego development is characterized by a process whereby an original state of infantile dependence based upon primary identification with the object is abandoned in favour of a state of adult or mature dependence based upon differentiation of the object from the self."

This state of infantile dependence is characterised by primary "identification." Now the author has defined primary identification for us in a footnote (p. 145): "I employ the term 'primary identification' here to signify the cathexis of *an object which has not yet been differentiated*" (our italics) "(or has been only partly differentiated) from himself by the cathecting subject. This process differs, of course, from the process ordinarily described as 'identification,' viz. an emotionally determined tendency to treat a differentiated (or partly differentiated) object as if it were not differentiated, when it is cathected. The latter process should properly be described as 'secondary identification.'"

Now if the object is not differentiated it cannot operate as an object. What Fairbairn is referring to then is an infant with needs, but with no "mechanism" by which to implement them, an infant with needs not "seeking" an object, but seeking de-tension, libido seeking satisfaction, instinct tension seeking a return to a state of rest or unexcitement; which brings us back to Freud.

The provision of a way out by the mother is not a part of the infant's mental activities, but something that may (or may not) be *given* to him. That *if all goes well* the individual infant may develop to a point at which he can begin to relate the object to his need, to seek it, to create it, to coerce it, etc. is well known.

As in many other instances we are left here with the feeling that Fairbairn's clinical and intuitive sense brings him all the way while his theory gets bogged down a few miles in the rear. His mother (of the schizoid type) who fails to give the feeling that she loves the infant as a person is surely the mother who cannot meet the infant's own individual needs as they arise at the very beginning, making the difference between the provision and the non-provision of a way out for the infant, at the start, over and over again, when libido seeks (not an object but) satisfaction.

Again Fairbairn, who does not allow for primary (psychic) creativity in his theory, could claim to have indicated his belief in it by quoting his comment (p. 141): "It (a house) is an object which is sought, even if, to be found, it has first to be made." Fairbairn nowhere states how the infant makes the (theoretical) first object. In his theory primary psychic creativity is not a human property; an infinite series of introjections and projections form the infant's psychic experience. Fairbairn's theory here lines up with the theory given us by Melanie Klein, which also allows no tribute to be paid to the idea of primary psychic creativity.

In strictly Freudian theory this point can be said not to have arisen, since the place in clinical work at which the question of primary creativity comes up for consideration has not been reached. The analyst is concerned with the whole range of reality and phantasy associated with inter-personal relationships and the gradual attainment of maturity in the instinctual elements in these relationships; nevertheless no claim is being made that these matters cover the entire range of human experience. It would seem that only comparatively recently have analysts begun to feel the need for a hypothesis that would allow for areas of infancy experience and of ego development that are not basically associated with instinctual conflict and where there is intrinsically a psychic process such as that which we have here termed "primary (psychic) creativity." It seems a pity that Fairbairn, who has so incisively described the schizoid character, with its sense of futility and emptiness, should in his theoretical constructs miss the use of a hypothesis which would have given a clue to the roots of this sense of futility and emptiness in infancy experience.

It would seem that while Fairbairn has been developing personally in accordance with honest psycho-analytic work, his theory has been adversely affected by the fact that he has not been in clinical touch with infants and with nursing couples. In consequence he fails to note the tremendous differences that exist between the needs of "whole" infants (however young) experiencing object-relationships of oral quality and those of infants at the theoretical start, who are emerging from a state characterised by primary identification by virtue of being mothered. On account of this he has had to waste his valuable study of dependency in infancy. In any discussion of the emotional development of the infant must it not first be decided whether or no the infant has in fact (through being treated as a person in his own right, with individual needs and tensions) become a separate being in respect of this matter of primary identification?

Fairbairn is almost in the position of one of those who do psychotherapy outside the psycho-analytic grouping altogether. His work is liable to be lost because of its not being integrated into the general body of developing theory. This, if it is true, weakens Fairbairn's position when he makes a special point that his body of theory supplants that of Freud, at any rate in certain important respects. While sharing many of Fairbairn's dissatisfactions, and while one is able to derive valuable ideas from his suggestions, one is nevertheless in the end left with the feeling that Freud's developing ideas provided and still provide a more fertile soil than the developed theory of Fairbairn.

Attention is particularly drawn to three details:

1. The section on emotional identification (p. 275), in which separation anxiety is correlated with identification. "So intimate is the connection between identification and infantile dependence that, psychologically speaking, they may be treated as the same phenomenon."

2. The "rehabilitation" (p. 292) as opposed to the "treatment" of certain war-neurosis cases and of sexual perverts, an idea which can be compared with the suggestion that has been made that a study of the management aspect of the psycho-analytic procedure in the treatment of acute regression states (preparatory to the correct interpreting of instinct-derivatives and unconscious phantasies in transference-neurosis) provides a fruitful line of research for the extension of the use of psycho-analytic therapeutic techniques.

3. The sorting out of two types of omnipotence (p. 213), the one being "represented in the omnipotence of mania and schizophrenia, whereas the latter type seems characteristic of obsessional and para-

noid states." It is as if in the first there is a regression and in the latter the patient brings forward early omnipotence and puts it into action as a defensive technique under ego-control. This still leaves room for a third and perhaps the normal use of omnipotence where it reinforces routine sublimatory activities, thus investing them with illusional potential that is both enriching and gratifying to the ego.

This is a most valuable and indeed stimulating book, giving the fruits of the life-work of a colleague; as such it will be widely read, and it cannot fail to be a stimulus to new thought.

51
John Bowlby

I. Review of *Maternal Care and Mental Health*[1]

1953

By the time that this review is in print this book will already have been widely read, and it has been rightly praised almost everywhere. I wish to join in with this appreciation of the book and of the work that it represents and of the specific trend in Dr Bowlby which makes him drive on towards a translation of the psycho-analytic findings of the past half-century into social action. I wish to offer criticism but without ceasing to admire and support.

The book is divided into two parts. In the first are described the adverse effects of maternal deprivation. It is here that Bowlby's special contribution can be looked for. Efforts must be made, he is convinced, to present psychological matters in statistical form, so that those who are accustomed to scientific papers (of the kind that are appreciated by scientists in all types of work) can assess the claims of those of us who are clinically minded and slightly scornful of figures. As in his previous monograph *Forty-four Juvenile Thieves: Their Characters and Home-life,* so here Bowlby justifies his thesis at least in respect of the subject under discussion, and he has collected together the reports of work that has been done in the various countries he visited which can be put in statistical form. He would be the first to admit that statistics are valueless unless based on data which are beyond reproach, and indeed it is just these data which are so difficult to collect in our specialty. One would guess that in nearly all the other types of psychological disorder there would be found to be not enough agreement over any simple statement of the phenomena observed for the statistical method to work. In this particular subject of maternal deprivation and its results there are certain justifiable simplifications, but

---

1. Geneva: W. H. O., 1951; also H. M. Stationery Office. This review appeared in the *British Journal of Medical Psychology* (1953).

clinicians will be all the time worried lest Bowlby has over-simplified in order to prove a point by statistics. Probably there would be general agreement on a statement like this, that *for the purpose of statistical inquiry* simplifications have to be made, but no harm is done provided that there is a return to the complex from the simplified before the construction of new theory.

It would be possible to overdo the deprivation theme. In order to keep matters simple, Bowlby has to leave out the whole consideration of *the resources normal children* have at their disposal by virtue of which they do not become deprived children when away from their parents unavoidably, and *not too long*. Probably some children are more hurt by the fact that the teddy they go to bed with could not be taken into hospital with them, or else by the fact that the teddy was taken in and there mingled with all the other toys, or sterilised or destroyed, than by the temporary loss of the actual parent. There is nothing in what Bowlby writes which contradicts such an idea as this, but I think it is necessary that we should remind ourselves that human nature is too complex for evaluation by the statistical method; certain types of *illness* can be dealt with in this way and particularly illnesses which are rather stereotyped.

In the second part, in which the prevention of maternal deprivation is discussed, Bowlby ranges widely over the subject, giving us the benefit of his experience which is enriched by his study of the literature. He is generous in his quotations. The whole set-out shows how much time and thought he has given to the subject and this part is of practical value and will be appreciated by the wide public of the world. With the opinions expressed one finds oneself almost always in agreement. I would specially single out the statement that "it is in the interests of the adopted baby's mental health for him to be adopted soon after birth." In practice it has become more and more difficult to bring this about. Also it is surely sensible for a baby who is to be handed over by the mother not to have the breast first, and to be handed over to the technique of the adoptive parent at the earliest possible moment; the idea that what happens for a few weeks after birth makes no difference to the psyche is something we shall have to give up, and the sooner the better.

I would like to make one criticism, and this must remain a personal opinion and it may be that other readers will not agree. I find one chapter, that on theoretical problems, very unsatisfactory. It seems to me it could have been left out altogether. Possibly it was inserted at a late stage, so that the author may be intending to re-write it. I would particularly ask the author to reconsider the sentence in which he says that "the psychic machinery which we develop within ourselves to harmonize our different and even conflicting needs and to seek their satisfaction in a world realistically apprehended *is our ego*" (my italics). I suggest that only confusion can result in the minds of those who are new to psychology by a statement that some psychic machinery "is the ego," especially as the word "ego" is used variously by various groups of people. The other way round would be more satisfactory for me, that the psycho-analysts call this psychic machinery the ego; others are at liberty to call it by some other name.

Apart from this awkward sentence there is to my mind a poverty of treatment in this theoretical chapter which lets the book down. Theoretical statements in the other chapters are much more satisfying though more popularly phrased. If there is to be a theoretical chapter at all then that is the place where it should be pointed out that there are very complex internal factors that cannot be dealt with in a book like this at all. At one point Bowlby attempts to be positive: "They [severely deprived children] are ineffective personalities, unable to learn from experience and consequently their own worst enemies. The theoretical problem is to understand how deprivation produces this result. The two main approaches to its solution are Goldfarb's discoveries regarding the impairment of abstract thinking in these patients, and the clinical findings regarding their inability to identify or introject. Each approach carries us some distance, but the day has yet to come when they lead to a unified body of theory."

I very much doubt whether Goldfarb's discoveries about abstract thinking take us very far. In fact it would be dangerous to spread around the idea that children who have a good capacity for abstract thinking are thereby enabled not to steal. One can quite see that in the whole "deprived complex" there can be found some specific impairment of the capacity for abstract thinking. The various phenomena have a common cause. What is to be feared is that readers who are new to this subject will think that the antisocial child can be largely explained by the presence of a thinking difficulty. In fact, the trouble is very much to do with affect, and to do with unconscious guilt and with such things as the fear of madness and fear of loss of identity and of contact with external reality. If the author really maintains what he has written in this chapter, then I must express disagreement with him, but I think that either I have got hold of the wrong end of the stick or else he has slipped up on this chapter, which he will re-write in the new edition which must be already due.

When reading this book one must have its purpose constantly in mind, and except in this chapter it seems to me that Bowlby has kept his audience in front of him. Because of this, presumably, although he has mentioned psycho-analysis, he has not quoted Freud in his bibliography. The unconscious is not ignored but it is not brought to the fore. This is understandable, but is it not a fact that the detailed day-to-day analysis of adults and children along with gradually developing psycho-analytic theory has been the thing that has made Dr Bowlby's work possible and timely?

There is now a film by Dr Bowlby and his team which excellently illustrates distressing facts about a child becoming deprived although happily able to recover.[2] Everyone who has worked in a children's hospital ward has had the chance to witness what this film briefly shows and to witness it over and over again. I could never make out why few people see this thing for themselves until I realised that if they did they would find ward work too painful. The film, used properly, could have a very big effect and we must not expect the team ever to make a better. The danger is that by forcing facts on a public that is not willing to suffer there may be reactions and counter-reactions and a new kind of muddle. The prevention of this rests with those who are in charge of the presentation of the film.

II. Discussion of "Grief and Mourning in Infancy"[3]

1953

A

I find it very difficult to take part in this discussion and yet I want to do so. Dr Bowlby has generously referred to me and my writings, and he has also studied the writings of many analysts and ethologists. What have I to complain about? The fact is that I do not feel he has

2. *A Two-Year-Old Goes to Hospital*, made with James and Joyce Robertson.
3. Dr Bowlby's paper was read at a Scientific Meeting of the British Psycho-Analytical Society in October 1959; it was subsequently published in *The Psycho-Analytic Study of*

understood some things that I consider important. I must try to make my meaning clear.

I could almost prefer that he should have given his own views regardless of other writers. This leaves us to use our own judgement about derivations. In any case there is no harm if then there be a genuine rediscovery of old facts or old theories. Something new and valuable always turns up when old things are stated in a new way. Dr Bowlby, however, seems to be anxious to show where he supplants the former analytic writers, and it is here I think that he is unconvincing. This is a pity because Dr Bowlby has some important things to contribute. I never tire of stating and restating the fact that his propaganda for the avoidance of unnecessary breaks in the infant-mother relationship has gone round the world, though I do also feel that the propaganda element necessary led to a fashion in child care and to the inevitable reactions which follow propaganda and over-conversion.

Then again, I want to join with Dr Bowlby in a move for broadening the base of teaching in child analysis, since I believe we are in danger from the fact that we pass out as trained child-analysts men and women who (some of them) have very little experience of children and of child care.

There is something in the way, however, and I do not yet know how serious is the block. In regard to this particular chapter of Bowlby's book which deals with grief, I feel most uneasy, and I want to examine the reasons for my uneasiness.

Let me say first that the idea of sadness was not one that was commonly referred to in the twenties. I got the idea from Merrill Middlemore who was working with me in the early thirties. She looked at the face of a boy patient of mine and said: "a case of melancholia." Up to then that referred to children who found life difficult, but suddenly I saw that the word "depression" was waiting to be used for the description of the clinical states of children and of infants, and I quickly altered all my language.

At this same time I was starting to learn about the mechanisms of depression and the contra-depressive defences from Melanie Klein, who had already been going strong for ten years or more, and who

---

the Child 15 (1960). Two typewritten versions of Winnicott's prepared contribution to the discussion were found among his papers, and as they differ substantially we have included both here. The first one was marked at the top in pencil with the words "Only extracts read actually," and the second with "More or less as spoken. DWW."—EDS.

had made it possible for me to bring into my analytic theory and work the observations I had made on many hundreds of children whose psychological disturbances started in the first weeks, even days, of their lives, and who were thorough-going psychiatric cases before the time that the Oedipus complex of those days was ripe.

Now it was in those early days of my work with Melanie Klein that I learned about the stages of grief, of protest, and of the denial of grief and depression which hardens into the manic defence. I was never a great reader, though I read Melanie Klein's *The Psycho-Analysis of Children* right through twice (on Dartmoor) immediately it came out in English. What I do know is that Bowlby is not the first person to discover the gradual transformation of grief into hardened indifference.

My differences with Melanie Klein are to do with my feeling that when she is telling us about early mechanisms she does so in terms that make us think she is talking about actual babies. But Bowlby makes me rally to her support, even if she doesn't need or want me.

I feel just the same about Anna Freud, whose work I came to know much later than I knew that of Melanie Klein. I really don't mind much what she and Dorothy Burlingham wrote down. It is a miracle that they wrote it down at all. The thing that was important was the work they did under conditions that demanded personal courage of a high order. I remember the conditions that obtained in London in the second year of the war, and the air-raid shelter in the War Nursery which had to satisfy the Ministries.

This work was not done in order that a book might one day be written called *Young Children in Wartime: A Year's Work in a Residential War Nursery*. It was done because Miss Freud knew that babies separated from mothers at an early age were unable to achieve anything so normal as grief, and that something had to be done. I sent Miss Freud the first case, and was I glad to have somewhere to send the child!

It can perhaps be seen from all this that emotions have been stirred in me by Bowlby's obviously genuine attempt to be fair to everyone.

What we may expect to get from Bowlby is the idea that human infants, like animals, may at the beginning be quite simply affected by some environmental condition so that they smile without first experiencing the mood that we (by projection) feel they must be in so that they smile. This is an extension of the idea that a baby's smile can be evoked by a touch on the face or by wind. I want to say that I have tried hard to use these ideas in my analytic work and I have not been able to see how they affect my work even with adults regressed to infantile dependence (which I regard as the best material for observations on the phenomena of infancy and infant care).

I take the risk of being one day thought to be an old fogey, and I say that I think that for the analyst the ethology contribution is *a dead end*. I like ethology because of what it tells us about animals. But I do consider that Bowlby has signally failed to show how he applies his views of early infantile reflexes to the area of development represented by the film *A Two-Year-Old Goes to Hospital*. By the time an infant is a year old we really do know a lot about him, and the complexity of two years is tremendous if we remember the whole elaboration of unconscious fantasy and of unconscious conflict. I consider that anyone who intends to add anything to what we know of the reactions of a two-year-old to loss of object must first show he knows what it is like to do the analysis of a two-year-old, or of the two-year-old that is in any patient of any age.

More specifically, I think Bowlby has omitted reference to the change-over from a relationship to a *subjective* object to a relationship to an object that is *objectively perceived*. This belongs especially to the period following the end of the first half-year, and (with tremendous variations from child to child) becomes something fairly complete at two or three years. This disillusionment process belongs to health, and it is not possible to refer to an infant's loss of object without referring to the stage of disillusionment, and to the positive or negative factors in the early stages of this process which depend on the capacity of the mother to give the baby the illusion without which disillusionment makes no sense.

All this is thrust aside by Bowlby's implication that there is a very simple object-loss phenomenon rather like the failure of a reflex because of the absence of the stimulus.

The matter which Bowlby is examining is so very much richer than he seems to suggest that I fear lest we may lose sight of all that reaction to loss can mean by getting engaged in some controversy about ravens or ducklings.

B

One of my difficulties is that Dr Bowlby says that his thesis is that "loss of mother-figure in the period between about six months and three or four or more years is an event of high pathogenic potential *because of the processes of mourning to which it habitually gives rise* and which all too readily at this age take a pathological course."

Would he consider rewording this?

Loss of the mother-figure is surely not pathogenic because of the processes of mourning. This would leave out the whole concept of mourning as an achievement. We have come to think of a long series of delicate mechanisms at the end of which the infant arrives at the capacity to mourn. When things go wrong we think in terms of a loss of the capacity to mourn, the loss of something that has been achieved in the emotional development of the individual. It is very specifically as a result of Melanie Klein's work that we have a great deal to say about the pathology of small children and older persons whose capacity to mourn has been over-strained. Melanie Klein's teaching under the heading "The Manic Defence" so impressed me with its importance that I wrote my Membership paper on this subject,[4] and as I understand it the term "Manic Defence" covers all the processes of the denial of mourning which is nevertheless retained as a theoretical depression. I myself have tried to take part in the development of the further concept of the deeper effect of object loss or neglect of ego support, and I have stated this in terms of the primitive emotional conditions and have used the terms "loss of contact with external reality," "loss of relationship between psyche and soma," and "disintegration." In my work on these matters I may have drawn heavily from the work of others. In the language I use in describing the emotional development of infants at the stages before and during the gradual establishment of their capacity to mourn I can find no place for these words of Bowlby's which he actually underlines, *"because of the processes of mourning to which it* [loss of mother-figure] *habitually gives rise."* Mourning implies emotional maturity and health. It would seem to me therefore that Bowlby has not been careful in the statement of his central thesis on which the whole of the rest of his paper depends.

I would like to choose one or two other points for comment. One has to do with Bowlby's assessment of Melanie Klein's theory of that which she calls the "depressive position." He seems to imply that Melanie Klein is referring to the infant's relationship to a part-object.

---

4. 1935; *Collected Papers: Through Paediatrics to Psycho-Analysis* (London: Tavistock, 1958, New York: Basic Books, 1975; London: Hogarth Press, 1975), ch. 11.

Now this seems to me to be a complete misconception of the whole theory. In the first place the part-object is a whole object from the infant's point of view except in so far as the infant is split or disintegrated. The whole point of the depressive position is, I believe, the gradual joining up in the mind of the infant of the limited object of instinctual desire and the whole object of the mother-figure's total personality. The infant's relationship to the part-object is very definitely only a part of the story. It is for this reason that some of us have tried to get Melanie Klein not to date her depressive position too early because it connotes a highly sophisticated state of affairs, that is to say, a full recognition of the mother as a human being and the linking up with this of the idea of the breast as a part of her. By the way, there seems to be no reason why the word "breast" should not be used when we are talking like this to stand for any kind of container, or part of the mother, with which the infant becomes familiar. In Mrs Klein's work there is frequent mention of the infant's attack on the body. This is the fantasy of the infant, but we are using our words, and we can say "body" or "breast" or what we like. Looking at infancy through older childhood, as we do in psycho-analysis, we come to the idea of a breast which is a body and a womb and a vagina and a bladder and a head and a biceps muscle. The main issue is not affected by these words which we use.

Briefly I would like to mention one or two other points. One is that Bowlby has not seemed to leave room here in his statement for symbolism and for the establishment (in health) of objects which stand both for the self and for the mother. He knows of course that the trauma when a child is separated from the mother is often not the loss of the mother but the loss of the thing that I call a transitional object. He also knows that if the mother is lost too long the transitional object begins to lose value as a symbol. These things are right at the very centre of the subject of a reaction to loss of mother, and are much more important to us than the study of animals, even of those animals that employ transitional objects.

It seems to me that Dr Bowlby is talking as if there were no such thing as fantasy in early infancy. Psycho-analysts are constantly surprised, however, to find how much fantasy has an early date. Unconscious conflict seems to have no place in Bowlby's psychology, and he seems to give us no room for the concept of the object dying and reviving within the infant, that is to say in the psychic apparatus, that which is lodged by the healthy infant in the functioning body. As a consequence of these omissions there seems to be no place in Bowlby's psychology for a description of those infants who because of gross mismanagement in the very early stages do not get near to anything as healthy as the capacity to mourn and perhaps do not even become integrated at any stage.

One other point. During the period to which Bowlby makes special reference, six months to three or four years, the child is in the process of change-over from a subjective object to one that is objectively perceived. Bowlby would be on very firm ground if he were to see that it is especially important for the infant that external changes are not made while this process of objectification or whatever we may choose to call it is taking place. This would be arguing along the lines that we are familiar with in the Society, and would link with the concept of the establishment of the reality principle.

I want to draw attention to the fact that in my view it would be wrong to deduce from this that the subjective object can be lost with impunity. This is a very complex subject and one that cannot be stated in a few words. It would appear that the subjective object of the first few months can be changed in the eyes of the onlooker and yet possibly not changed for the infant. For instance, one bottle can be changed for another; even a bottle can be substituted in the place of the breast. There is so much else that remains similar. Either the same person is feeding the baby or else there is a change of persons but the techniques overlap sufficiently. In spite of this flexibility which belongs to object relationships in the first months in which the object is a subjective one, I think that the loss of the subjective object is a major disaster, something which belongs to the order of things which are described by the words "psychotic anxiety," or the "basic fault" of Balint's nomenclature, or a failure of ego-support during the time when the infant's ego only has strength because of reliable support from the mother-figure, etc. This is the area in which we find ourselves discussing the origin of infantile psychosis and the origin of the liability to psychotic disorder which may show at any age in the individual's life.

52
Michael Balint

I. Character Types: The Foolhardy and the Cautious[1]

Dated 25 October 1954

It is often useful to examine the mixed qualities of the normal by comparing the opposed qualities that are to be found among the ill. Balint has suggested that there is value in contrasting two extreme types of behaviour pattern in the study of the admixture of dependence and independence in the healthy. He has applied names to these types but as I do not think these names are necessary I omit them here.[2]

There are those who seek and enjoy thrills, who let themselves go, and in the act of thrilling participation know of no danger. There are also those who like to have something to catch hold of, and who cling to almost anything when presented with a thrill situation, knowing it to be dangerous even when, in fact, it is not.

Balint usefully draws attention to the way that the problem of these contrasted types links up with that of regression.

It could be said that the foolhardy thrill-lover makes a regression towards the state of primary narcissism; there he is, or she, artificially placed in a situation that is part of himself or herself—as if a caricature were being made of the early state in which the individual only knows of environment as part of the self and has not yet repudiated the NOT-ME. We as observers see the dangers, but the individual concerned is blind to them. This blindness may be hidden in the devel-

---

1. On 20 October 1954, Dr Balint read to a Scientific Meeting of the British Psycho-Analytical Society a paper entitled "Funfairs, Thrills and Regressions," which later became part of the material for his book *Thrills and Regressions* (London: Hogarth Press, 1959). Winnicott was present at the meeting, and it seems that he wrote these comments a few days later, after thinking over what had been said.—EDS.

2. A full description of these character types appears in *Thrills and Regressions;* see also Balint, *The Basic Fault* (London: Tavistock, 1968).—EDS.

opment of personal skill; or it may be hidden in reliance on the technical skill of others, this being a subtle form of clinging.

In the second type of behaviour pattern, where clinging to an object is the main feature and danger is assumed, there is perhaps a flight forwards (instead of backwards) to a relationship to objects that have not yet, in the development of the individual, become properly external, repudiated, NOT-ME.

It will not surprise us if there is a state midway between the two extremes to which each is related, and from which each is a flight. I suggest that central to these two defensive organisations is the personal establishment of the state that is best described by the words I AM. This I AM state, as it becomes a fact, immediately develops into BEING or GOING ON BEING; that is to say, a time factor becomes included.

If these defensive organisations appear in relation to the establishment of the I AM state, it is necessary to look and see what anxiety belongs to that state. In health the maternal care which translates love into the necessary physical terms, and makes good-enough adaptation to varying need, carries the infant through the first I AM moments, and the early BEING experiences, enabling the sense of existing to become established. Maternal care that is inadequate shows up the anxiety that is potential in the I AM state. To BE implies an attitude to what is NOT ME. It could be said that the moment of I AM is immediately followed by an expectation of impingement producing reaction, in other words of a destruction of the I AM state. Essential to the I AM state are the innate processes of the individual and the continuity of those processes in time, and reaction to impingement breaks up continuity of being. Environmental failure at the critical moment brings threat of disintegration, and a new defensive pattern is along the line of reaction to impingement, which is the basis of the paranoid personality. (Actual persecution, repeated, is an essential part of this uncomfortable defence.)

These matters are obscure in the direct observation of infants, but become intensely important in the controlled regressions and progressions that appear in analytic practice.

Those infants who are lucky in their management at the beginning seem to come to EXIST and to feel real almost automatically. To the extent that an individual is unlucky and is mismanaged at the beginning (mother depressed, anxious, ill, etc.), so the individual is bound to organise a degree of defensive behaviour pattern, involving a regression to a caricature of primary identification, or a forward stretching to a relationship to external objects. In this way I personally find Balint's idea to be constructive.

The I AM state gathers new meaning as the infant develops, and is always under threat except in so far as environmental adaptation is adequate or becomes, as it gradually does, a matter that the child himself or herself can produce or partly provide. The problems of adolescence can often be seen to be a new variation on this basic theme of BEING, which comes under a new threat because of the biological drives which break up dependence on the home. At puberty, then, there is naturally found, even among those who will be healthy adults, a separation out into those boys and girls who seek the thrill and those who catch hold. In health, however, it must always be true that neither extreme is dominant; and for those who were most lucky at the beginning the I AM issue does not present difficulty. It is hardly necessary to point out that the I AM state and the state of BEING and the feeling of reality in existing is not an end in itself, it is a position from which life can be lived.

Eventually we find the world contains the three groupings; those for whom the EXISTENCE issue is not a difficulty; those for whom there is no hope of feeling real and who know no more than that feeling real comes at rare moments, as when a bomb is dropping; and those in the middle who are caught up in a life-long struggle in the establishment of personal existence, which they achieve in the company of others making the same struggle, and under the integrating influence of a philosophy.

To return to infancy, it can readily be seen that these same problems appear and reappear in all the various settings with which we are familiar. Infants who come through one ordeal may succumb at a later ordeal, but it is clear that in so far as the earliest ordeal is negotiated so far is the child in a good state for coping with mismanagement at later stages. Unfortunately (or fortunately) it remains true that at the earliest stage, that of the first I AM moment, dependence on environment is absolute. (No wonder that in the history of religion, we find this stage of personal development handed over to God!)

Very early in the history of any infant we find this same problem of dependence-independence displayed in the act of thumb-sucking (or some equivalent). In natural growth there is a long period in which the infant need not deal with the ME or NOT-ME aspect of the thumb.

The infant clings to the thumb and also enjoys separation from it. Or the infant, through the thumb, clings to the mouth and also enjoys separation from the mouth. And so on. In the course of time the thumb is found to be part of the self, and by that time a new capacity has developed, the use of fantasy. The thumb stands for an external or NOT-ME object, is symbolical of it as we would say. The external object being sufficiently available, the thumb can be used as substitute. This transition is itself allowed to take place slowly and gradually, in the infant's own time. Transitional objects are provided or are adopted which (when the infant is resting from the arduous process of sorting out the world and the self) are cuddled or pushed away, without being classified as thumb or breast symbols. In health, then (which means to imply healthy management), there is ample time for natural development.

Where through mismanagement the natural processes are interfered with the infant develops defences, according to the equipment derived from earlier stages. An example of gross mismanagement is the prevention of thumb-sucking. The infant whose thumb-sucking is prevented (assuming satisfactory management earlier, so that I AM moments have already been a fact) may organise defensive behaviour patterns along the lines suggested by Balint: denial of need for relationship, and excessive emphasis on relationships with objects more clearly external. I suggest that the alternation of the two defences can be easily observed clinically.

The same alternative defences may reappear, or be produced, at all the other stages. For instance, holding on to faeces may alternate with incontinence; or very early walking, climbing and the rudiments of truancy (dependence on personal technique) alternate with extreme dependence on care (dependence on the technique of those in charge).

In the much more complex state of the depressive position (Klein) in which the child has an inner personal world for which the child is responsible, in which the interplay of crude forces gives rise to moods of hope and despair, a defensive organisation is recognised (called the manic defence) in which the accent is on denial of depression. The defence gives a holiday from despair. Rycroft[3] has suggested that the study of the manic defence can be enriched by Balint's two extremes

3. Dr Charles Rycroft took part in the discussion of Balint's paper on 20 October 1954.
—EDS.

of behaviour pattern. By this suggestion, the quality of manic defence and perhaps a tendency to an adoption of that defence can derive elements from the early and very early defensive organisations that originate in threat to the I AM state or to integration. The tendency to manic-depressive swing certainly resembles the alternation of denial of dependence and exaggerated dependence (clinging) on NOT-ME objects. Balint's alternatives in this case both avoid the anxieties belonging to the establishment of the central I AM state and the central "depression" or concern, or sense of responsibility, belonging to the depressive position. There can be a holiday from responsibility. The manic-depressive swing in itself gives no opportunity for holiday, but is an alternation of two states each equally uncomfortable, the mania being unreal and the depression being intolerable.

In the matter of interpersonal relationships, as between whole people, with the central theme of the Oedipus complex and the child typically in the family circle, it is not so clear whether there is or is not a direct application of Balint's theme. At this stage, the child being 2–3–4 years old, there have developed vast new defensive organisations—and new anxiety types. The ideas of castration and of death have appeared, and instinct has become phallic and genital, and fantasy now enables the child to play at fathers and mothers and to dream of intercourse and to identify with each parent in turn as well as to tolerate being odd man out over short periods of time.

Nevertheless the relics of the contrasting types can perhaps be seen in the fantasy and play even of the most normal. The equivalent at this stage is probably to be found in the alternatives of killing the rival parent and of identification with him or her, in the basic triangular relationship. (I purposely omit crude intrusions of unresolved conflicts and behaviour patterns from the earlier stages into this forward stage of the Oedipus conflict proper.)

In adolescence there is a special new application of Balint's idea because of the new I AM difficulties, as I have already indicated. In consequence the activities of the adolescent, which are transitional between play and work, tend to be coloured by the phenomena of independence and dependence, of foolhardiness and of clinging, even in the healthy.

In health, however, foolhardiness is hidden in special skill, and clinging is hidden in well-justified respect for the skill and reliability of others, and for tradition.

II. Review of *The Doctor, His Patient and the Illness*[4]

1958

I am glad to review this book not only because it deals with a very important subject but also because I feel that the author expresses his personality well in this kind of work. It may prove that this is a pioneer's book.

It is not about psycho-analysis, but it does concern the psycho-analyst in his relationship to the general public. We are used to society's reaction to the idea of the repressed unconscious and of infantile sexuality, but we are not altogether alive to another danger, which is that if we are good we are also tantalising. We offer something, but we seem to withhold it. It might be that psycho-analysis would survive persecution and would yet be destroyed because in being good it reserves its benefits for those very few individuals who happen to be able to arrange to have an analysis.

In the work described in this book, Balint makes a specific attempt to widen the scope of analysis and to do so by using the potential that there is in general practice. Fourteen general practitioners formed a group with Michael Balint and Enid Balint under the auspices of the Tavistock Clinic. Gradually a statement of the problem was reached by this group, and perhaps the beginnings of a solution could be discerned. In what follows I shall attempt to show something of the content of the book and of the reasons why I feel that it is of importance to psycho-analysis.

General practice provides a good medium for the spread of psychotherapy along psycho-analytic lines. There are certain things about general practice which make the practitioner especially suitable for this work. It will be clear that it is not possible to act on the basis that every practitioner will have a personal analysis. Doctors must be used as they are, and if they are capable of a social life and perhaps are

4. London: Pitman, 1957. This review appeared in the *International Journal of Psycho-Analysis* (1958). Copyright © Institute of Psycho-Analysis.

married and have families, and if they can carry the immense burden of a general practice, they are likely to be mature in the sense which is important in carrying through psychotherapy. In fact, it is now generally agreed that a great deal of the practitioner's work is psychotherapy, whether he likes it or not.

It is pointed out, however, that many excellent doctors are potentially ill in a psychiatric sense, and these doctors are advised not to leave the field of physical medicine where they feel at home.

The first formulation made by the group was that the most important drug is the doctor himself. As Balint points out in the preface, there is no guidance in textbooks as to the dosage in which the doctor should prescribe himself. There is in fact very little literature on the "possible hazards of this kind of medication on the various allergic conditions met in individual patients which ought to be watched carefully, or on the undesirable side effects of the drug." The work of the group could be said to be an attempt at the compilation of a pharmacopoeia relative to the doctor himself as a drug.

There is one thing about the general practitioner which puts him in a very strong position for doing psychotherapy, and which indeed gives him an advantage over the psycho-analyst as well as over specialists of all kinds. This is his availability and the continuity of his practice over a number of years. On account of this there is no need for a psychotherapy to end except in so far as it develops an intensity which cannot be maintained for more than a limited period. The work of the Balints' group contributes to the psycho-analyst's problem in respect of certain patients whose analyses simply do not finish at the end of the set period. Most analysts have the experience of patients who in fact need to reappear from time to time. Analysts may feel that something has gone wrong when this happens, but to the general practitioner it would appear quite natural if their patients return from time to time, at critical moments or simply in order to get the reassurance provided by the continued existence and health of the doctor. The whole neighbourhood knows about the general practitioner and his family, and it is possible that his main psychotherapy is done on the patients who do not in fact come to see him but who use in a positive way the fact that they could see him should they feel the need.

So far I have referred to generalisations. The work of the Balints and the group is also more specific, concerned for instance with the psychotherapy which certain individual patients seem to demand. A principle that became enunciated is described under the term "the patient's offers and the doctor's responses." Examples are given making it clear that when the patient goes to the doctor he or she offers the doctor something, offers pains or anxieties or various symptom-groupings; the patient cannot predict how the doctor will respond. The doctor's response is "a highly important contributory factor in the vicissitudes of the developing illness." There follows an examination of the side-effects of the doctor as a drug. For instance, there is the effect of a physical examination which some doctors feel they must always make. There is the effect of the doctor who must reassure and whose own anxieties in one way or another dominate the scene.

Under the heading "collusion of anonymity," attention is drawn to a very important state of affairs which is also well known in social work. Sometimes it happens that many doctors are involved with one patient or one family, and they do not communicate freely with each other. No one person is assuming central responsibility. In social work the term "case work" describes the effort to gather together all the various elements and to place central responsibility on one social worker. It has been remarked in respect of social work that there may be many agencies interested in a case, so that the central problem tends to get pulled apart by these various agencies; there may or may not exist machinery for re-integration of the case. This state of affairs, or lack of case work, is described in this book under the heading "collusion of anonymity." It is a question whether this term does in fact convey what the author intends to convey. I would suggest that the group is describing *the scatter of responsible agents,* and is showing how in certain cases this scatter has as its cause a psychiatric disorder in the patient or in one of the central figures of the social drama. However, this alternative term fails to carry some of the author's meaning. A clear account is given of the effect of this collusion of anonymity on the evolution of the case.

Another matter dealt with is the training of the practitioner. Obviously, if the general practitioner has time, and there is teaching available, this is needed. The group did indeed have a modicum of instruction from other members of the Tavistock Clinic staff. It is important to understand, however, that lack of reliable theoretical knowledge is not the main problem. The main problem concerns *doctor usage*—the whole range of the use that the patient could make of the practitioner, whether the illness is in fact mainly physical, mainly psychogenic, or essentially a mixture.

The group begins to formulate "the special psychological atmosphere of general practice." There is discussion of some of the reasons for clinical success and failure, and also of the indications for the institution of a more formal psychotherapy. Formal psychotherapy produces its own problems of initiation and cessation. Balint never loses sight of the fact that it is not just a matter of specialised psychotherapy that constitutes the main task, but that psychotherapy passes imperceptibly into the whole of the work of the general practitioner, including his management of the case when the patient is physically ill.

Balint lays stress on what he calls the doctor's "apostolic function." This term, which is given considerable prominence in the book, might be misleading. Balint explains his use of it in the following way: "It was almost as if every doctor had revealed knowledge of what was right and what was wrong for patients to expect and to endure, and further, as if he had a sacred duty to convert to his faith all the ignorant and unbelieving among his patients." It obviously became very important for the general practitioners in this group to be introduced to the idea that *they must look at their own motives* and indeed *at their own personalities*. These doctors have something to contend with which is similar to, but not the same as, the analyst's primary need, which is to be analysed. If it were possible for the practitioners doing this work to become analysed, they would still need to undertake the special task which is examined under the chapters headed "The Apostolic Function," that is to say, they would still need to start from the beginning in an attempt to assess the premises of the medical practitioner's work. One could add that it would do no harm to any analyst if he should, from time to time, reassess the premises of his analytic work. It is not necessarily a matter of altering what is done. Whoever practises as a doctor needs to be able to look at what is being done and to become concerned with his own attitude and actions just as he is with the patient's presenting symptoms and responses to treatment. Balint evidently thinks of this as very important, and he makes the comment: "The study of the apostolic function is perhaps the most direct way of studying the chief—the therapeutic—effect of this drug" (i.e. the doctor).

Psycho-analysis surely has something to learn from the general practitioner's study of his attitude and of his prescription of himself. (The converse also is obviously true.) Balint claims that what the psycho-analyst knows about general-practitioner therapy is mostly contained in the literature on the theory and practice of interpretation, especially the part which refers to the management of the patient's tendency to "act out." The general practitioner is naturally caught up in the acting out of his patients, and perhaps it is true that in the majority of cases he can deal with the immediate problems that belong to a particular example of acting out and omit analysis of the central theme. It is interesting for the practitioner, however, if he can understand what is the unconscious or central theme while he is caught up with the acting out at the periphery.

The psycho-analyst is most aware of the role of the general practitioner when a patient in analysis with him needs attention on account of asthma, or giddiness, or a sense of impending death in the early hours of the morning. In other words, analysts do become aware of the part played by the general practitioner in the general management of the patient who is having an analysis. It is possible that analysts are not so well aware of the tremendous number of patients who are dealt with successfully by general practitioners without being in analysis at all.

53
Melanie Klein: On Her Concept of Envy

I. Review of *Envy and Gratitude*[1]

1959

Mrs Klein's recent book *Envy and Gratitude* draws attention to the subject of envy and stimulates consideration of the origin of envy in the human child. It would seem appropriate to use this detail in a book which contains very much else as an excuse for a personal statement. It is indeed interesting to take any concept such as that of envy and not only to think of its meaning in everyday life but also to try to trace it to the point of its origin in the developing human infant.

In this book Mrs Klein makes some rather definite statements about envy, and in my personal opinion she includes in what she says some degree of error. I find it very difficult exactly to point to the mistake which I believe she is making, and for this reason I find it an important exercise to try to formulate a view of my own.

It is valuable to the psychotherapist to be reminded of the importance of envy which of course he meets in his analytic practice as he meets it in life. Melanie Klein's use of the word "envy" is easy to follow when she describes the destructive elements in a patient's relationship to the analyst when the analyst is felt to be satisfactory. Naturally when the analyst is failing in some respect the patient can be expected to feel anger, but it is necessary to recognise destructive forces which do not belong to reactive anger. In health these destructive forces become aligned with those impulses which can be called loving. I personally feel completely at variance with Mrs Klein, however, when she takes the matter back to infancy itself, as when she says: "I consider that envy is an oral-sadistic and anal-sadistic expression of destructive impulses, operative from the beginning of life, and that it has a constitutional basis" (preface).

I feel that it is necessary to distinguish the description of an infant

1. London: Tavistock, 1957. This review appeared in *Case Conference* (January 1959).

from the description of the primitive processes as seen in the analyses of children and adults. As I write this, a patient who has recently started with me leads off in an analytic session with the following words: "At last I have found someone that I need not envy. I don't envy you if you are a good analyst. I may want to kill you but I don't feel I have to destroy the thing in you which makes you able to do my analysis." Later on of course this patient is likely to envy me, but she will have a reason. This envy will be associated with my failure to be available. Near the beginning of the analysis I have not yet been "found out," and I have been able to follow the needs of the patient closely enough so that there is no envy if I can do her treatment. From this detail it can be seen how envy is a vitally important recurring theme in treatments, and in analyses it can be studied in detail and its evolution can be followed. Envy turns up in the same way in the relationship of the social worker and clients and in all other professional relationships and needs to be understood. It is one of those things on which research must be done by the analyst and applied in work that is more general.

It would appear that the word "envy" implies an attitude, something maintained over a period of time. In this attitude of the subject to the object there is further implied by the word "envy" a perception of a property in the object, a property which is not a projection from the subject, an environmental factor, an external phenomenon, something belonging inherently to the object. Envy can here be compared with pity; the object really has something good or something bad about it, in which case the subject is involved in either envy or pity. For me the word "envy" implies a high degree of sophistication, that is to say a degree of ego-organisation in the subject which is not present at the beginning of life. It may be present in a matter of weeks or months, but we need a term (such as oral sadism) to describe the infant's relationship to an object, a relationship carried by an instinctual drive, and dating from almost the beginning. (At the beginning one must allow for a stage before there can be said to be a fusion of destructive and erotic impulses.)

Melanie Klein sees envy in her analytic work, and in this book she goes deeply into its significance there. It makes sense in referring to an analysis to bring in the word "envy." In an analysis, even when the patient is severely regressed and dependent, there is some part of the personality which is co-operating with the analyst and which is sophisticated and unregressed. In this way a patient may bring himself or herself to the analyst, and may even carry on a job or run a home, and yet be severely regressed and dependent at the place where the actual analytic work is being done. But Melanie Klein also carries this concept back to earliest infancy.

It is here that I want to express a personal opinion. If I accept as a fact that Melanie Klein is describing something true in regard to our analytic and other professional work I am left with an objection. For me, there is no description of an infant that leaves out the behaviour of the person caring for the infant; or in an object-relationship, the behaviour of the object. While I can get great value from seeing the primitive mechanisms of human nature from a study of the individual in analysis, I cannot transfer this to the actual infancy situation without bringing in the attitude and behaviour of the person caring for the infant. At the beginning, as I see it, the infant's relationship to an object is so intimately bound up with the presentation of the object to the infant that the two cannot be separated. In terms of object-relationships the infant is entirely dependent on the way each bit of the world is brought to the infant, so that one can say that the world is presented to the infant *either* in such a way that the object seems to be created by the instinctual drive in the infant *or* else in such a way that there is no link between the creative element in the infant and the existence of the external object.

If this view which I have often put forward is acceptable, it would seem that envy in an infant can only be part of a very complex state of affairs in which there is a tantalising representation of the object. Envy of the mother for something good about her could only appear if the mother is tantalising in her presentation of herself to the infant. "Tantalising" here means that the mother adapts just well enough so that the creative element in the infant is met and the infant begins to perceive that there is something good external to the self, and yet not sustained so that to some extent the infant feels deprived. Where the good qualities in the mother are available to the infant then envy has no place and the question of envy does not arise. According to this view envy has no deep root in the infant's nature and its appearance is a reaction to the failure of the mother's adaptation.

Here perhaps is a solution to the difficulty. The theme of envy could be stated in terms of a process of disillusionment starting with the mother's adaptation and including her gradual failure in adaptation matched to the infant's growing capacity to deal with such failure.

Naturally there must be failure of adaptation, just as I must soon fail to meet the needs of my new patient who has not yet "found me out." It would then be possible to see envy as a real thing in the infant's life. Envy would then be seen as a by-product of the developing mother-infant relationship and of the ego-organisation in the infant. If on the other hand envy is described as an infantile characteristic without mention of the behaviour of the object and all that that implies, then I consider that something is wrong. Talking about infants is not the same as talking about primitive stages in the emotional development of persons as seen in the study of patients. These two things are different because, as I have said, the patients bring to the analysis much healthy development and sophistication along with their illness and the primitive aspects of their own nature, and also because they cannot bring forward aspects of maternal care of which they were never aware.

In my opinion the word "envy" in the term "oral sadistic envy" weakens the concept of oral sadism. This concept has always had tremendous significance in the huge area of psycho-analytic thought and practice that has been explored by Melanie Klein. Oral sadism is valuable as a concept because it joins up with the biological concept of hunger, a drive to object-relationships that comes from primitive sources, and that holds sway at least from the time of birth.

II. The Beginnings of a Formulation of an Appreciation and Criticism of Klein's Envy Statement[2]

Dated 16 July 1962

In this essay I try to make personal use of Melanie Klein's Geneva Congress paper[3] and her book *Envy and Gratitude*.[4] Often I have expressed criticism of this part of her work, but my criticism is limited to two aspects, and no doubt these are inter-related. Firstly, I think the word "envy" cannot be used in the description of early infant life. Such a use of this word goes against the grain, and produces an unnecessary prejudice in me and in others against the general idea that is contained in the book. Secondly, the introduction of the idea of inherited aggression weakens the main argument of the book and challenges us to look at any weak spots that may exist in the total argument. The existence and importance of that which is inherited is something that no-one could doubt. The question arises, should a metapsychological argument go over into accounting for phenomena by reference to heredity until a full understanding has been reached of the interplay of personal and environmental factors? In my opinion there is a serious gap in understanding in Melanie Klein's argument and this gap is not acknowledged, but our sight of this gap is befogged by the reference to inherited aggression.

In a discussion in the British Psycho-Analytical Society[5] (following a paper by Dr Donald Meltzer) in which I challenged the ready assumption of Klein's work on envy in toto, Dr S. S. Davidson remarked that Melanie Klein had not just sat down and thought:

---

2. There is evidence that this paper, in which Winnicott was working out the details of his ideas, was written late at night and though later typewritten was never revised by him.—EDS.

3. Paper given at the Nineteenth International Psycho-Analytic Congress, Geneva, July 1955; see "A Study of Envy and Gratitude" (1956) in *The Selected Melanie Klein*, ed. Juliet Mitchell (Penguin, 1986).

4. London: Tavistock, 1957.

5. Probably at a Scientific Meeting on 15 February 1961.—EDS.

"What shall I write about?"; she had been moved to write because of her feeling that envy was an important matter needing examination on account of its importance in psycho-analytical clinical work, and because she felt she had a contribution to make as to its aetiology. This point is easily accepted, and for me as for many others it has been valuable to have attention drawn to the importance of envy in our psycho-analytic work, although the subject is not a new one, and it is unlikely that many analysts are habitually blind to envy when it becomes an important feature in an analysis. Moreover, it was important for us to be told that envy must be examined apart from the special case of "penis envy," a term that has been much used and that is not well translated from the German. Melanie Klein reminded us that we use the word "envy" outside the specific context of the female position at the phallic phase.

In effect, Klein showed us that patients envy the analyst when the analyst does good analytic work, work that is effectual, and from which the patient derives exactly the benefit which they could say they came to analysis to get. In the jargon of our psycho-analytic intercommunications, the patients envy the good breast.

I have no doubt from my own work that this is a true observation, and I value having it emphasised. At the same time there is much work to be done on this idea before it can be accepted as it is stated by Klein.

I suggest that Melanie Klein could not develop her argument of the analyst's "good breast" without going into the matter of the quality of the analyst's work, that is to say, the capacity of the analyst to adapt to the needs of the patient. Linked with this is the mother's capacity to make adaptation at the very beginning to the newborn infant's ego-needs (including id-needs). Klein's argument took her to a point at which she must either deal with *the dependence of the infant on the mother* (patient on analyst) or else deliberately ignore the variable external factor of the mother (analyst) and dig right back in terms of *primitive mechanisms that are personal to the infant*. By choosing the latter course Klein involved herself in an implicit denial of the environmental factor, and consequently she disqualified herself from describing infancy itself, which is a time of dependence. In this way she was forced into a premature arrival at the inheritance factor.

It falls on those who follow Melanie Klein to develop this rich theme and to restate the problem without resorting to an *implicit* denial of the environment. It must be emphasised that there has been no *explicit* denial of environment, and Melanie Klein herself was always distressed by the idea that a denial of the importance of the environment was always being attributed to her, especially by myself. But the fact remains that in this work on envy there is *implicit* a neglect of the behaviour of the environment.

It would be easy to illustrate Melanie Klein's main theme of envy of the good breast in the transference in psycho-analysis, as in nearly every case this becomes from time to time the main theme, and especially so towards the end of an analysis.

A male patient near the end of his analysis.

The analysis has been done very much on the basis of a positive transference, the negative transference always being expressed in terms of people in the environment. At first this involved the patient in almost delusional antagonisms, but for a long time now the patient has been able to use men fairly objectively in his acting out of the negative transference. There have been very acute examples in which the negative transference came on to myself.

The ending of the analysis has been very much worked through on the basis of first identification with the father at puberty and lastly destruction of the father and a supplanting of him. In the course of this the Oedipus complex has turned up in a simplified form which was important because of certain qualities in this patient's mother which distorted the picture. In the case of his mother he has always maintained that there are reasons why a boy needs to get away from his mother which are deeper and earlier than Oedipus complex reasons, preceding the Oedipus triangle.

The destruction of the good analyst came rather suddenly into the material and without the patient's understanding of the reasons for it. In the transference the patient now employed another split in the object, that between teacher and analyst. The analyst does no teaching, and the patient resists teachers. The patient has no difficulty in accepting the analyst but teachers are eliminated from the beginning because of his need to teach himself. This dates from childhood. There is an exception in the teaching relationship and that is that he has always found that when there is a really good teacher he has valued that really good teacher very highly. In his history, however, good teachers seem to die either from illness or war, etc.

In going over this material at this time the patient was very near to his own destruction of the good teacher. At this point it was necessary to interpret envy of the good teacher. The interpretation was a fairly long one and had to do with the patient's great difficulty in allowing someone else to be necessary. He can teach himself but in

450 On the Work of Other Analysts

order to get taught French he must lend to the French teacher the teaching role. He liked his good French teacher, but he was killed in the war. If the good teacher that is liked lives then he has to destroy him by ceasing to need him. It is as if he could only stand this handing over of the teaching to someone else for a limited time or in a limited way.

I then went back to the theoretical breast feeding. I said: "You could feed yourself better than anyone could feed you because you knew what you wanted; but in order to get milk you had to hand over the feeding to your mother. You could do this for a limited time and then you would wean yourself, so to speak. If this had happened in a satisfactory way you would never have had to know how angry you were at having to hand over the feeding role to your mother or to the breast. In the case of your mother, however, there was some tendency on her part to cling to her role and for this reason in your case you became aware of a tremendous need to get free, and this has dominated much of your life. Behind it is your anger with your mother or with a good breast for being necessary."

I recognised that in making this interpretation I am allowing for something which is almost exactly the same as Mrs Klein's concept of the infant's envy of the good breast. When all goes well it is a theoretical antagonism to the idea that the external object is necessary, something which is not true at the beginning because the object is a subjective object; but it gradually becomes true as the object becomes objectively perceived. In a very large number of cases it must be that the infant never knows about this which Mrs Klein calls envy of the good breast and which I call intolerance of the necessity for an external representative of that which is originally felt to be part of the self. When the mother relinquishes her role unwillingly or too slowly then the infant develops hatred and a need to get free, but this is not the envy of the good breast to which Mrs Klein refers; it is anger with the mother for her technical failure which brings into the living relationship a feeling which belongs to the latent theoretical primary unconscious.

A practising analyst has opportunity then for verifying this part of Melanie Klein's statement or for finding an absence of verification. It is a striking fact, however, that having completed a phase of this aspect of analysis the analyst does not find that the patient's analysis is finished. There is immense relief when this interpretation is given at the right moment, but something is left over, and undoubtedly it was this which Melanie Klein felt when she went on to state that some individuals who come for analysis inherit a powerful tendency towards aggression.

An attempt here will be made to illustrate the way in which there is a great deal of work to be done in the analysis of a patient *after interpretation of envy of the good breast,* and this would not be true if Melanie Klein's statement were correct. If her statement were correct, after the analysis of envy of the good breast there would be nothing more to be said about the patient's aggression except in terms of inheritance. This might have been found to have been correct but in fact this does not happen. It would be an important part of Melanie Klein's work on envy if it were to lead to a better understanding of that which she has perhaps wrongly named envy of the good breast in the living relationship of the infant and the mother at a very early stage.

In the case of the patient whose material has been used to illustrate envy of the good breast in the transference there proved to be a great deal of further work needing to be done.

A patient brought a dream near the end of his analysis. In the pattern of his analysis he had first of all had a long stretch of straightforward work in which he co-operated from a deep level. This made a great difference to him and it lasted three years. Then the analysis turned round into being chaotic and there was a clear reason for this, that the patient now needed to produce material which was not easily understood. This led up gradually to a certainty that there was no hope that he would get what he came for. In the first phase he had had no doubt whatever and now he became more and more certain that the analysis would terminate without being finished. In this hopeless phase good analytic work was being done as in the first phase and clinical changes resulted from this work. But the patient's expectations had altered. Envy of the analyst had always been evident and had been interpreted whenever it appeared for interpretation and had been related to the patient's childhood, according to his pattern.

The patient dreamed that he had unexpectedly acquired £20,000; it was not payment for anything and he had not even had to bet on a horse. He was annoyed with himself for not remembering anything more about the dream. The interpretation based on the available material was that he now knew what he had to come to analysis for, and he was telling me that in fact he had got it. He came for £20,000.

In the early stages he insisted on giving me a fee beyond his capacity to pay; and there had been many indications throughout the early phase of the analysis that this was a reaction formation, and that eventually it would be found that he came for money. There was stealing from me in token form from time to time. Interpretations along these lines produced a result and the patient said that in fact his analysis had increased his earning capacity to the extent that it amounted to the equivalent of a £20,000 increase in his capital value. Along with the interpretation of the dream came the feeling that the analysis would now be able to end instead of being artificially terminated. This meant an acknowledgement of what he had had from me, and this links with Melanie Klein's introduction of the idea of gratitude in the satisfactory resolution of these difficulties. Gratitude is dependence that is acknowledged. Further analysis was required of the need for money in its two aspects; firstly as a symbol of love, and secondly as a substitute for love carrying with it a recognition of a deprivation. In this case the deprivation was a relative one and very much bound up with the actual attitude of the father towards money which was in turn associated with the father's repressed homosexuality.

In terms of the emotional development of the infant this matter of envy relates to the environmental provision. When there is a good-enough mother, then the infant, at first absolutely dependent, does in fact get a "good breast"; the good-enough mother takes the infant's growing capacity to have a "good breast" personal quality which can be projected. The good-enough mother takes this projection. In this way in the course of weeks and months the good breast that the baby uses is not only a projection but is also available although external to the self. By the time the infant has come to perceive that the good breast is external and that it belongs to the environment and not to the self there have developed the germs of numerous mental mechanisms which enable the baby to allow the separation of the object and to make use of this separation in the start of the journey towards independence.

(The chief of these mental mechanisms I have tried to describe under the term "transitional phenomena," i.e. an intermediate area of experience which is both self and not-self, i.e. both baby and mother.)

It must be remembered that the patient dealing with the basic relationship to the breast in an analysis needs to come to terms with the *fact of dependence*. This involves, at one extreme, regression; and at the other extreme, where the ego can tolerate fact, gratitude (or blame).

For the baby in arms these conditions do not apply. Dependence is a living reality, and starts off with absolute dependence; gratitude and resentment as the acknowledgement of dependence have no place. Nothing else is known yet.

For babies there is a basic ration of "good breast" without which the early stages of the individual's emotional development do not get initiated. Various authors have attempted to formulate this. Balint in his concept of primary love, myself in my terms "good-enough mothering" and "primary maternal preoccupation." The "good breast" proves to be a jargon term for (a) "good-enough mothering" and (b) "satisfactory feeding" and (c) the joining together of (a) and (b) first in the environment and then in the mind of the baby.

In a matter of a few months after birth the baby is obviously capable of oral sadistic experience, that is to say, can experience primitive loving in which the motor impulses fuse in with the erotogenic zone satisfactions, and the infant arrives at the eating of the object, and of being eaten if loved. At about the same time this primary object ceases to be a subjective phenomenon, and if all experience becomes directed towards that which is symbolic of the primary object, the infant becomes able to play and to imagine, and experiences the use of the primary object only in dreams.

The main point is that there is a period of time, or a phase, in the life of the newborn baby, in which the main problems that concern the patients in analysis do not obtain. That is to say, there is a significant phase before the depressive position (to use Melanie Klein's term even if it is not a good name for a very important and real stage of development) can be reached and the development that this represents consolidated.

In this early phase the baby is developing a memory system and a self-awareness that become available for projection. The good-enough mother meets this projection; and in this way the baby's experience in relation to the good breast is a relationship to a projection from the self. *There is no room for envy here.* The baby whose mothering is not good enough never joins up that which was available for projection with this mother's good breast. The latter fails to take the projection. In the cases that come our way in analysis it can be assumed that there was a tantalising situation in which the mothering was good enough and not good enough, so that the baby knew of a good breast but did not get it, except as a thing that came as an impingement to disrupt the continuity of being of the self. In these circumstances, a baby envies the good breast, or destroys it when it comes in such a way that it does not take the baby's projections.

Here we have the paradox of a good breast that is a persecutor, a thing that must be destroyed. Thus aggression appears, directed towards the good object, but this aggression is reactive and is not the aggression of the primitive love impulse which represents an achievement, a fusion of muscular erotism and the sensory orgy of the erotogenic zones.

In other words there is no place in our theory for the baby's envy of the good breast when this is a projection, as it is when there is good-enough mothering. This concept of envy of the good breast is not valid except in the event of relative failure of mothering in the earliest stages.

In my view Melanie Klein's attempt to state the early history of aggression was doomed to failure since she tried to state it apart from the question of the behaviour of the environment. Between the hereditary factor and envy is primitive loving with eating that has not yet become ruthless because it is an achievement of fusion and the effect on the object is not yet a matter for concern. This is just prior to the depressive position, on the theoretical chart of human emotional development.

The following clinical observation illustrates this. It belongs to the analysis of a woman, aged 25 years. She described herself as one who has all her life cut her losses, and she has employed a successful defence, namely the full exploitation of substitute objects. This is a variety of false self, the falseness being rather in the acceptance of substitutes than in the setting up of a substitute self. The patient's motive for coming to analysis was to be got out of the employment of this defence which gave her no object-constancy, and which made her feel all the time uncertain as to the value of living.

In a crucial week of her analysis the patient arrived at the depressive position. She described herself as pro-bottle and anti-breast. She declared that she was a bottle. She threw the bottle down and broke it and watched it and gloated over its destruction. Her death was always an exciting idea, because of a dramatisation of this event which implied clearly that she was alive in all her other bottle-selves—enjoying her own funeral, so to speak. In fact she came to analysis to become able to die. From her material it could be seen that she was exploiting to the full her particular brand of manic defence and elation. But she had had an annoying dream. She was having analysis from M. How could M. give interpretations of the

Klein variety, with biting and messing into the good breast and all the attacking of the mother's body, when she was a maternal type, awfully boring? And so on.

The interpretation that was given on very clear evidence was that M. represented the Melanie part of Melanie Klein's name. In other words she had arrived at the thing she turned away from, the mother's dying breast. This came as a shock to the patient who said she had never thought of Melanie Klein as having anything to do with a good breast—only with the attack on the breast. Here was she now, getting Melanie—good breast—analysis (cf. Meltzer's "good breast brain"), and this led her to do the opposite to what she called cutting her losses. It led her to looking at the dying breast (failure in her own breast-feeding experience) and to be concerned about the part she might have played in the mother's failure. This could be said to be the "first time" this patient had ever genuinely felt concern in the infant-to-object relationship. At the same time she has well-developed concern for the mother-to-baby or child relationship.

At this point in her analysis, by chance, a damaged bird came into her life. On the way to analysis she came across a damaged bird and she had come to analysis in distress, conscious of once more "cutting her losses," turning from the bird which she feared. After a few minutes she returned to the bird, although this meant quite a long journey, but first she gave me time to interpret the bird as representation of the dying breast of her own babyhood experience. She did find the bird and restored it to life, and this was her analytic session that day. The experience marked a turning point in her analysis and perhaps in her life, though the changes involved a giving up of the elation that goes with a successful defence against concern. (One cannot exactly call this manic defence, since this term has been given to the denial of depression, in other words to a defence organised *after* arrival at the depressive position.)

Now this patient was exactly at the point at which envy of the good breast (good analysis) is liable to turn up. But this did not happen because the good-enough analyst was taking a projection of her own qualities. Not only had there been much material of the good-enough mother-to-child variety, but also on the very day that contained the main statement of a split between herself cutting her losses (dead breast) and her self infinitely involved with substitute objects (bottles), at the end of the session she said she felt sure I must think her an interesting case, and when she went away she felt empty but she had come to know that after a few hours, especially if she could sleep, she would recuperate. I interpreted here that I was in this way the baby and she was feeding me with her good breast, and she already knew about the breast's power to refill.

In this analysis more than in most in my experience there has been a need for the analyst to be someone who carefully does no more than meet or make real the patient's projections. In this analysis I have said very little, often nothing and seldom more than making one interpretation in a session. Very clearly here my good-enough analysis in this case is a projection, which I meet and try not to interfere with. In this way there is no envy of the good breast. Should I, however, by a technical error do or say something that is foreign to the patient's material that is available for projection, then I become a persecutor immediately, and must be destroyed, good or bad, and especially if good.

Conclusion

Good-enough mothering gives opportunity for the steady development of personal process in the baby. Here the mother's good-breast quality is a projection of a corresponding quality in the infant. The good-enough mother takes the good projection and makes it real. In so far as this happens the baby does not envy the good breast, but is able to identify with it and with the good-enough mother, and gradually to recognise that the mother who took the projection is part of the environment, or NOT-ME world.

In mothering that is not good enough the mother is not able to take the good projections, and then either there is chaos and the beginnings of psychosis, or else there is a tantalising condition in which the baby knows of a good external breast that cannot join up with that quality of the infant that is available for projection on to a good breast. In such a case the good breast is a persecutor and has to be refused or destroyed. The word "envy" is not applicable to this that the baby feels about a good breast that has failed to take the projection.

In the same conditions brought forward into the analysis of children and adults the word "envy" can be used, and used in the way that Melanie Klein does employ the word. The difference between the analytic situation and the situation in earliest babyhood is that the analytic patient must perforce deal with the fact of dependence, whereas at the beginning the infant is dependent and knows no other condition. In the same way the child or adult who is not capable of gratitude is ill, but for the baby there is no room for the idea of gratitude because a basic ration of good-enough care is a part of the baby, although it needs to be supplied by a mother.

In this way, although Melanie Klein's statement on envy is of great significance for the practising analyst, it is not something that can be applied to babies, and it is therefore not possible to draw conclusions from Melanie Klein's statement as to the origins of aggressive tendencies in an individual.

In fact, Melanie Klein's envy statement, in so far as her ideas are stretched to cover babyhood, seems to weaken her very important work on what she called the depressive position. The theory of the roots of aggression is not enriched by Melanie Klein's envy statement; it is confused by her falling back on inherited factors without seriously tackling the effect of mothering (or analysis) that is good enough or not good enough.

It can be assumed that inheritance is of utmost importance, but the psychologist cannot lean on the inheritance factor until everything that is possible has been done in terms of psychology.

Finally, the main point at issue is this. When an analyst (mother) does good-enough work (gives good-enough care) with a patient (baby) is this done on the basis of a projection onto the analyst (mother) of satisfactory internal factors in the patient (baby)? In my opinion the answer is in the affirmative, and unless this is made true by the analyst (mother) the good analysis (good breast) is essentially a persecutory object for the patient (baby).

This seems to me to be a modern statement of one of the main points in Freud's technique, that the analyst follows the patient's process, and interprets *only that which has already been presented by the patient for interpretation.*

Does the mother create the infant, or does the infant create the mother? In the metapsychology of psycho-analysis I hold that the infant creates the breast, the mother and the world.

III. Roots of Aggression

Dated 9 September 1968[6]

There is a need at the present time for psycho-analysis to take a new look at aggression. The recent book by Anthony Storr[7] has shown that the public is thirsty and hungry for a statement that indicates that due recognition is being given to the problem by science. In order to base ideas on objective observation the scientist must have the stage set for observing, and it is the psychotherapist who has the vantage point if only he can make use of his privileged position. And for me as for many others the psycho-analyst is of psychotherapists the one most likely to contribute something new, chiefly because of the analytic process which has got going in himself and which continues for life, that is, irrespective of the actual analysis which he underwent and about which he agreed with his analyst at a certain stage to say: this is the end.

No advance in psycho-analytic theory is made without nightmares. The question is: who is to have the nightmare? The further question—why does he need to have nightmares?—is not relevant and can be ignored. In our Society here, although we serve science, we need to make an effort every time we attempt to re-open matters which seem to have been settled. It is not only the inertia which belongs to the fear of doubt; it is also that we have loyalties. We associate specific ideas with peaks of achievement that mark the progress of our pioneers. In this way, when we look anew at the roots of aggression there are two concepts in particular, each of which must be thrown away deliberately, so that we may see whether they come back again of their own accord, or whether we are better off without them. One is Freud's concept of a death instinct, a by-product of his speculations in which he seemed to be achieving a theoretical simplification that might be compared to the gradual elimination of detail in the technique of a sculptor like Michaelangelo. The other is Mel-

6. This paper was prepared for the British Psycho-Analytical Society, but it is unfinished and was not, in fact, given.—EDS.

7. *Human Aggression* (London: Allen Lane, 1968).

anie Klein's setting up of envy in the prominent place that she gave it at Geneva in 1955.

It is not possible for us to go forward with scientific discussion unless we are prepared to cast aside both these concepts, unlinking the one from Freud and the other from Melanie Klein. In this way we get free from beliefs and from loyalties, and once more the only thing that we care about is truth.

Immediately, when we achieve this discipline, we see how much we have been indoctrinated by constant interjection of the words "death instinct" and "envy" in papers and statements. The essential thing is that neither concept could be discussed at the time because it was not the main theme, and a discussion of these terms must therefore distract and the discussant must seem, and indeed must be, rude. It is with relief, therefore, that we find ourselves here with no preconceived notions about the death instinct or about envy, and if either term is used it must be deliberately drawn in as part of the thing that is being discussed and about which we agree we are ignorant.

How easily these terms become clichés. For instance, Melanie Klein would not claim to have discovered envy or to have invented the concept. We must use the words "envy" and "jealousy" whenever they are appropriate in our talk and our writings, just as the words were used in the long years before Melanie was born. Indeed these two words have their own histories.

Melanie Klein took the word "envy" and gave it a specific use in a legitimate exploration of the origins of aggression in human nature in terms of the developing individual. But the word has now acquired an aura, so that there has probably been no paper by a Klein follower or by a student from the Klein group that has not included the word "envy," not as a descriptive term (the patient showed envy of the younger boys, this being a relic of the feelings she felt towards her brother at his birth, and in relation to the parents' attitude . . . etc.), but as a part of the label indicating place of origin (sea-island cotton guaranteed washable, drip-dry).

The sad effect of this awful thing about envy is that it holds up a true appreciation of Melanie Klein's contribution, which may easily have been particularly bold and rich just here. Something that feels wrong about her Geneva paper may turn out to be a small detail, and a truth may emerge if only we can get away from this loyalty to Melanie which makes scientific or objective appraisal out of the question. Here and now perhaps we can get behind this matter of loyalty (probably based, in its compulsive aspects, on envy) to the problem itself. We are discussing human nature, and we are particularly concerned with the developmental processess, and with that which would be called aetiology in the investigation of a disease.

Incidentally, I claim that it is legitimate for us to say that we feel there is something wrong with the Geneva statement. There is no trouble if we feel something is wrong with Freud's Death Instinct formulation because he himself seems to have had doubts, doubts proper to a scientist who knows that no truth is absolute or final, and that it is the thinking and the feeling and the freedom to speculate that counts. But Melanie Klein was served badly by her followers, who took what she said and stuck it up on a banner, when she would have profited more from being criticised. This tendency among Klein followers is best seen in Joan Riviere's sentence in her preface to the book *Developments in Psycho-Analysis*[8]—"She has in fact produced something new in psycho-analysis: namely, an *integrated* theory which, though still in outline, nevertheless takes account of all psychical manifestations, normal and abnormal, from birth to death, and leaves no unbridgeable gulfs and no phenomena outstanding without intelligible relation to the rest"—a sentence which Melanie would have disallowed had she been truly a scientist.

I have gone into these matters in some detail because I want to be able to arrive at any conclusion that may turn up without having to worry even if I should find myself saying just what Melanie Klein said. Should this happen it must come from me out of the objective data supplied by my patients, and not in any way from loyalty to a man or woman however much I may owe or feel in gratitude.

It can be said that Freud and Melanie Klein were both deeply concerned with aggression and its origin. In each case the concern had a depth of meaning that is rare and belongs only to special persons, persons who have a capacity for feeling in depth and who have become enriched by long experience and stabilised by the hard work without which personal fulfilment cannot be conceptualised and written down. Melanie, in particular, was affected by the rooted aggression she found in her patients to whom she had so much to offer that was good. Her patients went far and their antagonism could not be any more removed by analysis of anger at frustration. More and more it became clear to her that her value generated or touched off destruc-

8. London: Hogarth Press, 1952.

tive impulses in her patients, both male and female; a fair proportion of her cases she quite sensibly got rid of as unanalysable, and others stepped over into a fixed loyalty which unfortunately demanded too much of them. She was puzzled and applied herself specifically to this problem of the destructiveness in the transference that seemed to make no sense. At this point there was some sense of hurry, because she was getting older, and eventually because she was to have a physical illness that would prove fatal. She wanted to get over this hurdle and she made an attempt to do so at Geneva. The solution came along two lines:

1. To jump over everything backwards, and to state, without originality, that since everything is inherited, some persons might be born with a loaded inheritance on the aggressive side. This was a sterile statement, and it begged this whole question of aggression and its evolution in the developing individual baby and child.

2. To take the bull by the horns and to say out loud what was clinically evident, that her patients in the transference at a very deep level envied her, envied her for being valuable, or "good."[9]

One could say of these two lines of thought that the first although irrefutable should be brought forward and emphasised by a metapsychologist only after very careful exploration of psychological or emotional alternatives, and it is possible to argue that Melanie had not qualified in this respect. There are other considerations which she ignored. The second line of thought was bold and in conformity with clinical experience that all analysts can share; but it . . .

9. The word "good" itself was becoming a cliché, indicating an idealised object or perhaps an idolised object.—D.W.W. See Masud Khan, "Reparation to the Self As an Idolised Internal Object" (1968), in *Alienation in Perversions* (London: Hogarth Press, 1979). —Eds.

IV. Contribution to a Symposium on Envy and Jealousy

Written for a Scientific Meeting of the British Psycho-Analytical Society, 19 March 1969[10]

I feel very much inclined to take part in this discussion, especially as the idea of it probably arose out of a suggestion of mine to the Scientific Secretary. But I feel like taking part only if there is a possibility that I can say something constructive.

First I assume that we are not in this discussion concerned with envy and jealousy as these two words appear in nearly every clinical paper given in recent years by a Kleinian. Also I claim that in present-day usage of these two terms envy is a state of mind and belongs to a highly sophisticated mental organisation, while jealousy has the characteristic that its use implies that the whole person has already begun to mobilise revenge or theft.

The only thing that we are concerned with is the way that Melanie Klein brought in envy in her Geneva paper. I can readily forgive her this if she needed another word but could not find one.

As I have often stated, I learned a great deal directly from Melanie Klein in the decade before the war. It could be said that the new ideas that came from her in that fruitful period of her work impressed me and had a positive effect on the whole of my work. I found myself able to use the succession of new ideas. This never became quite so obviously true after the war and after the period in which Mrs Klein organised herself and her colleagues to defend her position. My feelings about Mrs Klein's work changed at the Geneva Conference during her reading of her paper on envy. It was not easy to see why it was that I could no longer accept her new statement of theory.

Quite briefly, while I could see that Mrs Klein was trying to reach to greater depths and to encompass a very difficult aspect of transference forces which may only develop at the end of a long analysis which seemed to be going well but which began to fail, nevertheless I

10. Read in Winnicott's absence by Mrs Enid Balint.—EDS.

knew that I had to make a protest and I did so immediately to Mrs Klein herself. My objection has to do with Mrs Klein's determination to make a complete statement of the individual development of the human baby in terms of the baby alone without reference to the environment. This, in my opinion, is impossible. True, it has been a main feature of psycho-analysis to get to the individual and personal factor and to see the way in which the environmental factor can be partly or even wholly a subjective phenomenon; nevertheless there is a stage at the beginning of the development of the individual when the environment comes into its own and has its proper place and a statement of its importance cannot be avoided. The new baby has not separated out the NOT-ME from the ME so that by definition the NOT-ME or the environment is part of the ME in terms of the ego of the baby. There is no way round this difficulty.

In the Geneva paper Mrs Klein jumped over this problem and landed herself in another problem. She went back to an exploitation of the hereditary factor, such, for instance, as an inheritance of an abnormal quantity of aggressive potential. The hereditary factor is of course real, but it cannot be said that psycho-analysis has tried to avoid this complication. Every tendency towards maturation is inherited and psycho-analysis is simply concerned with the interaction with what is inherited and what is environmental. It was a shock to find Mrs Klein avoiding something by exploiting something else. Incidentally, in terms of the ego-organisation of the very young baby, the inherited tendency is an *external* factor of a particularly gross kind. Possibly Mrs Klein may have thought that the hereditary factor was personal and not environmental, but this would be to leave out the whole problem of the immature ego, and dependence that is based on the fact that the NOT-ME has not yet been separated out from the ME.

What is needed from those who concern themselves with this subject is a study of the gradual change in the development of a baby at the beginning which belongs to the separation out of the NOT-ME from the ME. Envy of the NOT-ME object has a precursor which is the relationship to the not-yet-separated-out object which I have referred to as a subjective object. There is an area here for study which can occupy psycho-analysts for a long time to come, and without which there will be no effectual psycho-analytic understanding of schizophrenia.

I may say that my opinions were forged in my consulting room in the treatment, not always successful, but sometimes successful enough, of borderline cases in which regression to dependence was a marked and indeed an essential matter. I am only too keenly aware of the significance of the qualitative factor in the environment when this is my own understanding and behaviour and a patient is, for a period of time, merged in with me, the analyst.

In this exciting area for study the student will be involved in the concept of transitional phenomena, will need to be able to accept (not resolve) the paradox that the baby creates what is already there to be created, and will find himself fully strained in his belief in the reality of dependence as it obtains in the early stage before the individual ego has created NOT-ME elements. This is prior to anger at the frustrations that belong to the encounter with the Reality Principle.

There may be a place in all this for that which Melanie Klein is calling envy, but it will not have that name when its shape is properly delineated. Its name might be eagerness; but whatever name is found or invented, it will need to be seen that the quality is affected by the quality of environmental provision.

It is sad for me that Mrs Klein after all that she had contributed was not able to contribute at this point, and indeed by not contributing she seems to have handed on to her followers a peculiarly difficult task in that they have to proceed just here on the basis not of all the positive contributions that Mrs Klein made but on the basis of her denial of something which is nevertheless a fact. This is another way of saying that she too was human.

I would like to make reference to the fact that Dr Bion in one of his statements seemed to show himself to be free of this powerful tendency, which I suggest must be accepted as part of Mrs Klein's make-up, to deny the environmental factor even at the beginning.

As analysts we know only too well that in a transference setting in which work is being done which reaches to very early states it does actually make a difference what the analyst is like. In the same way at the beginning of every individual's development the environment has prime significance, being still part of the individual child. I contend that a study of the subtleties in this area can bring rich rewards to the student.

54
Joseph Sandler

Comments on "On the Concept of the Superego" [1]

Delivered at a Scientific Meeting of the British Psycho-Analytical Society, 7 December 1960

Before starting to make my contribution, I wish to make it clear that had I known what was expected of me I would not have agreed to speak at this meeting. Mr. Sandler's paper gives a very thorough statement of the subject of the superego, and a proper study of this paper would take me much longer than the time that I have been given.

I find the statement of the development of the idea of the superego in Freud's mind very useful and I am always grateful to anyone who will take the trouble to do this sort of research and to make this sort of statement. From this statement, one can see that, although Freud above all people knew that a great deal that is going on when the superego affects the id, and when the ego is at variance with the superego, or at one with the superego, he was talking in terms nevertheless which seem at first to refer to conscious life. One can be told by

1. Professor Sandler's paper was read at a Scientific Meeting of the British Psycho-Analytical Society on 7 December 1960, and was published in *The Psycho-Analytic Study of the Child*, vol. 15 (1960). It begins with a survey of the development of the superego concept in the writing of Freud, and goes on to show how the concept has gained complexity through the work of other writers, in particular of the ego psychologists and also of Klein, whose views on the very early development of a superego and of guilt are examined in some detail. Sandler believes that developments in psycho-analysis have resulted in a weakening of the superego concept through a "conceptual dissolution," as what had previously been seen as superego conflict now tended to be seen more in terms of object-relationships within the transference. In the second part of the paper he seeks, through tracing superego development from early infancy, to reformulate the concept. Here he emphasises the small child's "obedience to and compliance with the demands of the parents" and "identification with and imitation of the parents" as means of lessening the narcissistic insult inherent in acceptance of the Reality Principle. While allowing for a pre-Oedipal "pre-autonomous superego schema," he nevertheless places the crystallisation of the superego proper firmly with the resolution of the Oedipus complex. A more recent exposition of Sandler's ideas on the superego can be found in his *From Safety to Superego* (London: Karnac; New York: Guilford Press, 1987).—EDs.

a patient, as I have been told recently by a boy of 19, just the sort of things that Freud wrote down that are quoted by Sandler. To some extent this boy of 19 was influenced by the thought of this decade which is of course very much influenced by Freud's work. Nevertheless it was this boy himself who worked out in a self-analysis that he had an institution in his mind which was all the time influencing him. This was partly based on the idea of his father and of his parents in combination, and here he found he could manage by defiance. Part was based, however, on a very personal analysing and observing self, which studied everything that was happening in his life, and enabled him to get through without too much suffering. This which could be called a superego could be sadistic, and he recognised that his own sadism had gone into the sadism of the superego; he also recognised the masochistic perversion which was a way of dealing with the sadistic superego. He told me that he had tried to use the sadistic superego by turning it on to the part of himself that he loathed, which was a false self. He did not call this a false self because he was talking in his own language. He spoke of a very nice child which everyone thought he had been, but which he had come to see was not by any means his true self. He had been haunted, for instance, by the myth of the Doppelgänger, and he was all the time looking for the other self which would turn up at the moment of death when he would no longer be alive to keep the split operative. What he suffered from was the lack of spontaneity, and the only way that he could regain the spontaneity that he had lost was through the agency of alcohol which for a few hours would deal with this superego and release his spontaneity and his capacity to make relationships and to reach out towards heterosexuality. All this is superficial, however, if one thinks of what would appear in the boy's analysis.

It must have been from patients like this that Freud gathered the material for his work on the superego. Freud, however, was concerned all the time with the deeper aspects of this matter, and I want to suggest that in Mr Sandler's résumé he has not sufficiently reminded us of Freud's concern with dreams and with psychic reality and with fantasy. I suggest that he has spoken of the life of the individual in such a way that a reader coming to his statement without previous knowledge of Freud would think that everything went on in the mind rather than in the psyche.

I find it impossible to go any further in the discussion of this point without referring to the theme which I developed in my paper "Mind and Its Relation to the Psyche-Soma,"[2] joining this up with the concept of the true and the false self. I have referred to a false self living through a mind or intellectual life which has become separated off from the psyche-soma. Much as I admire those who can intellectually consider a concept, I am always on the lookout for a failure on the part of an analyst to deal with this problem of the patient who has a clear mind that is, however, not intimately related to the functioning body and the psyche, and the body ego. I think Mr Sandler is in danger of referring to human beings too much in terms of a flight to the mind.

I must now refer to the question: shall we study the development of Freud's thoughts as expressed (in the end) under the term "superego," and accept what we think Freud meant and limit our use of the term "superego" in such a way that we do not depart from what we believe was Freud's intention? On the other hand, shall we study similar ideas and try to drag the meaning of the concept of the superego over to cover other phenomena?

I hope that in this discussion the speakers will not get bogged down in a tug-of-war between those who want to keep the Freudian concept of the superego pure and those who want to enrich it or debase it.

We always have to be reminding ourselves when we are talking that a concept is not a thing. A concept is a way that we use for talking about a thing. We can use a word like "superego" in any way we choose, and we may choose to study Freud and to use this word as we believe he came to use it. If we do this it is simply because we want a common language. By contrast, if we take a word like "self," this is a word in the language; it has its history and it has its own meaning and we cannot muck about with it. This word "self" can teach us something but we cannot alter its meaning, not even if we want to. Mr Sandler has been rather careful in following this rule but even he makes one or two mistakes, referring, for instance, to the superego as a thing instead of to a concept about a phenomenon and a term that we are agreeing to use in referring to that phenomenon.

I would say that Mr Sandler's careful statement of the development of Freud's thought would make us say that if Melanie Klein had not existed we would have had to have invented her. This I believe is due to what I have described as Mr Sandler's presentation of the Freudian

2. 1949; in *Collected Papers: Through Paediatrics to Psycho-Analysis* (London: Tavistock, 1958; New York: Basic Books, 1975; London: Hogarth Press, 1975).

case, without enough reference to the unconscious and perhaps non-verbalised inner reality, the core of the dream world of the individual. In reading Freud's own work I do not get this feeling at all, because although Freud uses the mind and the intellectual processes and the verbalised part of feeling, he never lets us forget that he is talking about phenomena that have their roots in non-verbal material. In this way in Mr Sandler's paper we are left wanting some sort of statement like that which Melanie Klein eventually gave us on a psychic reality which is very closely related to the body and the body-functioning. I would have thought that Mr Sandler's statement of Melanie Klein's views could be accepted.

It would seem to me, therefore, that we are talking about two subjects, and perhaps we may decide at the end that they are one subject or that we like to leave them as two subjects. We are discussing Freud's idea of the superego as something which belongs to the passing of the Oedipus complex; we are also discussing the intra-psychic elements, mechanisms, phenomena, which date from the beginning of the individual's life. If we decide that there is a gradual build-up in health along the lines of these intra-psychic mechanisms, towards that which eventually becomes the superego of the Freudian concept, then we shall decide that we are all discussing one problem. We may choose to leave the matter open, but we may decide (and I personally would not mind at all if we did so) that these mechanisms of early mental functioning should not be called superego nor even given the dignity of the term "the pre-autonomous superego schema."

I would like to say that I do find it very important that a distinction should be drawn between the pre-autonomous age and the autonomous age if by this I understand that reference is being made to dependence and the gradual journey from dependence towards independence. In the same way I am impressed by the importance of assessing the subjective quality in the child's view of the parents and the quality of objective perception. Mr Sandler has thought out clearly the differences here.

At this point I would like to go to a comparison of the elements which in Kleinian conceptualising are called superego elements (but they need not necessarily be so called), and the classical superego of Freud which belongs to the passing of the Oedipus complex. I would like to make a comparison in terms of the analysis of patients. I would say first that the analysis of the Klein superego elements leads us back to the individual's instinctual life; it is the instinctual life that determines in the infant and the small child the build-up of benign and supportive elements and of persecutory or disruptive elements in the inner psychic reality, although there is also room for introjections which so to speak bypass the individual's instinctual living. By contrast the analysis of Freud's superego which belongs to the passing of the Oedipus complex takes us to the parents and to the effect that the authority of the parents has on the instinctual life of the child. At first view it would seem that there is a very big distinction between these two ways of looking at the same phenomenon through the analyses of individuals. But in the Freud superego concept there is every room left for the ideas of the subjective view of the parents, which introduces the idea of the parents as projections as well as of their use and acceptance as the individuals that they really are. In this way the work of analysis gets to the same place in the two cases, that is to say, to the instinctual life as experienced in the transference.

It is necessary that we should have a theory which covers the effect on the child of the absence of parents. The development of the superego in the child who lives without parental authorities and who lives in a community cannot be entirely dealt with on the basis that children find superego figures wherever they are. We have to take into consideration the fact that there is in healthy development of the healthy child a very great simplification of the whole of the superego development if the child does in fact live in the family and has the parents both available. The actual parents therefore contribute by being actual, as Mr Sandler indicates, even though the subjective view of the parents may be the chief elements in the formation of the individual's superego. In this way, and taking into consideration the psychic reality and the fantasy and the dream world of the child, we reach to the pregenital elements that contribute to the subjective view of the parents. Along with the consideration of pregenital instinctual life, we are also in the area of part-objects, dependence, primitive mechanisms of defence, defusion of instincts, etc.

If we take therefore Freud's superego arising out of the passing of the Oedipus complex we find elements that derive from the pregenital instinctual life and from the fantasy belonging to these areas of the experience of sub-human relationships, and in fact we find ourselves in the very area which is dealt with by Melanie Klein. What is this which Melanie Klein especially contributes here? My own way of putting it to myself is that Melanie Klein referred to the child's fantasy that his or her fantasy has a location within the self, inside the skin, inside the functioning body ego; in fact, in the belly or in the head. Philosophically of course fantasy that is personal to the individual and which we call the psychic reality has no location. In psychology, however, and in health, it is given location by the individual, and the wars between the benign and the persecutory elements in the inner psychic reality are played out in the body as well as projected outside the body. In other words, they belong to the whole body scheme of the individual, but the real place of origin of the conflicts is inside the individual, that is to say in the fantasy of the individual. The point under discussion really only concerns this intermediate area of our thinking process on the subject, this business of the child's fantasy that his or her personal fantasy is inside unless it is projected. In the analysis of the Freudian superego exactly as in the analysis of the hypochondriacal anxieties and the corresponding projections of the paranoid case, what ultimately makes the difference to the patient is the emergence of instinctual life in the transference. This is where there is a union of the analysis of the Kleinian hypochondriacal anxieties and the analysis of the Freudian superego; each is ultimately traced down in analysis to the instinctual life of the individual. Only the Freudian concept takes up the point that the actual parents have authority if they exist and play their part, and it rightly emphasises this aspect of superego formation. *Per contra,* the Klein concept underlines the superego elements that do not necessarily get to the point of development at which they can become whole and human. Surely it is in health only that the classical superego belonging to the passing of the Oedipus complex can be observed. By health I mean that the emotional development of the individual has taken place satisfactorily in the earliest stages of dependence, and the family exists, and the parents are present and playing their part in a fairly good way. It is a great relief for a child to be able to experience the anxieties that belong to the Oedipus complex. We have to say, this child is well enough to be one whole person amongst three, to experience the triangular situation, and to be able to work through in the presence of the parents all that is meant by the passing of the Oedipus complex and the setting up of a superego which has some relationship to the parents as perceived and the parents as conceived of. A very large number of children never have this relief. What happens in such cases is not that there is no superego but that the superego formation never becomes humanised and will remain rather like the polytheism before monotheism. It is then as if there are forces and mechanistic agencies that are feared and that must be magically countered, and that certainly cannot be defied. Every possible kind of frightening mechanism belongs to the lack of health in this area. In health the child may (to be sure) develop psychoneurosis, but nevertheless he or she has the great relief of a superego which is related to the human beings in fact, the father and the mother. The analysis can cash in on this. These human beings can be loved and hated, obeyed and defied, in the ordinary way that is well known.

I have to fit my theoretical views into the experience I had in my second child case, a successful, easy analysis of a 2½-year-old girl, who was what I would call normal. She had a severe feeding inhibition, and this started on her first birthday when for the first time she had a meal at a table along with both parents. She reached out, withdrew, and so started up her main symptom. The analysis (at 2½–3½) was very largely a playing out of the primal scene in terms of this meal, the two parents devouring the child, and in place of the inhibition there appeared extreme defiance, and an eating up of the parents and an oft-repeated overthrow of the table which was her world. Gradually identification with each of the two parents gave relief. Incidentally, as a mother she was sadistic towards her incontinent dolls, and also she was sadistic as a teacher, though her parents were very tolerant, and she herself had had no problem in regard to dryness and cleanliness.

This child, because she was normal, nearly employed the real parents in place of more primitive superego elements at the age of 12 months, and with my analytic help and support she quickly, at 2½–3½, became able to defy and to overthrow, and to identify, and even to obey. She now has two healthy children, born in holy wedlock!

In a big proportion of our cases the primitive mechanisms in the inner psychic reality get no such relief and we are needed to do the analysis of these hypochondriacal anxieties or of their projections; or often this statement is too advanced and we are needed in the management of still more primitive (or psychotic) anxieties when the child needs to become highly dependent and to manifest a delusional transference.

Although I disagree with four or five details in what I understand to be Mrs Klein's total theory, I realise how much I do accept her theory when I read Mr Sandler's alternative. As for my own work, I have been the leading figure in the movement towards a recognition of *need satisfaction* as earlier and more fundamental than wish fulfilment. And I have tried to get "internalisation" used for the imaginative elaboration of body function whilst reserving "introjection" for the magical process which can occur apart from eating.

I have also written in great detail about the correspondence between the mother's behaviour and the "cathected internal mother imago." To take up one point: when the mother's behaviour does not in fact correspond to the cathected internal mother imago the child does not "experience frustration, unpleasure and anger" . . . what happens is that the child tends to lose the capacity to relate to objects. If the capacity to be angry is retained, things are not too bad.

An important sentence is: "It is largely through the agency of the parents that the reality principle replaces the pleasure principle." Yes, but the parents do not act through introducing their idea of the real world to the child, they do it by adapting well enough to the child's needs, and then by graduated failure to adapt. All this precedes introjection and identification and imitation. The capacity for object-relationships having become established, the child can now proceed to such things as obedience, defiance and identification. I note that Mr Sandler leaves out defiance. He speaks of the child's need to feel loved, but the child must also feel real, and if defiance is omitted from the scheme and the child only obeys or identifies, then the child sooner or later complains of lack of feeling real.

Perhaps, however, we may find some value in the idea of the "representing" and "guiding" functions of introjects, building up to the human superego formation which relates to the passing of the Oedipus complex in children who are healthy and who get that far.

In the next few pages there are statements that need looking into. With many details I disagree, and I find an over-simplification of the subject. For instance, identification with the aggressor is part of a complex process: (1) introjection, (2) control, (3) threat of being controlled by (identification) and (4) tendency to re-project, etc. Mr Sandler relates this to reaction to loss. In dealing with loss the child (1) introjects, (2) subjects the introject to destructive agents (depressed mood indicates identification with dead introject), and (3) releases the introject to come alive again after sufficient expenditure of this inward hate. The two processes seem to me to have but little in common.

By the time I get to the end I simply make a note: what has become of fantasy? Maybe it is there but lost like the threepenny bit in the Christmas pudding.

There is a final quotation from Freud, in which Freud is talking about health and is assuming in the individual a capacity for identification with whole persons. This leaves aside, however, the growth of the superego out of the elements that belong to the primitive life of extreme dependence in which there are only part-objects.

55
Sigmund Freud

Review of *Letters of Sigmund Freud, 1873–1939*[1]
1962

It can safely be said that Freud as a young man had never heard of psycho-analysis, nor had he been even indirectly under its influence. His intimate letters to his fiancée, Martha Bernays (the first hundred or so of this collection), give us who value Freud for his contribution to science and to therapeutics a new chance, better even than the Jones's biography has given us, to judge Freud as a man. Does he turn out to be a human human being? These letters provide an answer.

Freud was born in 1856 and he became engaged to the 21-year-old Martha at the age of 26 in 1882. We are lucky to know so much about this young doctor when he was in love. As a man in love he shows all the usual signs, so that anyone who has been similarly affected must quickly recognise the affection.

We find he has a double allegiance, and he thus addresses himself to "lofty science": "Your Highness, I remain your humble, most devoted servant, but please don't hold it against me; you have never looked kindly upon me, never said a comforting word to me; you don't answer when I write to you, listen when I speak, but I know another lady to whom I mean more than I do to you, who repays my every service a hundredfold, and who moreover has but one servant and not, like you, thousands. You will understand if I now devote myself to the other so undemanding and gracious lady. Keep me in pleasant memory until I return. I have to write to Martha" (p. 29). Martha seems to have accepted this fact of the double allegiance. At a later date Freud refers to Martha's own ambition, and it is to be supposed that this found full scope in Freud's ultimate success. But one can see how easily Freud's scientific work could have been de-

1. London: Hogarth Press, 1961. This review appeared in the *British Journal of Psychology* 53 (1962).

stroyed had Martha needed more immediate satisfaction for her ambitions.

In those early days Freud collected round him a small social group composed of Martha's brother and her sister's fiancé and some of his own friends. This was called the Bund, and one wonders whether it might be possible to relate this social group with the later Bund, the professional one, which was composed of certain colleagues who helped to form a psycho-analytical society.

These letters show how Freud, very much a Jew, had a need and perhaps a tendency to find, day by day, the milieu in which he could have freedom, freedom to be himself and freedom to develop in his own way. So he was remarkably independent as a grown person perhaps because of his own dependence on a group, a group that was ever-changing, a group that ultimately depended in its turn at any one moment on Freud's own choice, and on his tolerance and on his intolerance.

But Freud had hidden away in him a terrific potential. It is true that he wrote in obvious sincerity: "I consider it a great misfortune that Nature has not granted me that indefinite something which attracts people. I believe it is this lack more than any other which has deprived me of a rosy existence. It has taken me so long to win my friends. I have had to struggle so long for my precious girl, and each time I meet someone I realise that an impulse, which defies analysis, leads that person to under-estimate me" (p. 211). Also, of himself ". . . who is still young and yet has never felt young" (p. 138). And again: ". . . in my youth I was never young and now that I am entering the age of maturity I cannot mature properly" (p. 214). But he was glad that Breuer said: ". . . hidden under the surface of timidity there lay in me an extremely daring and fearless human being. I had always thought so, but never dared tell anyone. I have often felt as though I had inherited all the defiance and all the passions with which our ancestors defended their Temple and could gladly sacrifice my life for one great moment in history" (p. 215). Added to this he could make a definite statement like that contained in his letter to Barbara Low after David Eder's death: "We were both Jews and knew of each other that we carried that miraculous thing in common, which—inaccessible to any analysis so far—makes the Jew" (p. 424). (By the way, he did in the end try to get behind this very thing when he put forward the thesis that Moses the Egyptian invented the Jew.)

So in this way we get from the letters the picture of a man establishing the personal fact: *I am;* and surely this is the original reason for the anxieties that are loosely called paranoid, and that lead to the necessity for a man to arrange for a circle of friends, both as a defence from all the others who are playing at the life-game "I'm the king of the castle," and in a positive way as a group of persons safe to love. This seems to be the task of the male half in Plato's fabulous division, and to correspond to the complementary task of the female half, which is to form a circle round the newly conceived.

It was into this pattern that Martha evidently fitted well. She retained the position of being Freud's other half. Freud was by nature the very opposite of promiscuous. Perhaps this one fact more than any other gave Freud the right to startle and disturb the world's mind, and made possible the launching of such ships as the Dynamic Unconscious, Infantile Sexuality, the Oedipus Complex, Psychic Reality, and many others that have proved to be not so much pleasure steamers as battleships in the Truth war.

For Freud surely this happy union with Martha to some extent solved his personal problem of bisexuality. He referred to Martha as Cordelia, and in so doing he found himself very happily in the same boat with Breuer (pp. 55, 56). But surely this leaves it for us to work out the place of Goneril and Regan. Lear had to suffer the machinations of his ambisexual first- and second-born before he could reach to the essentially female Cordelia. "Her voice was ever soft, gentle and low, an excellent thing in woman."

If Freud achieved this simplification in his life by the legitimate means of a happy marriage, he did also give us the instrument, the psycho-analytic technique, by which we might go further into the matter of the fear of WOMAN, as she can be in the unconscious of any person, man or woman.

Freud's last letters to Martha before their marriage are evidently missing. The reader suddenly finds Freud writing to his mother-in-law reporting the arrival of a baby. He has suffered during the birth, as men do, and now he is already very much loving his baby girl, who is only five hours old. He reports like a good pupil in infant-observation: "She weighs nearly 7 lb., which is quite respectable, looks terribly ugly, has been sucking at her right hand from the first moment, seems otherwise to be very good-tempered and behaves as though she really feels at home here. In spite of her splendid voice she doesn't cry much, looks very happy, lies snugly in her magnificent pram and doesn't give any impression of being upset by her great adventure" (p. 233).

All this feels very natural and normal, and forms a proper background for the other letters that gradually lead into the territory that has already been explored by Jones.

This reviewer finds immense wealth in this book, and in the insight it gives into the personality of so remarkable a man. Freud could talk about giving "free play to all the fountains of my irresponsibility" (p. 175); he could write: ". . . at heart I am still a child; I can be so happy simply because I am in another place, have different money in my pocket" (p. 92). He could laugh a whole evening at a Rome performance of *Carmen* (p. 275); and reading *Don Quixote* he could split his sides with laughing (p. 59); and on receiving a letter from Martha he wrote: "I leapt for joy—I never miss this exercise if there is the slightest reason for it" (p. 111).

And then, seriously, answering a letter from a friend who had suffered loss of a son, and writing on the anniversary of his loss of his middle daughter Sophie, he wrote: "Although we know that after such a loss the acute state of mourning will subside, we also know we shall remain inconsolable and will never find a substitute. No matter what may fill the gap, even if it be filled completely, it nevertheless remains something else. And actually this is how it should be. It is the only way of perpetuating that love which we do not want to relinquish" (p. 386).

Lastly, what of Freud's ideas about greatness in men? "Nor have I taken much interest in the whole species. It has always seemed to me that ruthlessness and arrogant self-confidence constitute the indispensable condition for what, when it succeeds, strikes us as greatness; and I also believe that one ought to differentiate between greatness of achievement and greatness of personality" (pp. 295–296).

One could claim that on the evidence of these letters Freud was human, and was a man of deep feeling, and he is already generally recognised as great in achievement. It may be that he could be said to have been great, too, in personality.

56
Harold F. Searles

Review of *The Non-Human Environment in Normal Development and in Schizophrenia*[1]

1963

Ideas, like the Word, can fall on stony ground, or they can be received into good soil and so bear fruit. An original idea needs an audience, and the good audience consists of those who have already had the idea; they are glad to find it formulated, and they are angry, too, that a chance for claiming priority has been missed. Thus, originality is tricky to assess and to attribute, and each originator is to some extent a copyist.

I like to be part of the audience, part of the good soil that makes this work of Searles bear fruit. The idea of a study of the non-human environment is a sound one, and long overdue in psycho-analytic circles. Searles discusses why it is that there has been this long delay, and indeed analysts may be expected to become suspicious of any trend that diverts attention from the theory of object-relationships, the object being human, or a part-object waiting to be allowed to become whole. This suspicion comes from the development of psycho-analytic theory on the basis of the id contained by the ego and controlled by the superego, or of the ego orientated both to the id and to external reality and permanently engaged in reconciling these two realities. When psycho-analysts became secure enough to explore ego-psychology and ego-relatedness, then new insight was gained both into the meaning of infantile dependence and also into the needs of those schizophrenic patients who carry along with their illness a tendency towards healthy though delayed emotional development.

Searles has made a whole book, and a very interesting one, out of this subject of man's relationship to the non-human environment—to

1. New York: International Universities Press, 1960. This review appeared in the *International Journal of Psycho-Analysis* 44 (1963). Copyright © Institute of Psycho-Analysis.

the dog as a dog, apart from its symbolism, and to the physical world apart from its meaning as mother, or as a place for taking projections. One could perhaps say that when Sechehaye gave that apple to that girl at that particular moment (symbolic realisation) Searles draws our attention to the fact of the apple, which presumably was suitably ripe, and also to the orchards from which apples come, and to Sechehaye's access to the products of orchards, and so on.

Certainly this theme develops very easily once consideration of it has been started, and even if the idea underlying what is written can be taken out and looked at here, it is the actual reading of the book that will reward the reader.

In regard to the idea, much of my own work has been related to this theme. I have had no fear that the theory of individual development will be interfered with by recognition of the part played by the environment outside the area of the individual's projections. One is reminded here of Hartmann's conflict-free area in the ego, which in no way interferes with the concept of conflict and anxiety.

It might be found that Searles's non-human environment comes round in the end to being the mother, but in a way that is different from the usual way by which environmental phenomena are seen as projections, and projections of introjections. I mean that this non-human environment may be looked at as an extension of the environment that is the mother, prior to the baby's arrival at object-relationships with id cathexes. I have developed this theme in terms of ego-relatedness, and in terms of double dependence. By double dependence I mean the relationship of the infant to environmental phenomena of which the baby could not possibly be aware, so that later as a patient the baby now grown to childhood or adulthood is not able to reproduce it as a pattern revealing itself in an analytic transference. In other words, the environment to which I refer in the concept of double dependence is one that is essentially not made up of projections. Later the individual may reach to a recognition of this in a sophisticated acceptance of "shared" reality. This acceptance of the reality principle is a matter of the intellect.

So some of the non-human environment of Searles is human, some is animal, some is vegetable, and some is purely physical. The force of gravity is an element of the non-human environment that distinguishes the period after birth from the prenatal period; on the positive side the infant knows this in the sensation of feeling heavy, and on the negative side the infant knows of gravity indirectly through the infinite panic associated with being held in an unreliable way. It took a Newton and thousands of years of sophistication for the concept of gravity to be formulated, and all the time in observation of developing babies we see the effects of non-human environment details, often never achieving the status of statement. Searles is attempting, I feel, to make a generalised statement, one that covers future developments, as for instance the possibility that one day psychology might contribute to physics in regard to some detail.

Would Searles agree to a change of name? It seems that his term is not good enough because his non-human environment may well be human, such as the colour of the mother's hair, the fact of her survival or death, or the profession of the father, who may be a miner and come home black, or a baker and come home white. I think Searles is referring to the non-projective environment, or all those aspects of the individual's environment that in fact take effect or impinge before the individual baby is ready to gain control of external reality by the mechanisms of projection and introjection.

The affinity between Searles's point of view and my own can be easily illustrated. For instance (p. 416) "The deeply regressed patient, more than any one else except for the infant, needs to have a non-human environment which is not only relatively stable and relatively uncomplex, but also beautiful." Leaving out the detail of beauty, which introduces more complex considerations, I find this idea of a relatively stable and relatively uncomplex non-human environment almost the same as my own insistence on the good-enough mothering without which the development that makes for mental health (in the sense of non-liability to psychosis) cannot take place satisfactorily. This is the non-human environment which is in effect the mother, the mother and father, the family, the place, affecting the baby before the era of control by projection and introjection.

The early oneness of the stage before the baby separates off the mother from the self, that which appears in psychotic illness as a merging, is a oneness not with a person, nor with an object; it is a oneness with the non-human environment, or, as I would like to call it, a non-projective environment. In this way Searles's study is of great importance for the understanding both of the needs of schizophrenics and also of the phenomena that are silently at work in ordinary good-enough mothering.

Searles may, however, prefer to stick to his term "non-human environment" and so to concentrate on referring to the fact that in the process of getting to control external reality by introjection and projection the developing infant (or regressed patient) is dependent on what external reality does in fact exist for use in the exercise of these mental mechanisms.

57

C. G. Jung

Review of *Memories, Dreams, Reflections*[1]

1964

The publication of this book provides psycho-analysts with a chance, perhaps the last chance they will have, to come to terms with Jung. If we fail to come to terms with Jung we are self-proclaimed partisans, partisans in a false cause.

Jung was a being, a real person, one who happened to live in Freud's time and who inevitably met Freud. The impact of their meeting provides material for serious study, and the manner of their parting is no less interesting to the student of human nature. Psychoanalysts can choose to line up with Freud, and to measure Jung against him, or they can look at Jung and look at Freud and allow the two to meet and to go together and to separate. In the latter case they must know their Jung, and the value of this book is that it allows us to know Jung as he was when entirely unaffected by Freud and all his works.

By "this book" I mean the first 115 pages. These first three chapters are genuine autobiography. Here is an autobiography to take its place with the other really convincing autobiographies; one has no doubt about the value of these chapters as a truly self-revealing statement. My review will concern itself with these important chapters, and mostly with the first chapter: "First Years."

I am sure that *every psycho-analyst must read* these first three chapters and so meet Jung as he was, and that no analyst who has failed to read them is qualified to talk or write about Jung and Freud and their meeting and their ultimate failure to understand each other.

In discussing these early details of Jung's life I put myself in the category of people who, in Jung's words: "always remind me of those

1. London: Collins and Routledge, 1963. This review appeared in the *International Journal of Psycho-Analysis* 45 (1964). Copyright © Institute of Psycho-Analysis.

optimistic tadpoles who bask in a puddle in the sun, in the shallowest of waters, crowding together and amiably wriggling their tails, totally unaware that the next morning the puddle will have dried up and left them stranded" (p. 28). In spite of this I must go ahead using the rich material Jung has supplied in order to look closely at the man Jung had it in him to be, and then was.

Jung, in describing himself, gives us a picture of childhood schizophrenia, and at the same time his personality displays a strength of a kind which enabled him to heal himself. At cost he recovered, and part of the cost to him is what he paid out to us, if we can listen and hear, in terms of his exceptional insight. Insight into what? Insight into the feelings of those who are mentally split.

I must ask the reader at this stage to understand that I am not running down Jung by labelling him a "recovered case of infantile psychosis." I may be a "tadpole amiably unknowing of my fate," but I am not besmirching Jung's personality or character. If I want to say that Jung was mad, and that he recovered, I am doing nothing worse than I would do in saying of myself that I was sane and that through analysis and self-analysis I achieved some measure of insanity. Freud's flight to sanity could be something we psycho-analysts are trying to recover from, just as Jungians are trying to recover from Jung's "divided self," and from the way he himself dealt with it.

In a way Jung and Freud turn out to be complementary; they are like the obverse and reverse of a coin; we can see when we know Jung, as we can now do, why it was not possible for him and Freud to come to terms with each other in those early years of the century, those early years in which Freud was struggling to establish a science that could gradually expand, and Jung was starting off "knowing," but handicapped by his own need to search for a self with which to know. At the end of a long life Jung reached to the centre of his self, which turned out to be a blind alley; and compared with this we may prefer Freud's groping and his gradual failure to finalise anything except that he had set going a process which we and all future generations can use for therapy, which is research into the nature of man, and for research, which is a therapy of man.

Let us say this about the relationship between Freud and Jung: they had to meet, but Freud could not have gone to Jung for analysis because Freud invented psycho-analysis, and also Freud needed to leave aside the area of insanity in order to forge ahead with the application of scientific principles to the study of human nature; and Jung could not have had analysis from Freud because in fact Freud could not have done this analysis, which would have involved aspects of psycho-analytic theory that are only now, half a century later, beginning to emerge as a development of psycho-analytic metapsychology. In other words, these two men, each possessed by a daimon, could only meet, communicate without basic understanding, and then separate. The manner of the meeting and of the separation is of interest but of little significance.

I can best contribute to a consideration of this book by making a preliminary study of the first chapter. It must be remembered, however, that when autobiography is under review no comment can supplant the actual experience of reading. I can only communicate with those who have read the author's own statement and have already absorbed it.

Because of my special interests I can bring more to the early chapters than I can to the later, and I come to the first chapter, "First Years," with a precise and detailed theory of the emotional development of the infant and with considerable clinical experience of all the various kinds of observation, direct and indirect, which are the stuff of child-psychiatry practice. Naturally I am excited by discovering this exceptionally rich source.

Jung's early memories are of a consciousness of beauty and happiness, and these show this only child's (a sister was born when he was already 9 years old) introduction to the world of beauty by those who cared for him. There is a negative to this sort of positive feeling experience, which in the end we must try to discover. It will turn out to be a distortion of integrative tendencies secondary to the mother's maternal failure due to her own illness.

By the age of 4 Jung's psychotic illness was established, and defences which were to be lifelong served him well; it is remarkable that in the end he was able to understand his own psychosis as deeply as he does in this autobiography.

I have stated elsewhere[2] that it is in the area of psychosis rather than that of psycho-neurosis that we must expect to find cure by self-healing. Jung provides an example of this, but of course self-healing is not the same as resolution by analysis.

Before the age of 4 Jung had had the breakdown which underlies the organisation of a defence pattern. This was remembered as a time

2. "Metapsychological and Clinical Aspects of Regression within the Psycho-Analytical Set-up" (1954), in *Collected Papers: Through Paediatrics to Psycho-Analysis* (London: Tavistock, 1958; New York: Basic Books, 1975; London: Hogarth Press, 1975).

when his father carried him round and sang to him. He was suffering, he thinks, from a generalised eczema, and he relates this illness to the estrangement between his parents that was taking shape at that time. In other words he was threatened by an ego-disintegration (a depersonalisation), a reversal of the maturational processes; and his defences settled down into a splitting of the personality, related at one level to the parental separation. We may guess that in Jung's case the splitting was not an inherited ego-weakness, if there is such a thing, and not entirely a primary failure to achieve unit status at earlier stages of emotional development, but that it was a defence organised at a time of dependence on parental union. There is evidence of an earlier external factor, namely the maternal depression, which affected his infancy and provided the negative for the positive qualities that he projected on to the landscape, on to things, and on to the world. His earliest memory is not of his mother. He made use, however, of women who were not his mother, and one of these women formed the basis for his conception of his own anima. (For me, the anima is the part of any man that could say: I have always known I was a woman.)

Jung is able to report a significant dream which gave the pattern for his life and lifework. *This is true Jung,* and it is legitimate to build on it tentative theories of Jung's personal difficulties and of his way of dealing with these difficulties.

I had the earliest dream I can remember, a dream which was to preoccupy me all my life. I was then between three and four years old.

The vicarage stood quite alone near Laufen castle, and there was a big meadow stretching back from the sexton's farm. In the dream I was in this meadow. Suddenly I discovered a dark, rectangular, stone-lined hole in the ground. I had never seen it before. I ran forward curiously and peered down into it. Then I saw a stone stairway leading down. Hesitantly and fearfully, I descended. At the bottom was a doorway with a round arch, closed off by a green curtain. It was a big, heavy curtain of worked stuff like brocade, and it looked very sumptuous. Curious to see what might be hidden behind, I pushed it aside. I saw before me in the dim light a rectangular chamber about thirty feet long. The ceiling was arched and of hewn stone. The floor was laid with flagstones, and in the centre a red carpet ran from the entrance to a low platform. On this platform stood a wonderfully rich golden throne. I am not certain, but perhaps a red cushion lay on the seat. It was a magnificent throne, a real king's throne in a fairy tale. Something was standing on it which I thought at first was a tree trunk twelve or fifteen feet high and about one and a half to two feet thick. It was a huge thing, reaching almost to the ceiling. But it was of a curious composition: it was made of skin and naked flesh, and on top there was something like a rounded head with no face and no hair. On the very top of the head was a single eye, gazing motionlessly upwards.

It was fairly light in the room, although there were no windows and no apparent source of light. Above the head, however, was an aura of brightness. The thing did not move, yet I had the feeling that it might at any moment crawl off the throne like a worm and creep towards me. I was paralyzed with terror. At that moment I heard from outside and above me my mother's voice. She called out, "Yes, just look at him. That is the man-eater!" That intensified my terror still more, and I awoke sweating and scared to death. For many nights afterwards I was afraid to go to sleep, because I feared I might have another dream like that.

At this stage we can already map out Jung's illness as follows:
Healthy potential.
Infancy disturbed by maternal depression, this being counteracted by father's motherliness.
Three years: psychotic breakdown, related to parental separation.
Temporary defence: psycho-somatic disorder eliciting father's motherliness (dependence continued).
Four years: main defensive organisation and the achievement of independence.
With the help of the rest of the book we can continue:
Various threats of breakdown in later childhood, with self-cure.
Defences include: True self (secret); False self; The forging of a life-work out of the defence organisation along with a permanent tendency to heal the split in the personality.
Eventually, in the arduous work of the autobiography, the remembering of significant details of infancy and childhood, the nearest possible self-cure of childhood schizophrenia. Here the true self is no longer secret, and the false self, which had immense value because it enabled Jung to lead a "normal" life in the world, has become relatively useless.

Seen in this way Jung's remarkable life takes a shape, and for us a valuable thing emerges, because we become able to understand the lie that Jung told to Freud. A dream was reported to Freud (pp. 155, 156) which ended:

Thick dust lay on the floor, and in the dust were scattered bones and broken pottery, like remains of a primitive culture. I discovered two human skulls, obviously very old and half disintegrated. Then I awoke.

What chiefly interested Freud in this dream were the two skulls. He returned to them repeatedly, and urged me to find a *wish* in connection with them. What did I think about these skulls? And whose were they? I knew perfectly well, of course, what he was driving at: that secret death wishes were concealed in the dream.

. . . I submitted to his intention and said, "My wife and my sister-in-law" . . .

And so I told him a lie.

In its place in Jung's life the telling of this lie is perhaps the nearest that he came to a unit self, until he was able, in old age, to write his autobiography.

When Jung deliberately lied to Freud he became a unit with a capacity to hide secrets instead of a split personality with no place for hiding anything. In this way perhaps Freud did perform some sort of a service for Jung, albeit without knowing it. We can see why Freud would not know, but it is for us to know and to understand as far as we can on the facts available. "Tout comprendre rend très indulgent."

It does not matter much what the lie was about. At some point, however, Jung had to lie to Freud, or else he had to start an analysis with him, one that could not possibly have led to cure, though it might have led to a flight from psychosis to sanity or to psycho-neurosis.

Could it be said that Freud's famous fainting turns tell the same story the other way round? It seems significant that in Jung's threatened breakdown at the age of 12 his symptom was fainting; behind the fainting was a "suicidal impulse," and behind this was infantile madness (disintegration, depersonalisation, reversal of maturational processes).

We may well be glad that Jung and Freud separated, and that each maintained a personal integrity and lived to enrich the world exceptionally.

Jungians and Freudians Now

It is now necessary to examine some of the effects of Jung's defence organisation against psychosis on the thinking of latter-day Jungians and Freudians. We cannot help noticing when we meet to discuss human nature that we are apt to use the same terms with meanings that are not only different from each other but that seem irreconcilable. The two worst offenders are the words "unconscious" and "self."

Unconscious

From the time of Jung's dream when he was 4 years old it was certain that he and Freud would not be able to communicate about the unconscious. Whatever Freud was, he had a unit personality, with a place in him for his unconscious. Jung was different. It is not possible for a split personality to have an unconscious, because there is no place for it to be. Like our florid schizophrenic patients (though he was not one) Jung knew truths that are unavailable to most men and women. But he spent his life looking for a place to keep his inner psychic reality, although the task was indeed an impossible one. By the age of 4 he had adopted the sophisticated theory of the underground of the dream, closely associated in his case with the burial of the dead. He went down under and found subjective life. At the same time he became a withdrawn person, with what was wrongly thought at the time to be a clinical depression. From this developed Jung's exploration of the unconscious, and (for me) his concept of the collective unconscious was part of his attempt to deal with his lack of contact with what could now be called the unconscious-according-to-Freud.

This gives us the idea of Jung's work as being out of touch with instinct and object-relating (except in a subjective sense). Jung's extravert No. 1 personality (False Self in my language) evidently gave a rather normal impression, and gave Jung a place in the world, and a rich family and professional life, but Jung makes no bones about his preference for his True Self (Jung's language) No. 2 personality which carried for him the sense of real. The only place for his unconscious (Freudian sense) would be in his secret True Self, an enigma wrapped in an enigma. This was dramatised in the secret contents of a pencil box secretly hidden, and then forgotten for several decades. Naturally the secret contents were significant and were eventually found to be closely related to common denominators in anthropological lore.

If Jung's special meaning for the word "unconscious" be understood and kept distinct from the various uses which Freud gave to the term, then it is possible for the psycho-analyst to join in with those many who find in Jung's writings a tremendous contribution to the study of people and to the correlation of facts gathered from far and wide. But the psycho-analyst would sacrifice essential values were he to give up Freud's various meanings for the word "unconscious," including the concept of the repressed unconscious. It is not possible to conceive of a repressed unconscious with a split mind; instead what is found is dissociation.

When Jung contemplated the idea of the erect penis in the place of the king on the throne in the underground chamber of his dream as a 4-year-old he did not connect this with, for instance, a projection of his own phallic excitements. He seemed to fear that a tadpole of an analyst would insist that he had seen an erect penis somewhere, but the thing an analyst would find lacking is any attempt to relate this with the 4-year-old Jung's instinctual life.

In this way there is but little Oedipus conflict in the split personality, nor is there a clash with the father in extravert living; and a clash with the father was in any case interfered with by the estrangement of his parents at that time, and by the fact that Jung's father became the reliable mother-figure in his life. He was therefore unprepared as a man to clash with Freud. An imaginative clash with Freud would alone have formed a basis for a friendship (sublimated homosexuality), and there is evidence that Freud would have welcomed some such imaginative clash.

Jung reached to his father's hate in an amazing way by having the idea of God's intention that his created men and women should sin, following the idea he had that God had shat from his golden throne on the beautiful new roof of the cathedral, breaking the walls asunder. Here again, naturally, Jung does not go one step further back and relate this to his own destruction of beauty. We could not expect to find Jung feeling God to be a projection of his own infantile omnipotence and the shitting as a projection of his own hate of the father in the mother; or at a more primitive level, his own destruction of the good object because of its being real in the sense of being outside the area of his omnipotence.

Jung describes his playing (which had to be done very much alone till he went to school) as a constant building and rebuilding followed always by the staging of an earthquake and the destruction of the building. What we cannot find in the material Jung provides is imaginative destruction followed by a sense of guilt and then by construction. It seems that the thing that was repressed in Jung's early infancy, that is, before the infantile breakdown, was primitive aggression—and we remember here that it is precisely this primitive destructiveness that is difficult to get at when an infant is cared for by a mother who is clinically depressed. (Fordham has referred to Jung's fear of his own destructiveness.)[3]

The Self

More difficult for me is a discussion of Jung's use of the word "self." (This has been discussed with clarity by Fordham.)[4]

The word "self" is not a psychological term, but it is a word we all use, and it is possible that Jung contributed more than did Freud to an understanding of what the word means or can mean. It was Fordham himself who jolted me into a recognition that I was using the words "self" and "ego" as if they were synonymous, which of course they are not; they cannot be, since "self" is a word, and "ego" is a term to be used for convenience with an agreed meaning.

The fact is that the term "ego" is used differently, according to whether Freudian or Jungian jargon is employed. Freud certainly used the term in differing ways, according to the era in which he was writing. In Freudian metapsychology the concept of the ego has its own evolution. The early idea of the ego as a part of the id has not stood the test of time. Ego-psychology in psycho-analytic circles began to develop in the thirties, and has now been carried a long way, so that the idea of there being an ego from the beginning (prior to and covering id-experience) is considered, especially if this be looked at as related intimately to ego-support given sensitively by the mother to the infant who is lucky enough to have an ego-supportive mother.

Work has been done in psycho-analytic literature on maturation in terms of the evolution of the ego, including the concept of the tendency towards integration and towards a capacity for object-relating and for the psycho-somatic partnership. Much expansion of theoretical understanding along these lines is to be expected in the near future. All this seems to be ignored in Jungian writings, and we cannot afford to ignore anything that is valid. Nevertheless the idea of the

3. M. Fordham, *An Evaluation of Jung's Work* (London: Guild of Pastoral Psychology, Lecture no. 119, 1962).

4. M. Fordham, "The Empirical Foundation and Theories of the Self in Jung's Work," *Journal of Analytic Psychology* 8 (1963).

self is very well dealt with by Jungians, and it is for the psycho-analysts to learn what they can in this field.

What must be remembered, I think, is that Jung himself spent his life looking for his own self, which he never really found since he remained to some extent split (except in so far as this split was healed in his work on his autobiography). In old age he appears to have dropped his No. 1 personality to a large extent and to have lived by his True Self, and in this way he found a self that he could call his own. Was he not clinically somewhat withdrawn in so doing?

Eventually he reached the centre of his self. As I have suggested earlier, this seems to have been satisfying for him, and yet somewhat of a blind alley if looked at as an achievement for a remarkable and a truly big personality. In any case he was preoccupied with the man-dala, which from my point of view is a defensive construct, a defence against that spontaneity which has destruction as its next-door neigh-bour. The mandala is a truly frightening thing for me because of its absolute failure to come to terms with destructiveness, and with chaos, disintegration, and the other madnesses. It is an obsessional flight from disintegration. Jung's description of his last decades spent in search of the centre of his self seems to me to be a description of a slow and wearisome closing down of a lifetime of splendid endea-vour. The centre of the self is a relatively useless concept. What is more important is to reach to the basic forces of individual living, and to me it is certain that if the real basis is creativeness the very next thing is destruction.

This is a matter that needs special treatment in a different setting. The fact remains that the search for the self and a way of feeling real, and of living from the true rather than from the false self, is a task that belongs not only to schizophrenics; it also belongs to a large proportion of the human race. Nevertheless it must also be recognised that for many this problem is *not* the main one; their infantile expe-riences took them satisfactorily through the early stages, so that a solution was found in infancy to this essential human problem. Gen-erally, the problems of life are not about the search for a self, but about the full and satisfying use of a self that is a unit and is well grounded. There are plenty of troubles of other kinds for the unit personality, though for the unit personality the word "self" has a clear meaning that does not need explaining.

It is truly difficult for those with healthy unit personalities to achieve empathy with those whose divided selves give them constant trouble. Jung has helped here, and among psycho-analysts there are some who are drawing our attention to the inapplicability of the so-called classical psycho-analytical technique to the treatment of schizophrenia.

Jung's life has shown, I believe, how psychotic illness may not only give a person a lot of trouble but may also push that person on to exceptional attainment. He has, of course, thrown a beam of light on the problem that is common to all human beings, in so far as there are common defences against intolerable or what might be called psychotic fears.

This is a book that can enable us to become objective in our assessment of Jung, in the same way that we wish to be objective about Freud. We ourselves undergo analysis, and we must be able to analyse our masters too; they could not have analysis by the very nature of things.

The whole book deserves careful reading. It is well translated. One word I question: "attained" as a translation of *erreichten*. "Ich konnte mich nie aufhalten beim einmal Erreichten." Could this not be "I could never stop at anything once I had reached to it"? "Attained" seems to imply assimilation. An error of translation here could queer the pitch for further games of Jung-analysis.

58
Erik H. Erikson

Review of *Childhood and Society*[1]

1965

"I have nothing to offer except a way of looking at things."

It is good to find this book now available in paperback. It is a hotch-potch, "a conceptual itinerary"; but I like it because of this, and because Erikson is a likeable person. His personality is free from bombast and he has a natural humility which makes him the right person to attempt to apply psycho-analytic findings.

The four parts of the book need to be joined together in the mind of the reader. The first is an Erikson statement of a psycho-analytic view of childhood, both the clinical problems and the general theory of development of the adult mature man or woman not out of a homunculus, but out of a dependent infant. This dependent infant is carried forward by inborn maturational processes. Part two might well provide the starting point for the reader who is new to this kind of reading matter. The descriptions of the childhood patterns in two American Indian tribes—which happen to be very different each from the other—is fascinating, and the author's main theme is best illustrated in this section.

Part three concerns the growth of the ego, and here one sees the foundations being laid for Erikson's main contribution, a study of identity problems (as in his *Young Man Luther*, 1958). Part four—recommended by me as second for the new reader—is on youth and the evolution of identity. This gives an interesting account of the American identity, and of the legends of Hitler's and Maxim Gorky's childhoods.

Erikson's main theme is that studies of societies seldom give proper place to infancy and childhood patterns: "a blind spot in the makers

---

1. London: Hogarth Press, 1965. This review appeared in *New Society*, 30 September 1965.

and interpreters of history: they ignore the fateful function of child-hood in the fabric of society." Every individual has been an infant and a child and brings to the social picture the drives, anxieties and mental defences that belong to every growing human being. Local societies, in the pattern of their attitude to their young, mobilise these drives, anxieties and defences to adapt their children to become not just adults, but adults in their specific community.

"Only an identity safely anchored in the 'patrimony' of a cultural identity can produce a workable psychosocial equilibrium," and "a fear of loss of identity dominates much of our irrational motivation; it calls upon the whole arsenal of anxiety which is left in each individual from the mere fact of his childhood. In this emergency, masses of people become ready to seek salvation in pseudo-identities." There is a feedback here into psycho-analysis. As an analyst one may not feel that Erikson's statement of psycho-analytic metapsychology is acceptable in all details. The main thing is that Erikson has taught us much, and now his special approach to individual and world problems will be read by many who are not actually students in the field of social psychology.

59
Virginia Axline

A Commentary on *Play Therapy*[1]
Undated; probably mid-1960s

This is not intended as broadcast material. It is simply just myself writing down notes in this way while reading Miss Axline's book on child therapy, actually called *Play Therapy*. There will be no attempt to make continuity and there will be long gaps.

An important paragraph for quotation comes on page 15. "Nondirective therapy is based upon the assumption that the individual has within himself not only the ability to solve his own problems satisfactorily, but also this growth impulse that makes mature behavior more satisfying than immature behavior." The reason why I am taking the trouble to make a comment on this book and on Miss Axline's work is that, it seems to me, her method and her attitude is one that can be communicated to suitable people in a relatively short period of time. There is no question about some modification of the training scheme for psycho-analysts and the theory of psycho-analysis must develop in its own way and be developed by psycho-analysts. Nevertheless, psycho-analysts miss something very important if they do not join up with the work of other psychotherapists and, in fact, they will find, as in the case of Miss Axline, that the work they read about corresponds closely to the modified analysis which they must do in certain cases if they are to get anywhere at all. The other thing is that psycho-analysis avoids the question of social need and social pressure. Psycho-analysts have to justify themselves socially in other ways than by meeting social pressure and they may be able to help those who are doing satisfactory work or very good work indeed by giving backing where they feel that the work is genuine and depends on the real

---

1. *Play Therapy: The Inner Dynamics of Childhood* (Boston: Houghton Mifflin, 1947). This commentary is a transcript from a tape recording. It is unfinished and was never edited by Winnicott.—EDS.

principles of childhood development and need. In my opinion, this work of Miss Axline is one of the really good applications of psycho-analytic theory and I am not put off by the fact that probably Miss Axline would not feel disposed to relate the theory that she uses to that of psycho-analysis. I do not know the answer to this at the moment, but I shall be seeing her and shall discuss this point with her. There is of course, the American antagonism to the idea of the training of non-medical people to be reckoned with and this must inevitably result in the sprouting of psychotherapy groupings where something is done that is not called psycho-analysis and that has not had the advantage of psycho-analytic training. Nevertheless, there are many people capable of doing this work and it cannot be expected that they will forever drown themselves in the American or United States rule that no-one but medically qualified men and women may be taught psycho-analysis as a technique. The time is coming when this rule is beginning to look absurd, as indeed it was predicted that it would look absurd. I say this without denying the fact that it may have been a good rule twenty years ago.

There is very special importance for me in Miss Axline's statement that she makes in her introduction, page 15, because it joins up exactly with the thing I have been trying to say myself in my lectures on child psychiatry meeting the challenge of the case, exploiting the first interview and so on. For instance, here is a statement: "This type of therapy starts where the individual is and bases the process on the present configuration, allowing for change from minute to minute during the therapeutic contact if it should occur that rapidly, the rate depending upon the reorganisation of the individual's accumulated experiences, attitudes, thoughts and feelings to bring about insight, which is the prerequisite of successful therapy." I am not quite sure about the accent on insight here, which at times may cramp the total theory because there may be cases, even in Miss Axline's book, in which changes occur without insight. It would seem to me that in infancy and in early childhood, a great deal happens without insight either from the parents or from the child. I could illustrate this: I went into a bookshop to buy a book and the assistant took me aside and asked me if I might discuss with him a child. He had a child of 2 staying in his house along with the child's mother. This was a little girl whose very young parents had already separated so that the child was only seeing the mother. This man himself had a little girl of the same age who was doing very well indeed. This little girl staying in his house could not bear to see him. Whenever he came near, she lay on the floor on her tummy and screamed and screamed. He, himself, was in a dilemma: should he try and make friends and so become a father substitute or should he just simply accept the situation and be glad that, at any rate, the child was having an open reaction to the absence of her own father which, evidently, he was reminding her of whenever he came into the room? Eventually, she became very attached to him but then she and her mother left his house and he then felt wicked at having become involved, although he couldn't help it, because he knew that the child would have to suffer another loss. What he said to me was that this experience had provided him with insights into what was happening with his own child. He and his wife would not have known how important their togetherness would have been for their own little girl had they not seen the terrible effect on the other 2-year-old girl of the separation of the parents. I would think that if they had not had this experience they would have been doing very good work as parents and the child would have been developing well, but without insight, and that the work would not be adversely affected by the fact that there was no occasion for insight. In any case, insight was not gained by the 2-year-old girl who was happy in her own secure home. It is unlikely that she was old enough, at the age of 2, to compare the state of the other little 2-year-old with her own. I think that in psychotherapy there is something equivalent, and in a statement such as the one that I have quoted room must be left for clinical improvement that is solid and permanent and yet not related to insight. Nevertheless, this statement contains essential elements where therapy starts where the individual is and bases the process on present configuration. When non-directive therapy grants the individual the permissiveness to be himself, it accepts that completely without evaluation or pressure to change. It recognises and clarifies the expressed emotionalised attitudes by a reflection of what the client has expressed. Here I find a very clear statement of something that I have tried to express in my own way in terms of the mirror, that is to say, in terms of the idea that the first mirror is the mother's face and that one of the functions of the mother and of the parents and of the family is to provide a mirror, figuratively speaking, in which the child can see himself or herself. The child cannot use the parents and the family as a mirror unless there is this principle of permissiveness to be whatever he or she is, to be himself or herself, accepted completely without evaluation or pressure to change.

The great thing that is different between play therapy of Miss Axline's variety and psycho-analysis is that the therapy stops short at the point where the therapist mirrors the child as he actually is. In other words, the complication of psycho-analytic interpretations is absent.

60
Willi Hoffer

A Tribute on the Occasion of Hoffer's
Seventieth Birthday[1]

Dated 13 June 1967

In writing this tribute to Willi Hoffer I start with a child psychiatry case description of my own, passing on from that to an appreciation of Hoffer's work.

Part I

In my hospital clinic I saw a baby boy aged 4½ months. He was brought by his mother, and his father's mother formed one of the party. This grandmother had arranged the consultation, but she left the mother and the baby and myself to ourselves.

There was an older child (a girl aged 3 years) who had been breast-fed for 10 months, and who had given no trouble. At the time of the birth of this older child the mother had had personal difficulties, including nightmares and also difficulties in relation to her own mother, but this anxiety state in the mother had not spoiled the little girl's early phase of infancy. Even a somewhat unfeeling attitude on the part of the nurses at the nursing home (pushing the baby's nose into the breast to make her start feeding, and, generally, not allowing for natural processes) had not interfered with the mother's early management with the girl baby.

Before the arrival of the second baby the mother had added to her personal experiences a certain amount of understanding through reading. After the boy baby's birth she behaved in a very sensitive way, allowing the baby to find the breast with his hands, and in every way the start was satisfactory. In spite of this, and the fact that the

1. Published in German in *Psyche* (1967).

mother was much less anxious than at the time of the first birth, this boy had been difficult.

For two months after the birth all went well. Then (at 2 months) the baby began to refuse the early evening feed. This passed, and then after a week he again refused a feed from the breast. The mother was now menstruating, but he took the breast milk from a bottle, and in this way showed that the trouble was not with the quality of the milk. It became clear that when he refused the breast this was motivated by powerful factors within himself: he just could not get near the breast. When in this state he would cry pitifully if he happened to touch the nipple. The mother tried squirting milk from her plentiful supply directly into the baby's mouth, but he reacted to this "as if he had been given poison."

All this time the baby was quite well and contented between the feeds and would take the bottle with satisfaction.

The mother was upset at finding her baby showed an aversion to her actual breast. She accepted the situation, however, and made arrangements for regular bottle feeding with her breast milk. She accepted advice to give up trying to overcome the baby's aversion to the breast.

At 4½ months, when I saw the mother and the boy together I was able to see that this boy was very much a person, and intelligently aware of his surroundings. He loved watching his sister and had recently become very much aware of his father. In fact, the aversion to the breast became a significant feature on a holiday Monday when the father was at home and was for the first time present at the baby's feed time. The relation to the father was positive.

Here then was an emotional disturbance in a healthy boy baby, starting at 2 months and fairly well organised at 4½ months. The people involved were:

The baby boy

The mother		The sister
(The mother's mother)	The father	
		The father's mother.

I made a note at the time that the mother could not be thought of as quite normal. Although not manifestly anxious she was rather excitable, and she was very much frustrated because she wanted to feed the baby and fulfil her function as a mother. I made a guess that she had to deal with a considerable quantity of a masculine element in her total personality make-up, which (if true) would complicate the fantasy of her breast-feeding function, and also her attitude to this boy baby, as compared with her attitude to the girl.

There was a further clinical detail of significance. The mother often felt, she said, that she could manage breast feeding the boy if it were not for the sister's very special attitude. The sister is intensely interested, but is unable to stand the baby brother's crying. Immediately he cries she shouts out: feed it! feed it! At the same time the other side of the sister's feelings were showing in her accident-proneness during the actual periods of the breast-feeding of her brother. Frequently the mother needed to interrupt the breast-feeding in order to deal with a crisis in the sister's life.

I was also informed that there were disturbances in the home (associated with other relatives) arousing considerable tensions, the mother being unable to prevent these, and the father seeming to be either absent or else unaware of the need that his wife had for him to create a calm atmosphere around her if she was to perform her delicate task well enough.

Experiment

I was able to make an experiment, applying what I know of the problems of babies who suffer intense distress through being unable to follow their natural instinct to approach the breast and the mother.

While the mother and the baby and I were alone together the baby went through one of these phases in which he was negatively orientated to the mother's breast, and intensely distressed. I put my hand between the baby's hand and the breast, thus producing an opposition. In response to this he temporarily lost his inhibition and struggled to get at the breast. This experiment was repeated several times, always with the same result. Eventually there he was lying in his mother's arms, sucking his left thumb, and with his right thumb in his left hand, and his right hand on the breast. The mother had not had a peaceful moment like this in her relation to this baby for over a week.

What I had done, no doubt, was temporarily to put outside the baby the controlling element in the baby's mind that otherwise obstructed the actual impulse to reach out and find the breast.

I find from experience that this limited clinical material can be used as a basis for a good theoretical discussion, and it is not my intention to exploit the material here or to give a dogmatic deduction.

This boy is now 9 and his sister 12. He had one psychotherapeutic session with me when he was 7 and has had a second one recently. The important point is that *his problem could be stated today in the terms that I recorded when I saw him at 4½ months.*

Part II

It is on innumerable experiences of this kind that I have based my own ideas regarding the theory of the emotional development of the human child. From this it could easily be guessed that I admire and value the two contributions made by Hoffer:

  1. "Mouth, Hand, and Ego-Integration," *The Psycho-Analytic Study of the Child,* vol. 3–4 (Imago, 1949), pp. 49–56.
  2. "Development of the Body Ego," *The Psycho-Analytic Study of the Child,* vol. 5 (Imago, 1950), pp. 18–23.

Here Hoffer was using observations of tiny detail that he made in association with Anna Freud and her other colleagues in the Hampstead War Nursery.

For me the important thing is the general fact that Hoffer was using these observations as a sure basis for theory. If observations do not fit in with theory, then theory must alter. Also Hoffer's two articles mark a change among psycho-analysts who went through a long initial phase in which it was thought that infancy could be seen through the analysis of adults or of small children, whereas, in fact, infancy can only be seen in analyses through the distorting lenses of defences organised at dates later than infancy.

I am reminded that in the years after the war (World War II) Hoffer was also showing a film he had made of a child eating away her own mouth. This was a deprived child. It interested him as it interests all of us to find out what it is in babies that makes them so seldom eat themselves, or even hurt their fingers with their teeth, though they do sometimes distort their jaws and their fingers by incessant sucking.

To these contributions may now be added Hoffer's Freud Anniversary Lecture 1966 entitled "Infant Observation and Concepts Relating to Infancy" (not yet published).[2]

2. Now published, together with the two other papers mentioned above, in Willi Hoffer, *The Early Development and Education of the Child* (London: Hogarth Press, 1981).

Here is a passage from "Mouth, Hand, and Ego-Integration" which gives the quality of Hoffer's attention to detail:

If we turn now to the Hampstead Nurseries infants, the most striking fact in their sucking behaviour was the directness and resolution with which from the twelfth week on the infant made the fingers approach and enter the mouth. This could be observed at any time during waking hours; it was of course more accentuated before and immediately after feeding. The hand may be introduced by the shortest route or by a wide circle of the arm while the eyes may follow the movements of the hand. At that age I could seldom observe vigorous sucking movements when the fingers entered the mouth, which was quite in contrast to the response when the bottle was brought to the mouth. The finger-sucking is mainly a rhythmic, intensive and pleasurable sucking. Length of duration seems to be more important than intensity. It may stop for a shorter or longer period while the hand with fingers bent hangs on the mandible. This indicates irritation of the gums due to teething.

In the example that follows, taken from the same article, Hoffer pleasantly describes what he observes:

Bertie, a boy of 16 weeks, is an experienced finger-sucker who suspends his ring finger in his mouth by bending the three remaining fingers and pressing them like a scaffolding towards the lower lip, thus preventing the hand from sliding into the mouth. One cannot overlook the high degree of adaptation the infant achieves in easing the oral tension. It is the hand which skilfully adapts itself to the needs of the oral zone, its shape and volume are changed from the fist to one small finger according to the need for stimulation. Finger or fist can penetrate deeply or slightly into the mouth, it can be directed toward the outer or the inner structures of the mouth. The versatility of the hand in the sucking process allows of originality and the elaboration of individual pleasure patterns in great numbers. Regarding Bertie's scaffolding, however, I have one reservation to make. Bertie was breastfed for the first seven weeks while he was still at home. It may be that a tactile sensation was aroused on his chin or lower lip by his mother's hand holding the nipple in his mouth. The position of his fingers while finger-sucking might therefore also be interpreted as a voluntary reproduction of an epidermic stimulation which he felt when sucking at the breast.

Likewise:

Another example of a genuine and self-directed hand to mouth movement was observed in Tom, when 16 weeks old. He had never been breastfed, but had been brought up with the bottle in a most satisfactory way. Filmed when sucking his thumb he revealed an unusual effort and exertion for a 16-week-old child. Tom held his arms slightly bent in front of the face, the fingers were stretched and those of the left hand tried to grasp the right thumb with a pincer movement. While both hands tried to get closer to each other with jerky movements, Tom's mouth was kept open, he made an effort as if he were trying to lift his head from the pillow, and his lips sucked in air like a turbine. When he succeeded in catching the thumb and introducing it into the mouth the left hand then was held over the mouth, locking it and preventing the right hand from sliding out again. Or if it did slide out, the left hand quickly pushed it back again and the thumb was pushed far back toward the palate, accompanied by quite intensive sucking. No other form of oral greed in connection with food was observed in Tom.

The content of the article justifies the conclusion: "We can therefore safely assume, that when entering the second year the infant has built up an oral-tactile concept of his own body and the world around him and regulates to a certain extent by this means his erotic and aggressive (active) drives."

In the second article to which I am referring, "Development of the Body Ego," Hoffer follows up ideas of the undifferentiated state as a theory supplanting the one by which the ego became differentiated from the id. What about "the ability of the infant to distinguish between the self and the world around him?" This question needs to be balanced with a study of the "response to stimuli from within the organ system."

Hoffer examines this subject again by making use of the detailed observations he had been making in the Hampstead Nursery. Quickly he notices that for the baby feeling the self involves two experiences, what the hand feels, and what is felt by the hand.

He observes "a striking difference between infants of up to ten weeks as compared with those of twelve to sixteen weeks."

An infant of four weeks when slightly hungry and waiting to be fed may display some oral activities, accompanied by movements of the head, arms and hands. The hands may still be kept in a position resembling the uterine position where the hands were nearest to the mouth. While the hand is moving over the face the mouth may get hold of it and finger-sucking will ensue. Until a few weeks old it will not make much difference whether the whole hand or one or two fingers slip into the mouth, whether a bottle or a comforter has been offered to the baby. The behaviour which it displays is (a) motor excitation, most probably due to hunger and influenced by former feeding experiences (searching for the breast) and (b) attempts to relieve the excitation by mouth activities which may lead to finger-sucking.

Quite different is the behaviour observed in a sixteen-weeks-old infant. Little is left to chance gratification. During the state of expectancy before being fed or after a successful feed the infant may insist on a definite form of oral-sucking gratification and the activities leading to this gratification comply with almost all the criteria by which we assess ego functioning.

Here follows a list of functions of ego-integration:
1. Genuine perceptual activity.
2. Motor control.
3. Functioning of memory.
4. Reality testing.
5. Synthetic function of the ego.

In this way the reader is led by Hoffer to the complex ego concept from a clinical position. This must surely have set a standard for much of the work that has since been done in various parts of the world. It is on close observation of this kind that we know we must base our ideas about object-seeking, relating to objects, excited and unexcited sensual satisfaction, exploitation of satisfaction in defence against anxiety, the beginnings of control (as compared with omnipotence, and even the experience of omnipotence through successful adaptation to need) and many other matters of vital significance.

Summary

I have given an introductory specimen of clinical observation. My main aim will have been achieved, however, if I have brought readers to a re-examination of Hoffer's two contributions which will bear repeated reading and which should be closely studied by all those who attempt to formulate ideas relative to the very early stages of the structuring of the human personality.

61
James Strachey

Obituary[1]

1969

When James Strachey died in April 1967 he was 79 years old. Naturally, there are but few alive now who knew him in a personal way, and it is therefore not easy to find the material for a biographical comment. At the time when his death was announced we were so near to the fact of losing him that I think we did not want to talk or write about him. Perhaps now we can get pleasure from beginning to remember what he was like.

Strachey was the product of what used to be a very definite grouping in English society, the Indian Civil Service. His father was Sir Richard Strachey, G.C.F.I., F.R.S. (b.1817, d.1908). He was secretary to the governor of the Central Provinces at the time of the Mutiny.

Sir Richard and Lady Strachey had a large family, twelve children, I believe, two of whom died. The ten who lived, I am told, grouped themselves as if into two generations, with James coming as one of the younger five. I know nothing yet of his early life.

When the time came, James went to Hillboro Preparatory School and there he had as his friend the poet Rupert Brooke. The fact of this friendship gives us a pointer to the nature of Strachey as a boy.

At the next stage Strachey was a success. He was a day boy at St Paul's School, London, and was in the scholarship stream. It seems that he lived up to expectations. From St Paul's he went to Trinity, Cambridge, where I am assured he did absolutely nothing for three years, except of course that he met everyone who was interesting and talked about everything that seemed to him to have importance. I would be surprised to learn that the talk was of politics. The only question was, would he get a degree? and I am told that he was given

1. Published in the *International Journal of Psycho-Analysis* 50 (1969). Copyright © Institute of Psycho-Analysis.

a pass degree in law, which I should have thought was about the bottom except perhaps a pass in history which at Cambridge could at that time be achieved by one hour's reading a day during term time. It is difficult to think that he read law for even an hour a day.

Perhaps after Cambridge he was somewhat at a loose end. This was just before the First World War when his sister was already head of Newnham. The First World War came and found James a conscientious objector. He was of slight build and the opposite of pugnacious, and although not in any way effeminate he might be said to have been delicately made and the wrong person to be in the fighting line. It was fortunate that he had an elder brother who was a regular army colonel and who strongly upheld James's objection to fighting, so that permission was given to James to work for a Quaker organisation. This had to do with the feeding of the English wives of German interned civilians. Alix ventured the opinion that in doing this work James underwent a sort of "conversion to the idea of the value of love," this coming through his contact with the Quaker motive. There was no church religion in his life.

After the war there was an opening for James in journalism because his cousin St Loe Strachey was editor of *The Spectator,* and he became St Loe's private secretary. He also did work for *The Nation* (which was later incorporated into *The New Statesman*). During this phase he wrote many book reviews. Alix described to me the way that James always left everything to the last possible moment, and she illustrated this with a picture of a holiday at Lyme Regis. A review had to be posted. She went with him to the post office and he was writing the review as he went along in the street; this was possible because he was always quite certain what he wanted to write. Just as the box was about to be emptied he put down the last word, sealed the envelope and posted it.

There were those who said of Strachey at this time that he would never settle to any one thing. Evidently he was groping for something; he knew not what.

I understand that he was positively influenced by a quotation from Freud in a book by C. G. S. Meyer. From here he developed the idea of becoming a psycho-analyst. At that time Ernest Jones was recommending all who applied to be analysts to become medically qualified, and Strachey actually entered medical school. After a few weeks of dissecting frogs' legs (as Alix put it) he found himself once more without aim and direction. Perhaps it is characteristic of Strachey that this time he dealt with his personal difficulty by writing direct to Freud.

To his surprise he received a letter inviting him to Vienna, Freud being pleased to find an inquiry coming from England so close on the heels of the war. It was then that Alix and he got married and they went out to Vienna together and it appears that something halfway between an analysis and a conversation broke out between Strachey and Freud. On his return he got in on the ground floor, so to speak, of the psycho-analytical edifice that was under construction, and he was accepted as an analyst because of his personal contact with Freud.

I would say that Strachey had one thing quite clear in his mind as a result of his visit to Freud: that a process develops in the patient, and that what transpires cannot be produced but it can be made use of. This is what I feel about my own analysis with Strachey, and in my work I have tried to follow the principle through and to emphasize the idea in its stark simplicity. It is my experience of analysis at the hand of Strachey that has made me suspicious of descriptions of interpretative work in analysis which seem to give credit to the interpretations for all that happens, as if the process in the patient had got lost sight of.

Gradually Strachey came round to his main psycho-analytic contribution, a series of lectures in 1933 (*International Journal of Psycho-Analysis*, 1934) in which he formulated the concept of the mutative interpretation. Here he made explicit the principle of economic interpretation, interpretation at the point of urgency, accurately timed, gathering together the material presented by the patient and clearly dealing with a sample of transference neurosis.

I knew nothing of Strachey as a man, of course, till 1933, when I stopped my ten-year analysis with him. Then I slowly discovered that he was just about as shy as I was. I longed to get to know him but always I had the awful feeling that he was nothing if not erudite and sophisticated, which I was not. He was at home in an area which I had discovered too late, since I did not meet the cultural life (except in the form of an evangelical religion) until I was at public school. Strachey had grown up in it, in this third area of living, the area of cultural experience.

Strachey's familiarity with literature, music and ballet filled me with envy and made me feel somewhat boorish when in his company. Incidentally, Strachey undoubtedly had a very good brain, which is a help.

I think what one noticed about this shy man was his unaggressive nature, yet there is no need to think he had no aggressive feelings, and in any case he could be stubborn. His wife knows about his indignation and indeed his anger, which was often not obvious at the point of urgency. Often he was angry in committees, and he hated the way in which the commercial side of publishing influenced matters, especially following the retirement of Leonard Woolf. I think he may have felt that the integrity of Freud's work and of his own work of translating and editing ought to have been automatically given pride of place over commercial questions.

Already in the thirties it was quite clear to anyone who had thought Strachey would never stick at anything that he had found something to stick at, apart from the practice of psycho-analysis which indeed does involve perseverance. He had become vitally interested in Freud's writings and loved to speak about the links which showed the workings of Freud's mind, links that could be made because Freud reported his dreams and wrote very many letters. There were also Freud's errors of fact, reflecting feelings or conflicts that could sometimes be tracked down.

Strachey was very bored with all the controversies that led to the splitting of the Society around personalities rather than around the difficulties inherent in Freud's contribution and out of the scientific developments based on clinical psycho-analysis. For him the political strains and stresses in the Society, which could not be avoided if the Society was to remain a unit, were unbelievably irrelevant; in fact, it is possible that the main thing about Strachey is *unassailable intellectual honesty.* Is it not true that intellectual honesty is only possible in the area which was Strachey's own life, that is the area of cultural experience? Intellectual honesty in living leads to the stake and did nearly lead Strachey as a conscientious objector to prison. In terms of mysticism and psychedelics, intellectual honesty takes one only to a personal view of the bird of paradise. It is perhaps only in the cultural sphere that intellectual integrity becomes actual, and can be a permanent feature. This was James Strachey as I saw him.

I have no intention to try to do what in any case I am certainly not qualified to do, which is to assess at this point in time the value of Strachey's main work, the Standard Edition, but I suggest that what Strachey has done is to take Freud's writings and to place them in literature where intellectual honesty reigns supreme and even a printer's error is a disaster.

The last twelve years were definitely happy ones in the Strachey family. When he and Alix took over Lords Wood which Alix's mother, herself a considerable artist (Mary Sargent-Florence) had so long dominated with her forceful personality, they settled down to concentration on this one huge topic of Freud's writings. The house helped by providing isolation; Strachey spent most of his waking life in one of the large rooms. Everything that he did was shared by Alix, whose familiarity with the German language had an obvious importance. Strachey's devotion to a cause once took him on what must seem to us to be a side-issue, though indeed there may be a connection between the two facets of devotion. James as a child had been very close to his brother Lytton, who was some years older, and this did not cease when Lytton went to live in the *ménage à trois* with a friend of Alix. (This was an artist who called herself Carrington because she did not like her first name. There are two sensitive and remarkable oil portraits of Lytton by Carrington in Alix's possession.) James had to go through the sad experience of Lytton's slow death from cancer of the bowel, which for a long time was not properly diagnosed.

It happened that a biography of Lytton was in preparation, and during these twelve years of concentration on Freud's writings James was at the same time much concerned with getting the facts right in this biography which he was not really happy about. Work on this had to be (so to speak) stolen from Freud, and possibly James overworked as a result of his urge to get finished both in regard to Freud and his brother.

The honours that came to him included the Schlegel-Tieck Award, given for translations. I myself accepted this award, after Strachey's death, on behalf of Mrs Strachey, at a reception given at the German embassy.

It was a great thing for James to go with Alix for a Caribbean holiday on the royalties received from work done.

To end this informal account of James Strachey, I want to say that he was a good sample of an Englishman. He was not a great man, I think and hope, although who can say to whom posterity will give this award? But he was a man who was so infinitely enriched by what he had gathered in from the cultural inheritance that he did not depend on distractions for feeling glad to be alive. Those who shared his life undoubtedly shared with him this same richness which came from friendships, from literature, from art. He will always be my favourite example of a psycho-analyst.

62
Anna Freud

Review of *Indications for Child Analysis and Other Papers*[1]

1969

This book is the eightieth volume of the International Psycho-Analytical Library. The first fifty numbers were edited by Ernest Jones; the present editor is M. Masud R. Khan. Although the book is long (690 pages) it is not heavy reading because of the way the material is presented. The Hogarth Press has very successfully helped the reader by a beautiful use of paper and print.

The book represents volume four of a series of seven books that will give the total of Anna Freud's contribution in lectures and writings. This volume covers the period 1945–1956 in which Miss Freud's writings were intimately related to her clinical work and teaching activities, and while she was still very much under the influence of her experiences at the Hampstead War Nurseries.

In reading such a book it is not necessary to agree with all the details. What is important is that one is confronted with a true picture of the evolution of the theoretical position of a particular person, and it can be seen that Miss Freud is consistent, while at the same time growing and allowing herself to be influenced by clinical experience and by the writings of such colleagues as Ernst Kris and Heinz Hartmann whose work interwove with her own.

The book also provides a very good opportunity for the newcomer to look at psycho-analytic theory through the eyes of one who was intimately associated with the later Freud and who carried on after his death according to what she has always felt to be the main principles for which he stood. As she is basically a teacher, I think teachers will find her presentation agreeable.

1. London: Hogarth Press, 1969. This review appeared in *New Society,* 21 August 1969.

I never cease to be fascinated by the details observed in the Hampstead War Nurseries. Reports of this unique experience are as fresh today as in the 1940s, and the student has much to learn from this well-documented work. In the same way there is good material for discussion in other clinical work—as, for instance, the special investigation made in respect of six young German-Jewish orphans whose parents died in the worst manner of the Hitler regime.

Miss Freud in the Hampstead War Nurseries and in all her work at Hampstead has been able to keep in touch with the observers while herself remaining relatively uninvolved with the children themselves. This position of detachment may have given Miss Freud the freedom to use the observations as material for the support or correction or development of orthodox theories of child development which were of course constructed originally from the analysis of adults. Whether Miss Freud would feel that she had this relative detachment at the time I cannot tell, for there is no doubt that the whole of this important practical work in which a psycho-analyst went out to meet a social need meant a great deal to her.

Those who knew her when the war was in progress and when there was so much anxiety in the air were amazed at the way in which she was able to be a brilliant organiser as if no bombs were dropping and as if no one was in danger. No doubt bombs are not as bad as persecution, which affects the mind and threatens one's personal integrity, and Miss Freud makes a reference to this in a footnote: "It would be unfair to ascribe responsibility for any shortcomings of the work to the very severe war conditions which reigned in England at the time. On the contrary, the experience of common danger, common anxiety and strain, created in the staff an atmosphere of enthusiasm and exclusive devotion to the common interests which it would be difficult to duplicate under peacetime conditions."

Obviously the reading of a book of this length must take time, but it is possible to promise the reader that it will be easy to read this book right through and that at the end a great deal will have been learnt; it will have been learnt in the right kind of way through watching the development of Miss Freud's conceptualisation which is based on her personal view of Freud's work and her freedom to be influenced by observation and by the original thinking of colleagues. This book is one for the shelf and for enjoyment. It is full of observation and objective evaluation, and it is worthy of its position as the eightieth volume in the International Psycho-Analytical Library.

On Other Forms of Treatment

Physical Therapy of Mental Disorder: Convulsion Therapy

Towards the end of the Second World War Winnicott became very much involved in the issues surrounding the use of the physical treatments of mental-hospital patients that were at the time gaining acceptance in psychiatric practice. This chapter and the next contain most of his writing on the subject, divided into two sections dealing with the treatments about which he was most concerned, namely convulsion therapy and leucotomy.

The first public expression of this concern appeared in his letter to the *Lancet*, 10 April 1943, on prefrontal leucotomy. During this year he also prepared the paper entitled "Treatment of Mental Disease by Induction of Fits" with a view to publication (possibly in the *British Journal of Medical Psychology*), though in fact it never appeared. In 1944 he organised a symposium on shock therapy at the British Psycho-Analytical Society, which took place on 15 March. Papers were read by Hans Thorner, Helen Sheehan-Dare and Clifford Scott; and Winnicott himself started it off with the Introduction reproduced here. The paper entitled "Kinds of Psychological Effect of Shock Therapy," which was found after Winnicott's death, had also evidently been prepared for the symposium; across the top was a handwritten note saying "The paper I did *not* read. DWW."

The leading article from the *British Medical Journal*, "Physical Therapy of Mental Disorder," is an abridgement of a paper read on 27 November 1946 to the Medical Section of the British Psychological Society. This article, like Winnicott's first letter to the *B.M.J.* (25 December 1943), resulted in prolonged and sometimes acrimonious debate in the correspondence columns of the journal, an indication of the deep-seated feelings of medical practitioners and particularly of psychiatrists about the issues he raised.

During the early 1950s there was a further burst of activity on Winnicott's part, mainly connected with ethical considerations surrounding the practice of leucotomy; and in 1951 he was invited by Professor R. M. Titmuss to open a discussion on the subject at the London School of Economics. This took place on 13 November and was attended by members of the staff and post-graduate students in the fields of sociology, psychology and social work. The "Notes on the General Implications of Leucotomy" were prepared for this occasion.

Further public letters written by Winnicott on these subjects but not reproduced here are to be found in the *British Medical Journal* of 22 December 1945, 13 December 1947 and 25 August 1951; the *Lancet* of 18 August 1951; and the *Spectator* of 12 February 1954.

EDITORS

I. Treatment of Mental Disease by Induction of Fits

Dated July 1943

The problems that cluster round the treatment of mental illness by fits are of three kinds, which I will indicate by questions.

A. What does the *idea* of being given fits or of having a fit mean to the patient? (I am not, of course, just asking for the conscious answer of the patient, though even this can be valuable to know.)

B. What does the uncontrollable internal thing happening, the *actual fit*, mean to this patient? (Here I mean to the patient's unconscious.)

C. What physical effect does the fit have on the brain tissue? (Presumably this is thought to be slight, otherwise how can it be held that it certainly does no damage? And in any case the answer to this question is relatively uninteresting to the psychologist because the fit is the same whether the patient is depressed or schizophrenic or neurotic. Any physical effect must be of the shot-in-the-dark variety, comparable to the "alternatives" of mediaeval medicine.)

It is with the first of the three questions that this paper is concerned.

What is the present position? A large number of men and women have been improved by fits therapy, so that instead of being chronic cases in an asylum, they have become more or less independent and have returned to home and to work. Some ill patients, even ones who might not have recovered spontaneously, have been cured by having been given fits, or at least have been returned to the state they were in before they broke down. Further, asylums being all over-full, anything which enables patients to be discharged is valuable to the state.

Although it has not yet been proved that the fits are harmless to brain tissue, I can quite believe that they are, for after all, the convulsive features are of muscle, not of brain, and probably only the congestive part of the fit endangers the delicate brain tissue itself. In any case, it is simplest to base this discussion on the assumption that the fits have no physical effect whatever, which may well be the case.

Unless I have missed something in the considerable literature, no research worker in this field has satisfactorily explained the therapeutic action of the fits, nor has much concern been shown over this lack of knowledge, which makes the treatment to say the least unscientific, even if it is most beautifully done by a team whose skill and technique are beyond praise. I think I can assume that any light that can be thrown on the mode of action of treatment by fits will be welcome, and for this reason I am writing this article although I do not give the treatment myself.

The question is: *What does the treatment and what do the fits mean to the patient?* As I have some evidence on this point, I wish to present it. The evidence comes from my psycho-analytic practice, the type of research which is in the best position to provide the clues to this type of problem.

Psycho-analysis enables the patient and the analyst to get very deep into the unconscious meaning of things, at least in so far as the particular patient is concerned. In fact so much detail becomes understood in an analysis, that it is very difficult indeed to convey what happens in the course of the treatment to those who do not happen to have experienced analysis themselves. Moreover it is difficult, in reporting a case, to make absolutely certain that nothing is written that could possibly give away the identity of the patient, for which reason no attempt can be made to describe the whole case which so clearly illustrated for me the meaning of treatment by fits for at least one patient. The work involved was considerable. The analysis lasted one year (a short time, not long enough for completion of treatment) during which I visited the patient five times a week in a mental hospital, and each time I stayed with her an hour.

The patient was a girl of 25; intelligent, and from a cultured family. For some years her life had been becoming more and more involved, in a political way, and the outbreak of war had complicated her personal problem by making the available intrigues less wide in scope.

To ordinary people war brings about a simplification of issues, and is therefore a relief. For her this very simplification made her less able to hide her own divided personality, so that she had no alternative but to appear mad. She was admitted to a mental hospital in a state of acute confusion and labelled (rightly I think) schizophrenic. Later on she was certified.

While in various institutions she was given first insulin treatment and later cardiazol fits, but in her case no good result followed. It happened in this case that the patient, although consciously hating psycho-analysis all the time, co-operated fully with me, and responded very satisfactorily. Her personality changed towards the normal in relation to the work done in the analysis, and at the end of the year she was able to be de-certified and discharged. Since this time she has returned to secretarial work in connection with politics with some success, and although I do not claim such a case as a "cure," I do claim that a fits therapist would be pleased to get such a result.[1]

In the course of this analysis, which was incidentally a piece of highly complex and detailed research work, I became able to see some of the meaning of the fits and of this type of therapy to the girl. This may be difficult to describe in a way that is easily intelligible to a non-analyst, and therefore I will approach the subject by recording an indirect observation. If this can be understood, it will provide a stepping-stone to further understanding.

The girl had been asked to give her permission for the fits therapy. In analysis it became clear that the giving of permission was an expression of the patient's suicidal wishes. She understood the treatment as something that was to make her forget. It appears that one of the doctors actually explained the process in these words, but in any case she would have felt this to be true. For her the treatment aimed at destroying part of her brain, and *for this reason* she gave permission. *For this reason* also she controlled the phenomena that can follow the fits and did not let any effect follow, either good or bad, because she could not admit that she had expressed suicidal wishes by agreeing to the treatment.

---

1. The cessation of the analysis was chiefly due to the advice of a well-known psychiatrist who reported: "Psycho-analysis does not help in this type of case; therefore although it seems to have helped here, I do not advise its being continued."—D.W.W.

This patient had a high valuation of the mind and brain, for reasons which I can give, and for her the important part of the personality, without which life is useless, was this brain, or mind. Intellectual exercise had always meant more to her than bodily exercise and experience, and in fact this might have led to her having reached a high academic standard. Unfortunately her brain was not above average (I should say) in capacity, and the brain which she overvalued was her father's which she (unconsciously) "nursed" in her own head.

I must say, at this point, that this girl's father had died before she was born. The only way he was known to her was through his writings, and these meant a very great deal to her. It was his brain that she had been able to meet, and love, and incorporate, and this idealised father, with whom she had never been angry, she had lodged in her own brain.

Somewhere, of course, was the hate of her father of which she knew nothing in actual experience, and this hate of her father was represented by a fear or conviction that someone would destroy her brain, or part of it (namely her father, lodged in her brain).

In her illness she was struggling with her acute need to be the cleverest person (in political intrigue, for instance, preventing the war), and she was confused at discovering her inability to do what she set out to do, and at her increasing tendency to "miss the boat" as an adolescent girl and a young woman. She had to cope more and more with her hate of her father because of his having died before she knew him, and also because of his not having given her a good enough brain and enabling her to solve world problems as if by magic.

In this state of confusion she saw a psychiatrist, and she was conscious of a fear that people were plotting to destroy her brain (i.e. that part of her with which she felt identified with her father).

She had the impulse to do this herself by suicide, but her love for her idealised father made her protect him successfully from her own assaults on him.

At this point she was asked to consent to fits therapy. She gave permission, and then saw to it that this form of therapy should not work, for the only result she could *imagine* from the treatment was dementia, representing severe depression in connection with the death of all that was left of her father within her, absolutely her responsibility.

From all this it can be seen that if a patient is asked for permission for fits therapy it is always possible that the positive answer can be, and is very likely to be, a suicidal act. That is to say, the understanding doctor might, if he knew exactly what he was doing in every individual case, offer the patient a suicidal attempt which actually does not kill. It is well known that genuine but unsuccessful attempts at suicide can have a beneficial, even curative effect, and treatment by fits could perhaps be used in this specific way. But it is not so used. It tends to be used as a blunderbuss treatment with no theory to support it.

This patient of mine tended to regard all psychotherapy as an attack on the brain, and her conscious opposition to psycho-analysis turned out to have this basis too, in that it was an expression of her delusion that people were plotting to make her unable to remember. The fact that this analytic treatment enabled her to remember some very important experiences of childhood which had become repressed had no effect on this delusion, which had to be treated as a delusion, that is, analysed, and not argued with. The psychiatrist who finally advised her to leave off treatment when she was de-certified seemed to her to be right because he seemed to share her delusion that psycho-analysis was part of the plot to destroy the good brain she believed she had received from her father, that which she protected from the hate which she owed her father, but which she did not know anything about until she came to analysis.

I have left out very much. For instance, I have said nothing about the girl's very deep love of her mother, which she discovered after finding out how much more than she knew she had hated her actual mother and had suffered under the actual mother's depression and repressed hate of the father who died before the patient's birth. Rivalry between mother and daughter was expressed in no better way than in their depressions—who has the dead father (husband) inside? My patient had never been allowed to acknowledge depression, this being the mother's perquisite. With me she became depressed, finding the new experience valuable. She became able to become depressed because she found that her analyst, unlike her mother, could tolerate her becoming depressed. Her mother would have cheered her up into a false happiness, spoilt her in every way, and would have become frankly depressed herself.

The main point is that almost any violent therapy, and fits therapy in particular, tends to feel like an attack on something inside one, something towards which one has confused and conflicting feelings—great love mixed with great hate. This has special significance for a patient with paranoid delusions. The good thing inside is dead, then an aperient ought to help; it is alive, then better let a doctor attack it by giving fits, or by cutting the brain about. The intolerable thing is to find that anything is hated and loved at the same time.

Treatment by fits cannot but mean a very great deal indeed to a patient, and also to a normal person if it were proposed to give such treatment to a normal person "for prophylactic reasons." The fact that healthy persons would not consent to undergo this treatment is another way of saying that normal people are the opposite of suicidal, that is, they want to preserve the things inside them, which they value.

It is of very great importance that these psychological considerations should be understood, and given full recognition. Not only is it bad for the profession that psychiatrists should be willing to go on giving shot-in-the-dark therapy (of so violent a kind, too), but also a fillip is thereby given to the old die-hard belief that insanity is a physical disease of the brain.

In these, the 1940s, it ought to be axiomatic that mental disorders are essentially independent of brain-tissue disease, that they are disorders of emotional development. The fact that brain and other physical disease is related to mental disorder does not alter this axiom. The next cry is always for new treatments directed at the brain tissue and function, and surgeons are now exercising their ingenuity at prefrontal leucotomy. Yet we are not impressed, because no one has published adequate research on what it means to a patient to have an operation on his brain tissue. Insane people often cry out for someone to remove their brain, along with their heart and lungs and other localisations of dead internalised things, once loved and now beyond mourning. These insane persons' cravings are more easily to be excused than the new devices of eager and sincere therapists.

I realise that this bit of research is a drop in the ocean. But it does perhaps indicate the need for more research, and the kind of research needed. And although it only concerns one patient, it involved about two hundred hours of solid work, and this work was an application of much similar work done with other patients who did not happen to have had treatment by fits before coming to me, and would be of value in the analysis of other schizophrenic patients, regardless of whether they had had insulin or treatment by fits, of course in co-operation with psychiatrists who are not antagonistic to analysis.

The work was a direct application of the therapeutic technique and theory devised by Freud and developed by his followers, especially by Melanie Klein. I also owe a great deal to many discussions with Clifford Scott.

II. Shock Treatment of Mental Disorder

A letter to the editor of the British Medical Journal,
25 December 1943

SIR: The even course of medical evolution has been interrupted and
set back, according to my view, by the treatment of mental disorder
by the induction of fits—a short cut to psychotherapy and a wonderful way of doing psychiatry without having to know anything about
human nature. I do invite general practitioners to state clearly
whether they favour this treatment, which has features that remind
one of the more violent of the mediaeval attempts to drive out evil
spirits.

Actually I do not see how permission is ever obtained for the treatment to be done, as there is good evidence that when an adult gives
permission for it to be done on himself he does it out of an impulse
which is akin to a suicidal one. What makes a man feel like hurting
himself makes him feel like allowing and even asking for shock treatment. The ethics of collaboration with this suicidal impulse is doubtful. It must be remembered that the treatment is certainly not being
given only to hopeless cases; it is being tried in all types of psychological illness. Personally, I would never give permission for this shock
therapy, simply because I see no way of proving that it is harmless.
But I think that the profession as a whole could reasonably oppose
the treatment on the grounds that it offers a by-pass to true understanding of human nature, just at a time when we are becoming able
so tremendously to enrich our medical practice through the assimilation of recent researches in psychology.

I would go further. Planning, if it is to be as good as jogging along,
must take into account unconscious factors. There is such a thing as
a doctor's unconscious antagonism to ill people who do not respond
to his therapy. In my opinion shock therapy is too violent a treatment
for us to be able to make use of it, at the same time being sure that
we are not unconsciously intending it to hurt the patient. Psychiatrists
must know themselves very well indeed to feel happy when adminis-
tering the treatment, and to withstand criticisms and even antago-

nism, which we must expect sooner or later in the lay press. (Attention has been drawn by your correspondent Dr Martin Cuthbert [Nov. 20] to one type of public reaction.)

This letter is intended as an invitation to the profession generally to discuss this matter, which, on account of its ethical implications, cannot remain a purely psychiatric or scientific problem. And I should very much like to know how many there are who feel as I do that no one could have the right to sanction the giving of fits to a child.—I am, etc.,

D. W. WINNICOTT

III. Shock Therapy

A letter to the editor of the British Medical Journal, *12 February 1944*

SIR,—I should be grateful if you would allow me to reply to the letters that have followed mine of December 25. Most of these letters have been from psychiatrists, and this has disappointed me, since my aim was to sound the opinion of the profession as a whole. The general practitioner is probably too busy at present even to read letters, and yet I think his opinion on specialist practice should constantly be sought by specialists, if for no other reason than that the G.P. himself lives among his patients, among the therapeutic failures as well as among the successes.

I am well aware that a certain number of psychiatrists who are students of human nature are using various kinds of shock therapy as an adjunct to their psychotherapeutic work. These have nothing to fear from a letter from me to the medical press. They will continue their work, retaining, modifying, and discarding according to their careful observation of effects. Quite different from this is the idea which is developing that the treatment of mental disorder is shock treatment of one kind or another, and that this is something which can be ordered and given like chemotherapy in the case of septicaemia. No treatment of mental disorder will ever be invented which can be properly practised by anyone but a student of human nature. My letter has had some value in that it has produced an authoritative statement that shock therapy (of whatever kind) is not a treatment in itself. The opinion which I expressed— that shock therapy of mental disorder (even if it can be valuable in good hands) is a serious setback to the health of psychiatry—is strictly a personal one, and it is only fair to my psycho-analytic colleagues for me to make it clear that my letter expressed only my personal feeling.

Several of those whose letters were published assumed that I had psycho-analysis in my mind as an alternative to shock therapy. As a matter of fact I did not mention the word, though it is true that my training has been in the psycho-analytic discipline. The alternative which I am advocating is good general management, good personal doctoring and nursing, with toleration of therapeutic failure. This is extremely difficult to put into practice in the case of hopeless psychiatric material; but for every hopeless case there are hundreds, or rather thousands, of hopeful cases, and it is for them that we must plan psychiatric practice. This may sound surprising to some institution psychiatrists, but general practitioners will understand what I mean when I say this—that when medical science is able to control the physical part of certain common conditions, such as influenza, rheumatism, and high blood pressure, a great deal of serious depression, paranoia, and chronic hypomania will be revealed. This will have to be treated as flu and rheumatism and high blood pressure have always been treated—by personal doctoring and nursing. One of the really useful things the psychiatrists used to teach us was that depression phases tend to pass spontaneously with no more than an intelligent toleration of the condition on the part of those caring for the patient, watch being kept for suicidal attempts, deliberate or accidental. Freud made this teaching understandable by pointing out the relation of melancholia to normal mourning, which has its term and from which recovery can be expected. If the psychiatrists are really concerned to give help they can do so very much more than (with notable exceptions) they do now about occupation therapy. Perhaps the term "occupation therapy" is unfortunate, because it reminds one of the proverb about "idle hands," whereas a better term would indicate that what is wanted is a specialised form of vocational guidance which gives subjective reality its proper place alongside the patient's relation to the external world.

One might have been content to let research into the value of shock therapy take its own course if it had not been for a certain communication which I received with regard to post-war planning. I was told that when peace comes an institution will be set aside for psychiatric illness in childhood, in which psychotic children will be treated by shock therapy. Just like that. Now my friend Dr Rogerson may be gravely in error in thinking that psychosis in childhood is rare. In my opinion it is common. What schizophrenia and depression and paranoia and hypomania look like in childhood is a matter outside the scope of this letter, but the point is that the vast majority of cases recover spontaneously with right management, or, at any rate, manage to find some way of life which suits the type of personality. Those who use shock therapy in the treatment of adults generously admit that they have no idea how it works when it does work. I hoped by mobilising general medical opinion to make it impossible in England for this research to be done on children.—I am, etc.,

D. W. WINNICOTT

IV. Introduction to a Symposium on the Psycho-Analytic Contribution to the Theory of Shock Therapy

Read at the British Psycho-Analytic Society, 15 March 1944

On 7 October 1942 this Society devoted one evening to the subject of shock therapy, a paper being read by Dr Freudenberg, illustrated by a film. (I was personally unable to be present, owing to illness.) I think it is true, however, to say that the full reaction of the Society was not shown at that meeting. Indeed, it could not be, since the subject is a wide one and many members had not given the matter much thought before hearing Dr Freudenberg's valuable contribution. Even now it is not certain that the Society as a whole is aware of the extent of the application of this form of treatment, which now includes the giving of fits induced by an electric current to out-patients attending one of the London teaching hospitals, and elsewhere.

In the *International Journal of Psycho-Analysis* last year (1943) Dr Cyril Wilson published what he called "An Individual Point of View on Shock Therapy." It may be taken for granted that this article is known to the Society and therefore Dr Wilson is not reading a paper today. In this article the psychological aspect of shock therapy theory is opened up, and my idea of arranging this symposium was to continue Wilson's work, attempting to develop a psycho-analytic contribution to the subject. I should consider the symposium a success if it encouraged the Scientific Secretary to set up a research group for the purpose of collecting the fruits of analysts' individual experiences bearing on shock therapy. Psycho-analytic experience is so very much deeper than any other of its kind that it may well be true to say that through our analyses of a few patients who have undergone the treatment in one of its various forms we have a collective understanding that is more important than that of the many psychiatrists whose job it is to administer the treatment to large numbers of patients.

Some members have expressed themselves as unwilling to offer their opinions because they have not personally administered shock therapy, or have not witnessed it. I suggest that there is no need for such diffidence. If we have had the opportunity for analysing one patient who has had the treatment we must not waste the valuable material we have gained in this way. But I would suggest further that each analyst can contribute, apart from actual analysis of shocked patients. He has come to know many patients intimately, so intimately that he could guess what it would mean to any of them if they were to be given the experiences that these shocks give. It would be quite logical for a psychiatrist who had invented a new form of therapy to consult with the psycho-analysts as to the expected results of such new therapy before applying it.

It seems to me to be very much within the scope of the Psycho-Analytical Society to study the psychological aspects of this physical treatment of mentally ill people, and we should be as interested in helping the psychiatrists to understand why they get good results as in pointing out to them the limitations and the dangers. We ought even to be able to help them from the theoretical end in their choice of cases and in their choice of one form of shock rather than another. If I am right, it is because of our belief in the unconscious as much as because of our knowledge of the structure of the personality that we have value. That is why we cannot wait to be asked to help. It may be that the current explanation of the results of this therapy on a physical basis is a serious error and one which no-one but the psycho-analysts can correct. In any case, if there is a physical explanation this does not eliminate the need for full examination of the psychological mechanisms at work alongside the physical.

In this discussion it might be thought wise to assume that no physical brain damage is done through the treatment. No-one can be certain that this is true, but it is unlikely that we in this room bring proof either way. However, if we assume that no physical brain damage is done some might think that we must also assume that physical changes do not occur in the brain at all, not even changes for the better. Of course there is the momentary electric or chemical change brought about by the excitant, but it is difficult to believe that physical changes, that can be relied on to do good and not to do harm, could be brought about in the brain by this blunderbuss method.

I must remind members here that some doctors administer the treatment because they believe that it *does* damage the brain, and so cuts out irritating suppressed memories. The next step is the operation of pre-frontal leucotomy, in which the association fibres between the frontal lobes of the brain are actually *cut*.

In my opinion it would be out of place to argue here about the ethical considerations which I raised in a letter to the *British Medical Journal*, because in this Society we are concerned with the subject as something for scientific study, and we assume that if the profession could be shown that the treatment were bad, then the profession would automatically drop it in practice. I have no personal doubt as to the integrity of any psychiatrist practising shock treatment, but I must reserve the right to interest myself in his motives, as we do always interest ourselves in our own motives as analysts. In a scientific discussion ethical considerations cannot usefully be brought forward until considerable progress has been made with theory. In the *practice* of psychiatry, however, and it was to this that I referred in my *B.M.J.* letter, ethical considerations have to be given due weight from the start.

If I may refer to the *B.M.J.* correspondence I think several points emerged from it which have value in a scientific discussion. One is that no claim is made that anyone really understands how the treatment works. We are therefore treading on no-one's corns if we have our own theories. From the correspondence and also from an impression gained at a recent meeting of the Medico-Psychological Society it is evident that thousands of treatments are being given yearly, and that the claim that the treatment makes patients accessible to psychotherapy should be taken as valuable only in certain instances, for each practitioner of this form of therapy reports too large a number of cases treated for us to believe that he has made use of the increased accessibility in more than a small proportion of the total. On the other hand I have evidence that certain psychiatrists are really only using the shocks as an adjunct to their psychotherapeutic work, and it seems to me that these workers in the field are in a very different position from the majority who rely mainly on the shocks.

I gather that it is now conceded that the best results are gained in involutional melancholia, and in the depression phases of milder type that tend to recover spontaneously with good management. The results with the severe melancholias are no doubt striking, and if we are to contribute usefully we must examine the ways in which these good results might be obtained through psychological mechanisms.

In order to clarify discussion I have suggested working out the following three problems, which of course overlap:

a. The effects of the various shocks on the anatomy, biochemistry and physiology of the brain and of the body in general, and the meaning of such bodily changes to the patient.

b. The meaning of shocks, and more specifically, of fits, and of the idea of being given shocks and fits, to normal and various types of ill people. Here I mean conscious and unconscious, and repressed unconscious.

c. The meaning to the patient of the actual fit or uncontrollable bodily happening. Here I refer to unconscious meaning (not specifically repressed unconscious).

V. Kinds of Psychological Effect of Shock Therapy

*Written for the Symposium on Shock Therapy
held at the British Psycho-Analytical Society,
15 March 1944*

I wish to discuss this under five headings:

1. *The effect of the therapy on the staff and the atmosphere of the institution.* I think it would be a mistake when examining the psychological effect of any new treatment to ignore the difference that the introduction of this treatment can make in the general atmosphere of an institution and in the attitude of the doctors and nurses. It is perhaps especially important to take into account just this sort of thing in considering work done in a mental hospital. In a mental hospital there is a large number of ill people, severely ill and chronically ill and ill in a way that means they cannot avoid being a severe burden on people. The burden of the psychiatric case has to be borne by people and not by machines and it sometimes amazes me that we are able to find doctors and nurses who are willing to do this work. It is well known that in the past cruelty has flourished in mental hospitals, one reason being that some of the patients "ask for it" and another being that in caring for so much incurable human material attendants must develop a special attitude owing to there being but little relief of the kind that psycho-analysts are used to when they see patients improving directly as a result of their work. Mental hospital work carries an immense frustration and this must apply also to ordinary psychiatric consultations which lead only to good management of cases and not to cure of people. In parenthesis I should like to say how important it is that I, as a psycho-analyst, should recognise the special burden of pure psychiatric work because in the analysis of psychotics the psycho-analyst periodically needs the co-operation of the mental hospital doctor and he won't get it if he can't understand the special nature of that work.

The introduction of a form of therapy that can be applied to a large number of otherwise untreatable patients may easily have made a big difference to the feeling that prevails amongst mental hospital staffs.

If this is so, I think it must be true that doctors and nurses and attendants have become better doctors and nurses because of the new hope and the lessening of the sense of frustration through the introduction of shock therapy. Also the high degree of skill and knowledge required for proper control of, for instance, insulin therapy, brings to the mental hospital medical men and women who have knowledge and skill in bio-chemistry and other subjects and this must all tend to awaken or keep alive a spirit of scientific enquiry which I think was generally lacking in mental hospitals a few decades ago.

It would seem to me to be relevant to this discussion to take into account the possibility that the attitude of the mental hospital staff towards the mental patients has improved as a result of the introduction of new therapies including shock therapy and, assuming this to be true, to instigate research into the effect such improvement would be expected to have on the various types of psychiatric case.

2. *The effect of the treatment through its being thought of by the patient as part of the doctor's emotional relation to him.* Psychiatrists do speak of the importance of the emotional relationship of their patients to themselves and do to some extent examine the results of shock therapy in the light of this which they call "transference." I think they feel they have learned about transference phenomena from psycho-analysis and to some extent they do refer to the same thing that the psycho-analysts mean when they use this term. They do see that the emotional tie between the patient and the doctor is based on a re-living of past experience or is a dramatisation of fantasy. I think, however, that there is usually only a limited understanding of the psycho-analytic view that transference feelings are abnormal only in so far as they are unconscious. It is probably very rare for psychotherapists to base their treatment as the psycho-analysts do on the gradual making conscious, through interpretation based on material presented day by day by the patient, of the repressed elements in the transference. Dr Wilson deals with the question of transference in psychotic cases in his recent paper in the *Journal*.[2] I quote one of his sentences: "I suspect that some psychiatrists who use shock therapy tend to place too much reliance on their insulin or machine and too little on their own personality."

He develops this theme fully, and gives the impression that he himself values shock therapy only as a method of treating patients who

2. Cyril Wilson, "An Individual Point of View on Shock Therapy," *International Journal of Psycho-Analysis* 24 (1943).

would otherwise remain untreated, without giving up the idea that the results may possibly be achieved through purely psychological mechanisms.

To develop this theme I should be repeating much of what Dr Wilson has written.

3. *The effect of the treatment according to conscious and pre-conscious ideas and fantasies.* From reading some of the literature and from listening to discussions, I have been struck by the way in which some psychiatrists seem to ignore even the most superficial psychological aspects of the problem. This may be a mistake on my part, or it may be that it is not thought to be worthwhile to report the ordinary discussion of the subject with the patient. I should like to be told by a psychiatrist reporting cases what kind of a discussion he has with each patient before he starts. An illustration might help here, though I am not claiming that it proves anything. A patient who had had electrically induced fits in an institution told me: "We haven't been told that the treatment gives us fits, and I am not sure that we are supposed to know, but we actually do all know because the rumour spreads round in secret." This would seem to show that in this particular instance the patient was not getting information which she could easily have made good use of. When I asked her if she knew from first-hand experience what a fit was like she said she had never seen a fit, and then she suddenly remembered that, as a tiny little girl, she had been frightened by seeing another child have a fit in a nursery school. I give this instance only to illustrate the way in which, perhaps only in isolated cases, ordinary conscious and pre-conscious feeling can be ignored or wasted when large numbers of mentally ill patients are being treated by a physical treatment. I take it with a grain of salt when psychiatrists report that they give psychotherapy, using shocks only as an adjunct to the psychotherapy, unless they are contented to report having treated only a few cases. If one man has given several hundred treatments I cannot see how he has followed up each case with adequate psychotherapy.

4. *The effect of the treatment according to the expectation that can be predicted in various types of ill people.* It should be possible to make a statement of what each type of patient tends to expect from the world. Shock therapy could be thought of in relation to these expectations. I have been unable to satisfy myself at all in making such a statement and if this line of approach should be thought to be fruitful I should like to get help. For instance, some hysterics expect people to express ambivalence towards them. Perhaps they are not

surprised when doctors who are caring for them give them fits that are painful and unpleasant. Other hysterics expect a sexual assault, and perhaps these would tend to think of the shock treatment in this light. Masochists would certainly be liable to turn the treatment to their own account in their own special way. Doubters and other obsessionals are always expecting to feel guilty about something and I know of at least one who felt equally guilty at refusing shock treatment and asking for it. Anxiety cases are such a mixed group that they do not admit of generalisation, but I should think that any anxiety patients who were not too anxious to be given the treatment would experience an immediate, if temporary, relief because their fantasies are always worse than reality.

Depressed people feel they ought to destroy something in themselves and they can be relied on to use any dangerous thing that comes along as a self-punishing or a suicidal act. They get relief if they try to commit suicide but do not die. They expect to have to kill themselves in destroying the bad part of themselves, and so shock therapy, which can easily feel to the patient as if it kills something within the body, can easily be made use of by the depressed patient who finds he survives the treatment.

People whose personalities are built on a contra-depressive basis, hypomanic personalities with a central core of depression that is not acknowledged, might be said to expect to be able to ward off everything, and I guess they can defend themselves from being fundamentally altered, one way or the other.

Introverted personalities tend to expect nothing from the external world, at least nothing of importance. They may, however, feel the fit to be an assault on their world that they locate inside themselves, and that is another matter altogether.

Paranoid personalities are always expecting to be attacked and for them all treatments tend to feel like a return of their projected hate. Shock treatment would easily become a dramatisation of the delusion, and there have been cases reported of patients who first of all welcomed the treatment and later blamed the doctor for having tortured them. (Wilson, Hardcastle.)[3]

5. *The effect of the treatment according to a patient's fantasy about his personality and his body.* I will only mention this aspect of the

3. Wilson, "An Individual Point of View on Shock Therapy"; D. N. Hardcastle, Letter to the Editor, *British Medical Journal*, 29 January 1944.

problem briefly, although I believe it to be the most important of all.

In all patients and indeed in all people, the personal fantasies about the body are important, but the psychiatric patient's fantasies about his own body and personality are vitally important. Whereas it is possible to do a great deal of the analysis of a neurotic person on the basis of the recovery of the instinctual life in the transference analysis without using the patient's rich fantasy about his body, it is impossible to do the analysis of a psychotic patient without being prepared at any moment to find that the patient's fantasy about his body is the important thing. In fact, the reason why psycho-analysts are supposed to be unable to treat psychotics may be because, whereas it is known that psychotics are very much concerned with their fantasies of insides and outsides, it is not generally known that psycho-analysts are now able to take into account these, the patient's fantasies, about their bodies and do so without becoming mystical and without ceasing their main task which is to relate everything eventually to instinct, to experience and to reality. In other words, we have not only to take into consideration any pictures *we* may like to draw to illustrate our conception of a patient's personality structure; we also have to know that there is a real personality structure, rather a rigid one if the person is ill, one which we could see if we had the eye and which we can discover and modify in the course of analysis, this being the individual's own unconscious fantasy of his own self. In terms of psychic reality, nothing could be more real. It has been built up in the course of instinctual experience, and in its structure can be found powerful defences and careful arrangements; and the individual's external world may also be abnormally affected for him by whatever he holds there, projected, belonging to his inside (according to his own fantasy).

Here indeed is food for thought. Psychotic patients with complex and rigidly defended personality structures and arrangements find themselves becoming convulsed. Before anyone can assume that changes resulting from such treatment or any other treatment are produced through physical mechanisms, research will have to be done on the way these shocks are isolated by the patient or are allowed to produce alterations in the internal arrangements which are so tremendously important in every detail to these patients, to the extent that they would die or spend their lives in asylums rather than loosen control.

VI. Physical Therapy of Mental Disorder[4]

1947

The full title of this talk was "Some Reasons for a Personal Prejudice against the So-called Physical Therapies of Mental Disorder." By representing my ideas in this form I admit that I prejudge the situation. This may be an unscientific approach, but perhaps it is a suitable one in the case of such unscientific methods of treating the disordered mind. My objections are not to the brutality of the methods. Compared with psychiatric illness, even a broken back is not much, and a broken leg nothing. Moreover, with good care these accidents can be so reduced as to be negligible. I of course assume the good faith of those who practise the arts against which I am prejudiced. I know of no case whatever in which I would ascribe the giving of physical therapy to any but the ordinary motives of the practising physician.

Science in Medical Practice

A doctor is consulted because someone suffers. Patients, and especially relatives, demand therapy; but the doctor is trained in the scientific method, and his job is to apply science. By so doing he disappoints even if he gives relief to his patient. But he serves the community by being part of a bulwark against superstition. It is open to anyone to go to a quack for magical relief, but it is the doctor who is expected to represent science, or objectivity, and to be not afraid to do nothing if science cannot help. Diagnosis is based on scientific knowledge; the basis of therapy should be the same.

Scientific Psychology

A scientific approach to mental phenomena follows on acceptance of the theory that mental disorder is a disorder of emotional development, that the basis of mental health is laid down on what is inborn,

4. From the *British Medical Journal,* 17 May 1947.

from birth, by the course of development of the personality and development of the individual's emotional contacts with external reality. Through Freud's formulations and work, especially his method for objective investigation of unconscious phenomena, there has been a steady development of psychological insight.

The development of scientific psychology could briefly be described in three stages: the first bringing understanding of neurotic ambivalence, the second bringing understanding of depression and hypochondria, and the third bringing understanding of the more primitive mental states which reappear in the insanities.

First came the elucidation of the disturbed relationships between people and the disturbances in people of their instinctual functions as a result of their unconscious conflicts. The work was done from the sorting out of love and hate as it emerged in the transference situation. Following this, as it appears to me, the patient's conscious and unconscious fantasy about himself began to become analysed: his depression and conscious sense of guilt became his sense of something wrong inside himself, and the psychology of hypochondria became the psychology of the results of loving and hating. The incorporation and discharge of objects came into the analytic interpretation. Melanie Klein's work made all this possible, and mania as an alternative to depression was seen to be an extreme example of hypomania as a denial of depression.

The new work on depression naturally linked up with the examination of the integration of the personality itself, and phenomena of integration and reality appreciation, etc., began to be able to be dealt with in the transference developments and to be brought into relation to instincts. These developments have enabled psychology to encroach on the domain of the alienist, the doctor who manages the insanity case.

Convulsion Therapy

Along with this steady progress of psychological science there has been a development of the practice of convulsion therapy. My main objection to convulsion therapy is that it comes as *an escape from the acceptance of the psychology of the unconscious* and from the implications of the psychological developments of the past fifty years.

It is well known that there are several techniques, but from my point of view the electric technique is worse than the others because of the ease with which it can be done. Moreover, electricity has special significance for the unconscious, and paranoid and schizoid persons are well known to mix up the idea of electricity with ideas of magical influence. Such considerations do not necessarily make E.C.T. bad, but they certainly put us very much on guard when we interpret results, and when we meet the prejudice in favour of E.C.T. that is common among psychiatrists today. Whatever the technique, convulsion therapy is empirical. No one has the slightest idea how it works, when it does work. It is true that empiricism carries no final objection. However, scientists hate empiricism and regard it as a stimulus to research.

Our responsibility is great. What is done here in England tends to be done blindly in many parts of the world, especially where there is no access to libraries or training in psycho-analytic method or free scientific discussion. The sociological ill effect of a therapy has to be considered as well as the immediate effect on individuals.

Theory of Mental Health

The march of psychology, because of psycho-analysis, is towards the completion of the theory of mental disorder as a disturbance of emotional development. The basis of mental health is being laid down in infancy, in the developing relationship between infant and mother, and even in a more primitive way between the infant and his subjective mother, and more primitively still in the infant's self-establishment. The result of this theory is the fruitful one that the prevention of mental disorder is a new task of paediatrics. In contrast, the result of the empirical therapy of mentally ill people by physical methods is a relatively unfruitful one; it is that more and more neurologists must be found who are qualified to give people fits. These are two sociological results that can be compared one with the other.

Many besides myself have deplored the fact that convulsion therapy inevitably leads away from the psychological approach to a biochemical and a neurological one. Convulsion therapy attracts to mental hospitals people with first-rate qualifications for dealing with the complexities of insulin shock and of all the biochemical changes that need study in this kind of work. The physical therapies in general draw to psychiatry physically minded young doctors, and it is always unlikely that men and women who have reached a high degree of postgraduate training on the physical side will be willing or able to start again and to go into psychology at its beginning. Leucotomy in an extreme degree attracts the wrong kind of doctor to psychiatry. To my mind the modern acceptance of leucotomy is the direct result of the acceptance of empirical shock therapy.

If the sociological results of convulsion therapy are bad the sociological results of leucotomy are deplorable. I think leucotomy is the worst honest error in the history of medical practice. In mental hospitals the result of leucotomy is a new accession of power to the neurosurgeon, an unqualified practitioner from the point of view of the psychologist. Let us not be deceived by his very high degree of skill as a neurosurgeon, this having nothing to do with the case. If one deplores leucotomy and its collaterals one must deplore the convulsion therapies that paved the way for it. The feeling against leucotomy is too great to find expression—the general public and doctors alike are too appalled by this application of empirical method to do anything about it. And they are afraid that if they raise objections the psychiatrists will cease to relieve them of the awful burden of insane relatives and patients.

Let me apply the formula I devised earlier on. Now, instead of private suffering with demand for magical treatment being met by the doctor who applies science, it has become true to say that society's suffering (on account of its mentally ill members) leads to the use of the doctor (because of his being supposed to act according to scientific principles) to cover a panic application of magic. Leucotomy should be a quack remedy, available for those who ask for "cures."

From this subject of leucotomy with its irreversible brain changes I come back to convulsion therapy with a feeling of relief. At least here no damage is done (so we blandly assume). If it should turn out that the effects, good and bad, of E.C.T. are, after all, psychological effects, no one individual has been really hurt, and the convulsion subject can still employ psychotherapy if it should come his way. He can even recover spontaneously in the course of time, with good management, if he is so disposed.

Objections to Convulsion Therapy

To condense my views so far expressed I would say I would not give convulsion therapy, because (1) I would not have it done to myself; (2) it draws to psychiatry the wrong kind of doctors, skilled in the wrong way; (3) it undermines the public's justification for relying on doctors to keep their scientific heads in face of the demand for magic; (4) this form of therapy done here in England leads to mass treatments by the same methods of treatment all over the world; (5) physical methods of treatment represent a tendency away from scientific psychology. Here I would like to add a new point—which is that the chief indication for E.C.T. seems to be involutional melancholia and the lesser depressions.

Now, *depression is the illness of valuable people*. At the borderline depression is the breakdown of people who are overburdened with responsibility or loss. On this side of the line is the valuable person, often a good mother, who burdens herself with too much concern. On the other side is the same phenomenon, but less conscious, and this is depression. In depression at least the patient suffers for her own illness. E.C.T. is at present being applied to the valuable people, and if this is recognised it no doubt makes the psychiatrist very concerned indeed as to his own suitability for his task. Few of us are innocent of depression, and if we have escaped it we may have done so by a contra-depressive defence which is more abnormal than the frank depression phase of a patient.

Psychological Effects of Convulsion Therapy

Having thus summarised my prejudice I would like to give my guess as to the future developments in the psychology of convulsion therapy. I think that psycho-analysts and those trained in that sort of way should work at present on the assumption that all the results of E.C.T.—good, bad, and indifferent—are psychological results. The immense field of the psychological effects of the idea of E.C.T. has been seriously neglected. To discuss this it is not necessary to have given E.C.T. to a thousand patients, or indeed to have given any at all. What we need to do is to pool experiences of the feelings and ideas found during analysis of patients who have had convulsion therapy, and of patients who are in touch with fellow patients who have undergone convulsion therapy.

Need for Research

I give two lines of approach. The subject that urgently needs research and discussion is that of the patient's conscious and unconscious reactions to (a) the idea of E.C.T., etc.; (b) the experience of submission to convulsion therapy; and (c) the actual fit. Here are some suggestions.

(a) *Reaction to the idea of being given a fit.*—I suppose a *normal* person hates the idea. It must be for this reason that psychiatrists do not have fits given to themselves whenever they feel a bit depressed. *Anxious* people are likely to be able to become frightened at the *idea* of the fits, in the same way as they can become frightened at the idea of anything. In contrast they may be especially brave in relation to the actual experience. *Obsessional* patients' difficulties are greatly increased when the idea of convulsion therapy is put before them. The organised defence against spontaneity and uncontrol is liable to be strengthened. Obsessional doubt is liable to find a setting in the problem whether to give or to withhold permission. Guilt will be felt whichever line is taken. In organised *paranoia* the fits are easily felt to be part of the hostile attack that is expected. In one patient, a girl who had a delusion that someone was trying to destroy her brain, this form of therapy was felt to be absolute confirmation of her delusion. In cases with thought-transference delusions and the fantasies that so readily get mixed up with theories of electrical phenomena and malicious influence, it can well be imagined that electrical shock therapy has a special significance.

(b) *Reaction to the experience of being given fits.*—In cases with a tendency to *conversion hysteria* a partial knowledge of brain-functioning is easily used in rationalisation of paralyses and paraesthesiae following convulsion therapy. *Depressive people* equate the convulsion with dying, and easily feel absolved by having experienced what it is like to meet death. They hanker after convulsion therapy. In some cases each successive convulsion becomes more dreaded, and the last one is equated with death, and recovery from it gives a new lease of life because of the emotional experience. *Suicidal* impulses can be met by the convulsion. By this seeming experience of death a suicidal patient can use convulsion therapy as an alternative to suicide. This is comparable to the relief that a suicidal patient can get through a genuine suicidal attempt—one from which the patient recovers through successful intervention.

(c) *Reaction to the fit itself.*—In what may be called *introversion neurosis* the patient has organised a secret inner world in which relationships are good, and this has been done at the expense of trust in the external world in which are placed the bad relationships. It is probable that in these cases the actual fit is felt as a threat to the artificially good inner world, and in consequence a rearrangement has to take place with less complete secret hoarding of good relationships within.

This approach is tentative and admittedly incomplete, but I give it to indicate the way the results of shock therapy may be examined as psychological phenomena. It is just here that research is most urgently needed. Curiously enough, it is also just here that there is an unwillingness on the part of practitioners of convulsion therapy to investigate. Much of the objection to convulsion therapy would disappear if the mechanism by which results are obtained were understood. The main trouble is that false theories are built around the assumption that the mechanism by which change is brought about is a physical one, and these theories have already paved the way for the wide employment of leucotomy—and who knows what may follow?

Society's Unconscious Reactions to Insanity

I also want to put forward the idea that these physical therapies express society's unconscious reaction to insanity. This is by far the most difficult thing I have to say. I have reason to believe that the good results that can come from these physical therapies depend on this—that by them expression is given in an acceptable (because hidden) form to the unconscious distress society experiences in face of mental illness. By unconscious I really mean unconscious, and I mean repressed and unavailable to consciousness. Massive guilt feelings and fear and consequent hate are roused in people who are concerned with mentally ill persons, and I think this unconscious hate also underlay the cruelty to mental patients that notoriously coloured the management of the insane up to recent times.

Tail-piece

As a last word I would like to say why I have no hope that these arguments will make any sudden difference to the now established practice of psychiatry. Mental disorder can be maddening to nurse. Abolition of shock therapy tomorrow would place on the doctors and nurses of mental hospitals an emotional burden which they could not suddenly take, and there will be those who claim that this alone justifies the method. I see this argument, and respect it. Nevertheless, there seems to be a need for someone to register a strong objection to easy and seductive methods which tend to lead away from the difficult path that must be walked by those who try to understand human nature and to eschew magic.

Physical Therapy of Mental Disorder: Leucotomy

I. Prefrontal Leucotomy

A letter to the editor of The Lancet, *10 April 1943*

SIR: Dr Fleming and Mr McKissock have described fifteen cases treated by prefrontal leucotomy and Dr Hutton fifty cases. It is precisely because their work is of a high order that I take this opportunity of drawing attention to the special objection that is easily felt to the treatment of mental disorder by any method that leaves a permanent physical deficiency or deformity of the brain, even if favourable results can be shown to follow in certain cases.

The theory that schizophrenia, manic-depression, psychosis and melancholia are diseases with physical basis is still held by some; but the alternative theory that these mental diseases are disorders of emotional development (with varying degrees of hereditary factor) has not been disproved. I suggest that until this latter theory has been disproved, it is a very serious matter indeed for a doctor to subject patients to an operation in which the actual tissues of the brain are cut. It is for those who wish to try to cure mental disorder by operative measures, or by the induction of fits, first to prove that the insanities are actually brain-tissue diseases.

I hold the view that ordinary insanity is a condition closely allied to genius and special talent and to personality of exceptional value, and naturally therefore I feel disturbed when I hear of treatments which absolutely preclude full recovery, even if these treatments can be shown to cause a shift towards sanity in a proportion of cases.

Moreover, it is a very great help to people with mental difficulties for them to be able to contemplate or even to have a period of breakdown. The idea of the voluntary patient seems to me to be partly built on this rock. But the public is getting to know that a breakdown will mean a course of fits, or perhaps a permanent deformity of the brain, and I think this is not the sort of thing to encourage that early report of symptoms which is rightly sought by those who treat the psychoses.

D. W. WINNICOTT

II. Leucotomy[1]

1949

In many respects the medical student is out to learn, postponing till after qualification the attitude of inquiry which belongs to maturity and health. Perhaps leucotomy, the treatment of mental disorder by a surgical procedure that is destructive of brain tissue, provides a good example of a therapy that is open to question, and that need not be accepted even for the purpose of satisfying the examiners.

In the medical press I have expressed my personal criticism of leucotomy in the strongest possible terms, because I believe it to represent the worst possible trend in medical practice; but this criticism has always been made in respect of the opinions held by those who use the method, and never in respect of the medical men themselves, who are known to me as ordinary people doing the best they know for their patients, and experimenting only when they genuinely believe they see justification for experiment.

It should be remembered that there exist in large numbers insane people in asylums in the British Isles, and this represents a tremendous drain on medical and nursing man-hours. No one could be criticised for trying to lessen the burden on the community provided by the hopelessly insane. Leucotomy does make some very difficult patients less difficult, and relieves some acute sufferers from prolonged suffering. No wonder the neurosurgeons turn from the very highly skilled technique which enables them to remove rare brain tumours to the far less skilled cutting of nervous tissue in respect of a common condition. In any case, it could be argued, the brains of the worst

1. From the *British Medical Students' Journal* 3 (1949).

mental cases are already diseased—syphilitic, arteriosclerotic, scarred after inflammatory processes.

What, then, are the reasons which make it seem to me that the operation should be abandoned?

First, I would say that if it is intended to relieve the community of the burden of the hopelessly insane, why not a more complete cut, say of the brain stem, or a deliberate policy of euthanasia? The answer is that this puts a responsibility on the medical man that he should not have—the responsibility for deciding as to life or death in respect of a fellow human being. This is a different matter from the decisions doctors make every day in respect of their opinions as to diagnosis and treatment to cure from disease.

The simple argument, that anything is justified that relieves the community or relieves personal suffering, is not good enough. Argument in favour of leucotomy can start with the claim that it is a good treatment for a patient who is mentally ill, that is to say, on the likelihood of its effecting a cure, but it must go further and show that it is not harmful to people in general.

It should be remembered, here, that it is one thing to cure a patient of cancer of the breast by removing a breast, and quite another thing to "cure" a patient of mental disorder by removal of a part of the brain function. In the first case the person is left intact, and in the second it is the person that is maimed.

The theory of today is that it is the brain tissue that is needed before the mind can even start to be, and any other theory must first displace this one if it is to be accepted. Those who practise leucotomy have not tried to give a new theory, but have let it be assumed that the brain is the physical organ which is needed for the functioning of mind and consequently the organisation of personality.

At this point in the argument we must consider the fact that certain very ill patients have been considerably helped by leucotomy, have even left hospital and returned to work and to family life. If the treatment has only been given to very ill patients, then no harm has been done, and to some there has been benefit.

Unfortunately, a treatment cannot exist in a circumscribed way like this. It soon becomes applied to less severe cases. Theories arise and (in the case of leucotomy) the possibility of treatment gives power and direction in the mental hospital to the neurosurgeon, whose skill is in surgery of the brain and who is not trained to be a student of human nature.

First, in regard to the wider application of the treatment, it is natural that each unit should wish to do its thousand cases in order to have a round number for a report, and some of the thousand will be diagnostically at the less ill end, and in fact it will be seen in the reports that patients have already been leucotomised who have been diagnosed as suffering from depression, obsessional neurosis, etc.—certainly the cases are not confined to the brain-diseased.

This raises the vast question of the psycho-genesis of insanity. It can be said that it is impossible to be a brain-surgeon and also to be well informed psychologically. The two disciplines are too exacting for one doctor to grasp both fully, at one and the same time. And it would be easier for a really first-rate psychologist to learn to be a neurosurgeon than for the latter to learn to be a psychologist, simply because psychology can only be learned over a period of time in which the learner has to grow to meet the emotional demands that psychology puts on himself. No medical student, however brilliant, can just *learn* psychology; he has to spend years maturing and developing his own personality, while gradually coming to grips with the subject. In fact, experience shows that psychology taught to medical students can easily upset even what appeared to be stable personalities. The psycho-analysts' rule is undoubtedly sound: that the psychology of the unconscious can only be taught to people if they are themselves being analysed or if they have had previous successful analysis.

Reports on the psychology of patients before and after leucotomy and given in good faith by neurosurgeons are apt to look naïve in the extreme to the psycho-analyst, who is perforce used to the extreme complexity of human material, and who is more aware than most people of the areas of ignorance in the understanding of persons.

There is a vast amount of evidence available to those who care to study the deeper aspects of psychology that the ordinary insanities—schizophrenia, the depressions, paranoia, as well as obsessional neurosis and delinquency—are disorders of emotional development, *not disorders dependent on brain-tissue changes*. Obviously, brain-tissue changes produce personality and behaviour changes, but people who are ill mentally on the whole are ill in spite of having healthy brain tissue. Mental illness that is not just a confusional state is an organised pattern, an organisation of defences, and of resistances, and of postponements of forward emotional development. This pattern would appear logical to the investigator if the whole truth were known. If an insane person is studied in sufficient detail the course of the illness becomes intelligible as an expression of the difficulties inherent in life, difficulties in personal development, in environmental influence, and in the interaction of the two. It cannot be argued that because brain syphilis produces ideas of grandeur and because arteriosclerosis produces perseverance of ideas or narrowing of intellect, therefore emotional disturbance spells underlying brain-tissue changes. In fact, the whole evidence points the other way.

The neurosurgeon, however, who starts off with a readiness to see insanity as a collection of separate illnesses, with brain-tissue changes, is not easily persuaded that his patients are still human beings. Even when they are withdrawn, degenerate and incontinent, they are still struggling with the problems of life which for the more fortunate of us have merely been a little easier to solve. When those who are not psychologists see symptoms and resistances disappear after leucotomy they feel supported in their theories, and have no idea that the removal of resistances can mean the final loss of the individuality of the person concerned.

It is really only the psycho-analysts who respect resistances, and see in them the unconscious struggle of the person to find himself. The whole tendency of modern (non-psycho-analytic) therapy is to bypass resistance.

Perhaps the best example that there will ever be of the bypassing of resistance is the operation of leucotomy. In fact, every person who feels he is going ill in a mental way in these days cannot be sure that he or she will not be insulted by physical interference with the brain tissue. This is not exactly the best way to get people to apply to be voluntary boarders in the early stages of psychiatric disorder. Many who would recover spontaneously with a few months of being tolerated, and if possible cherished somewhere and kept from suicide while in a depressed state, do in fact struggle on in their ordinary life through fear (well founded) that they will not recover without having at least been given a series of fits, and perhaps having had the brain irreversibly altered. After interference with the physical brain no man or woman can be sure of his identity: he is not there to be sure, because the person built up over the whole time since birth is not there.

If I behave today in an acceptable way this is a build-up of all my life, and a positive social contribution, an infinitely complex and actively meaningful example of the relation between all of me since my birth to all my environment. If I behave still better because I have had a leucotomy I am not making a better contribution, because it is not me behaving.

Human beings are entitled to all manner of dreams, including the most sadistic, and our job as medical practitioners with a scientific training is to provide the public with a reality against which they can match their dreams. Patients dream that their doctors are in love with them, but the doctors' oath forestalls this, and it very seldom happens that a doctor abuses his opportunities for intimacy. Dreams can be matched against reality.

In the same way patients dream of bad doctors doing fantastic and mutilating operations. On the whole doctors do not operate except under very highly controlled conditions, employing scientific principles in complete justification of their actions. Leucotomy seems, to me personally, to be on the borderline between science and superstition. I think people should not have to undergo this ordeal of which they are frightened even to dream. Those who practise leucotomy are frightening patients very much more than relieving the suffering of a few individuals under their care, they are producing a fear of doctors and increasing the fear of madness. This has far-reaching effects. Fear of madness leads to a flight to an extreme of sanity which is a false step in civilisation; it means a flight to the logical and the conscious and the easily planned, and a loss of contact with individual integrity, and the hidden depths of the personality of each person.

In my opinion the responsibility taken by those who blindly cut about the brains of persons just because they are insane is tremendous, and it is for them to take much more trouble than they have taken hitherto to show that they recognise the wider implications of their practice.

III. Notes on the General Implications of Leucotomy

Used to open a discussion on leucotomy held at the London School of Economics, 13 November 1951

Preliminary Survey

1. The fact of mental illness
2. The actual problems of management
3. The revolution in mental-hospital nursing
4. The value of the physical treatments
5. The gradual evolution of professional opinion about the various treatments

Statement of present position of the physical treatments in psychiatry.

Personal Standpoint

Consider a series of types of physical treatments: at one end, physical care, permission to regress
then: added narcotics
then: drugs aiding reliving of forgotten situations
then: insulin shock (skilled team work)
then: electric convulsion therapy (relatively unskilled)
then: leucotomy
then: euthanasia

Philosophical Considerations

1. E.C.T.—being unskilled has an effect on the practitioner's theories of human personality growth and abnormality.

2. Leucotomy alters the seat of the self, puts a premium on relief of suffering and creates teams of skilled neurosurgeons who constitute a type of vested interest, which can affect scientific evaluation. Theory of insanity as an organisation of the self appropriate to the circumstances.

Influence of Emotions on Judgement

Separation off one from another of two themes (inter-related of course): (a) Efficacy of (say) leucotomy compared with that of (say) psycho-analysis. This involves discussion of meaning of word "efficacy" in this setting. And (b) Philosophical considerations, ethics of interference with brain functioning, ethics of therapy involving irreversible changes.

Observation In psychiatric papers at the present time (a) is being fully discussed without reference to (b).

Relative Importance of Various Body Organs for the Existence of an Individual Psyche

Obviously the healthy psyche needs a healthy and intact body. Nevertheless, it is possible to examine the relative values of various parts of the body to the psyche.

Mutilation of brain vis-à-vis castration:

anxiety about brain mutilation, anxiety about castration (conscious, unconscious)

brain mutilation as *symbolical* of castration

False implication: that brain mutilation is *only* symbolical of castration, i.e. not in itself deserving fear, avoidance, condemnation, etc.

Illustrations (for simplicity, considering only males):

a. *Mutilation of main motor nerves to upper limbs.* Result, helplessness. It might be done (let us suppose) as a cure for masturbation, or stealing, or aggressive acts toward people. *This is unthinkable, we know no surgeon would perform this operation in this country.*

Yet it would leave the psyche intact. A biographer could write "he bore the insult with dignity." Perhaps the victim might have said "Forgive them, for they know not what they do!" Circumcision is often performed to cure or prevent enuresis, masturbation, sexual aberrations—showing that surgery can easily become the handmaid of superstition and unconscious hate.

b. *Castration, i.e. removal of testicles.* Here we know about the results. To some extent the psyche is affected, in that the instinctual drives are modified. The effect on the psyche is more direct therefore than the removal of other (so called) internal glands, i.e. glands producing hormones.

At the present day castration would never be performed as a treatment of behaviour disorder, nor at the request of the individual (though it is part of the masochistic organisation for exactly this request to be made). The operation leaves the psyche to some extent intact, but the change is irreversible unless a testicular extract could be prepared exactly to replace the internal hormones lost, in which case the psyche would be again intact, though the individual would have to adjust to being unable to procreate. Surgeons sometimes tie the two ducts that carry spermatozoa from testicles, so that the patient need not fear he will impregnate the woman with whom he compulsively cohabits. This is not necessarily irreversible. (Cf. women after removal of [a] womb, [b] ovaries, adding ovarian extracts replacing hormones.)

c. *Subsidiary considerations.* Removal of both kidneys can be said to leave the psyche intact, except that gradually uraemia develops, and there is an increasing toxic distortion of the personality up to death. Removal of a limb naturally affects the individual, the cause of the removal of the limb being important. But the psyche is intact. Blindness, deafness, etc., all affect the individual, but leave the psyche intact; it is the person himself or herself who adjusts or fails to adjust to the mutilation.

As far as can be told there is not usually any injury to the brain tissue as a result of electrically induced fits, though it is very difficult to prove this. Few of us would voluntarily undergo a course of ten fits. (We can ignore the accidents that belong to this form of treatment as to any other—overdosage, fracture of the spine, etc.—as they do not affect the main problem.)

d. *Surgical treatment of the brain* has now to be considered. Brain tumour can often be removed, the operation being one of the most remarkable in surgery. It may in some cases be completely successful. In other cases more or less brain substance is involved, so that after the operation the patient is not able to make a complete return to normal. Something of the personality has gone or altered. This is unavoidable. The same can be said of other operations on the brain tissue for *surgical cure of brain abnormalities.*

It is not this group of phenomena that is under discussion. Consideration of these phenomena is important, however, as it brings forward the axiom that *the brain tissue* by and large *is the somatic (or physical) prerequisite for the existence of the psyche.* Some parts of a brain are more important than others in this respect (the motor and sensory centres are less, for instance), but there is no other organ that has comparable importance for the psyche's existence.

Question: Is this self-evident, or is it something that needs to be established?

Main Theme

What is being discussed is *the mutilation of normal, healthy brain tissue for the treatment of disorders of the psyche,* i.e. to alter an individual's behaviour, to lessen suffering, to make nursing easier, to restore *functional efficiency.* Here something is being done which attacks the psyche itself, by disturbing its physical basis.

Of a person so treated we can no longer say: "he bore the mutilation with fortitude," because the meaning of the word "he" has altered. We cannot say "she suffers less now than before," because "she" is not the same as before. All we could say would be: "whereas the total he or she suffered (or misbehaved), the new sub-total he or she suffers (or misbehaves) less."

I have said that it is unthinkable that (a) or (b) would be performed by a surgeon today in this country. Yet this infinitely more terrible operation has been done on thousands of people in the last ten years, and the advocates of this treatment are claiming a wider and wider field for their activities. At first it was only the hopeless mental hospital case that was leucotomised. Then gradually, obsessional neurotics were so treated, and melancholics whose own suffering could not be tolerated by the doctors in charge of them. Now the treatment is advocated for all sorts of psycho-somatic disorders. Soon the only symptom not qualifying a person for this treatment will be the obsession towards treatment by leucotomy, a contagious disorder to be found chiefly (alas!) in psychiatrists.

Effect on the General Public

This is a subject for research by the social psychologist. Does the fact that leucotomy is practised make one more afraid of madness, or less? Can it be that the apathy of the public to this problem, which is like that of euthanasia if it were being daily practised, is due to fear?

Fear Associated with the Leucotomy Problem

1. Conscious fear that some dependent who is insane will be sent home from the mental hospital.

2. Fear that if one becomes a voluntary boarder in a mental hospital one will be irreversibly mutilated.

3. Fear of the wish to be mutilated (masochistic, unconscious guilt, etc.); cf. fear of suicide.

4. Fear of the idea of a malevolent doctor; this fear always lurks behind the usual belief in one's doctor when one is ill. A malevolent doctor is unthinkable when one is ill.

5. The question of the soul and its relation to the psyche-soma. Does a newly conceived baby start at par in respect of soul, or at some degree above par? Very deep religious convictions are involved in this problem, and most people like to take it for granted that the soul is implanted, in the same way that God is not conceived of but perceived.

The Crude Issue

To put the matter crudely, either I or the psychiatrist in question is mad.

In the former case Dr X will sign me up (i.e. certify) and order my leucotomy (with the very best of intentions) and there will no longer be a D.W.W.; the resulting yes-man will be a sub-total D.W.W., no doubt much happier and free from missionary zeal and social sense, and released for the pleasures that belong to lack of true aim.

In the latter case, the psychiatrist is mad and I psycho-analyse him. He, of course, does not want to be psycho-analysed, so he remains unanalysed, and I remain a frustrated analyst. But he retains his psyche intact. This is the difference between the two awful alternatives.

You can see why for me it is a very serious matter, this which is the world's choice. For society of today must decide, not the psychiatrists who are cluttered up with immediate clinical problems. Who is to be considered mad? But whereas I am fighting for the very existence of my psyche my adversary knows that his psyche will be left to him intact and he knows that when he resists psycho-analytic treatment it will at least be himself resisting. I envy him.

IV. Prefrontal Leucotomy

A letter to the editor of the British Medical Journal,
28 January 1956

SIR: The correspondence on leucotomy that has restarted reminds one that there is no place other than in your columns where this subject can be discussed in a broad sense.

Some years ago I expressed my view that leucotomy was the worst honest error in recent medical practice, and I am often asked whether time has led me to alter my view. Actually it has not. My opinion does not carry much weight because of the fact that I have not made a special effort to examine leucotomised patients, and my objection is not based on direct clinical study. It is based, however, on indirect study such as the analysis of patients, some of whom have been patients in mental hospitals. If I were to find a case undoubtedly improved by leucotomy my view would not be altered. Actually, I have only come across distress due to the existence of leucotomy as a method of treatment.

It must be remembered that leucotomy is a deliberate disturbance of healthy brain tissue, the aim being to bring about mental changes that, in the view of the psychiatrist, are good. There is nothing comparable here to the attempt to remove a brain tumour or to relieve a subdural haemorrhage. The whole matter therefore revolves on the psychiatrist's view of what is good, and no attempt has been made by psychiatrists to discuss the meaning of the word "good" in this context.

The letters of Drs D. W. Standley (3 December 1955, p. 1390) and Clifford Allen (17 December 1955, p. 1502) make me wish to re-state my view: (1) There are many distressing post-leucotomy cases now in the community, and relatives are concerned now not with breakdowns of human endeavour, which are understandable, but with after-effects of very questionable neurosurgical procedure. Irreversible changes have been produced in patients whose illnesses were at any rate *theoretically* capable of remission prior to this operation. The emotional burden of these cases is not likely to be taken up by the psychiatrists, who are responsible for throwing back on to the community something worse than the awful burden of a defective child. (2) All mental-hospital patients, voluntary or certified, become quickly concerned with the problem: Will I be subjected to E.C.T., to insulin shock, to leucotomy? For some reason or other, psychiatrists do not seem to know this. Mental patients talk of very little else. They are in a dilemma that they should never be in, by which the doctor seems to be coming in on the side of the self-destructive impulse, and in this respect leucotomy is much worse than the other physical methods. They are permanently under the shadow of a threat of leucotomy which they come to know as a surgical procedure which changes them from themselves into something else, they know not what. Those who are capable of artificially getting well organise themselves on to a pseudo-recovery out of *fear,* and so escape to the world outside psychiatry. There are now almost no asylums for those patients who need and can make use of a period of breakdown; there are only mental hospitals for the quickest possible cure of the mentally sick; and unfortunately fear of leucotomy has become a real factor in the production of a rapid turnover in mental hospitals. This rapid turnover looks well on paper. (3) The existence of leucotomy as an accepted procedure is very bad for the doctor and nurses. It provides the extreme example of a psychiatry that by-passes the study of human nature and of mental health as a matter of maturity of emotional development of the individual. Nothing better than leucotomy divides psychiatry as a blind therapy from psychiatry as a complex but interesting concern for the human being who finds life difficult and whose problems we can feel to be represented in ourselves.

If the medical profession were to give up the practice of leucotomy a great deal would be gained. So substantial would be the gain, according to my view, that the possible loss of therapeutic relief in certain cases would be an insignificant consideration.—I am, etc.

D. W. WINNICOTT

65
Occupational Therapy

Review of Adrian Hill's Book *Art Versus Illness*[1]

1949

I think this book is good. Adrian Hill, himself an artist and art teacher, had a period of enforced idleness as a phthisical subject in a sanatorium, and he discovered a new reason for drawing and painting. It made him feel better, and perhaps indirectly affected the physical healing process. What could be more natural than for him to become, on discharge from the sanatorium, a militant protagonist of Art versus Illness?

The book tells the story of his adventures. In order to sell the idea that burned holes in him when he had to hang round for various kinds of permission, he needed much self-control and patient understanding of the mentality of doctors and nurses and committees of management.

The main idea is that when ill people are not too ill they absolutely need help in the management of their souls, or inner worlds, or whatever you call it. The time of enforced idleness is either a time wasted or else time for inner growth and development. It is well known that children as well as adults can develop depth and poise during an illness with rheumatic heart disease, or when immobilised by tuberculosis or a fractured femur; but it is touch and go, whether the strain of simple contemplation may not prove too great, and the result be disruptive rather than productive.

Adrian Hill clearly sees that a good teacher can make all the difference between disruption and integration, by personally sponsoring art interest and activity. In some cases he does no more than provide a frame on the wall opposite the bed into which a series of interesting prints can be inserted, whereas in other cases he organises actual

1. London: George Allen and Unwin, 1948. This review appeared in the *British Journal of Medical Psychology* 22 (1949).

556   On Other Forms of Treatment

drawing and painting, but he always aims at finding the true personal contribution that the individual patient has the capacity to make.

One wants to know, can the author see that his idea, though original in one sense, is not new, that many, indeed, have had the same idea and have put it into practice, although not perhaps on a wide scale? If he can, then we can be glad of his personal enthusiasm and wish him well in his crusade.

What is the relation of all this to occupation therapy? This question may have been answered somewhere, and the answer is not in this book. I would say that at its worst, occupation therapy is an organised attempt to keep people from themselves, and that this is opposite to the aim that Adrian Hill sponsors. Some think that the official occupation-therapy teaching is dangerously veering towards a training in skills, an immense number of skills, the training being enough to put off the true artists, potters, musicians. Yet, of course, there has to be an official course and qualification, and there would be chaos if occupation therapy were to be handed over to artists.

In the war my wife, herself an artist, potter and modeller (working in the occupation therapy department at the Maudsley Hospital, then at Mill Hill), found that constructive clay work could be used in this same self-revealing way with men and women who had various kinds of psychiatric disorders. In psychiatric work there is a need for close co-operation between the artist (potter, etc.) and the medically responsible psychiatrist, and this is not always forthcoming. It is more likely to develop if the artist is a qualified occupation therapist.

At its best occupation therapy is in fact just what Adrian Hill is describing. An artist, potter, musician, sculptor, modeller, who lives in his own chosen medium, takes the trouble to reach a group of bedridden or immobilised patients, and by personal contact enables each patient, in his or her own way, to create a bridge between the unconscious and ordinary conscious living, a bridge with two-way traffic. Much happens, but the main thing is that the patient, by gradually discovering his or her creative urges and positive integrative forces, is enabled to look at what is inside the self to see whatever is there, the chaos, the tensions, the death, as well as the beauty and the innate liveliness.

As an example of the use of music I remember a long-term convalescent home for rheumatic children in Warwickshire at which all the children were making pipes, playing them, writing original themes, conducting, or in some other way contributing to the musical pool. A musician (not an occupation therapist) was on the staff. This was an immensely enriching experience for the children, and it is of no significance if none of them later became musicians. It would, of course, be a nuisance to be forced to become musical if one happened to be ill in a music-mad institution.

The wireless can be a tremendous help to the ill person, provided the knobs and the *Radio Times* are within easy reach. One can use the various programmes for personal growth. On the other hand, to be subjected, when ill, to a programme chosen by the engineer in the hospital basement is to be "occupied," and prevented from finding oneself or from growing.

This book can be used, then, as a corrective to the bad tendencies (if they exist) in the official occupation-therapy outlook, and as a support to the good tendencies. It is unfortunate that the words "occupation therapy" seem to divert attention away from the enriching experience to the manufacture of an article that can be shown on view day.

66

Behaviour Therapy

A letter to the editor of Child Care News, *June 1969, replying to an article advocating the use of behaviour therapy in the treatment of maladjusted children*

Dear Editor:

Behaviour Therapy

No doubt an appreciative comment could be made on Carole Holder's article on Behaviour Therapy (*Child Care News*, May 1969, no. 86). To write this one would need to stand, however, on a platform that is different from the one on which I both live and work. It would be important to me to have the opportunity to let my many social worker colleagues know that I wish to kill the tendency of this article. I would like to go further, and at any rate to start to say why I want to kill it.

It could be a good idea to give this statement of behaviour therapy to social workers who are self-selected, selected, and trained for case work. It can only be good to be reminded that local morality systems are taught not only by example but also by slaps on the bottom and sanctions. But are we likely to forget this basic fact, since a great deal of our work arises out of the *failure* of behaviour therapy as practised at home and in institutions?

I might claim to have earned the right to make this protest since I have never accepted the word "maladjusted," which was shipped across the Atlantic in the twenties as part of the Child Guidance Package Deal. A maladjusted child is one to whose needs someone failed to adjust at some important phase in his or her development.

Imagine a social work group based on behaviour therapy principles. Such a group would soon be filled (through self-selection and selection) by those who naturally adopt the behaviour therapy attitude. The training would simply deepen the grooves and the ridges of personality patterns already set in the behaviouristic manner.

This would truly be a battle lost, because these people that I am describing in terms of grooves and ridges *will not know* that there is another kind of social work, one that is orientated to the facilitation of development processes; they *will not know* about the positive value of containing the strains and stresses of individuals and groups, and of allowing time to heal; they *will not know* that life is in fact difficult, and that it is only the personal struggle that counts, and only this that feels to the individual to be worthwhile.

The article of Carole Holder shows with clarity that it is possible to look at life with extreme naivety. The trouble is that this amazing over-simplification of social work must appeal to those who are needed to give support to social work in terms of money. Behaviour therapy can easily be sold to committee members who in turn sell it to the other members of municipal councils whose skills are in other fields. There are always those who claim that they derived benefit when their fathers imposed the family morality on them, or when a strict teacher at school made it hurt to be lazy or to steal. *This is what people believe in to start with.*

Unfortunately, doctors and nurses, by and large, have to be included here because their work is also based on an essential over-simplification: disease is already present, and the job is to eradicate it. But human nature is not like physiology and anatomy, although based on it, and doctors are again, by self-selection, selection, and training, unfitted to do the social worker's job of acknowledging and containing and believing in human conflict and suffering, which means tolerating symptoms that give evidence of deep distress.

Social workers need just now to look at the philosophy of their work all the time; they need to know when they must fight to be allowed (and paid) to do the difficult and not the easy thing; they must find support where it can be found and not expect support from administration, from rate-payers and tax payers, or from parent-figures generally. In fact, in this localised setting social workers need to be themselves the parent-figures, sure of their own attitude even when unsupported and often in the curious position of claiming the right to be worn out in the exercise of their duties, rather than to be seduced into the easy way of inducing conformity.

For Behaviour Therapy (I give it capitals to make it into a Thing that can be killed) is an easy way out. All that is necessary is for the therapists to be agreed on a morality. It is wicked to suck the thumb, it is wicked to wet the bed, it is wicked to mess and to steal and to break windows. It is wicked to defy parents, to criticise school regulations, to see faults in university curricula, to hate the prospect of a life at the conveyor belt, or to boggle at a life ruled by computers. It is open to anyone to have a personal list of good and bad, and for a company of behaviourists with more or less identical moral systems to get together and set about producing symptomatic cures.

There will be failures, but there will be many successes, and there will be children going about saying, "I'm so glad I don't wet the bed any more thanks to Miss Holder, or an electric bell apparatus, or some other 'response-shaper.'" All that is necessary is for the therapist to exploit the fact that human beings are a kind of animal with a neurophysiology like that of rats and frogs. What is left out is this, that human beings, even those with intelligence of quite low grades, are not just animals. They have a great deal that animals do not have at all. I personally would think of Behaviour Therapy as an insult even to the higher apes, and I would include cats.

It is sad that there are not enough case-workers, and that there never will be. It is a far sadder thing to think that Miss Holder's last paragraph should perhaps be used by those responsible for Children's Departments to justify handing this "economic and sensible procedure" to the child-care officers, a procedure designed to make naughty clients good.

Obviously I am trying my hand at response-shaping. I want to kill Behaviour Therapy by ridicule. Its naivety should do the trick. If not, then there must be a war—and the war will be a political one, as between the dictatorships and democracy.

Yours faithfully,
DR D. W. WINNICOTT

67

Physiotherapy and Human Relations

1969[1]

The term "psycho-somatic disorder" is in common use. The public understands fairly well the sort of illness to which people are commonly liable which is not simply a bodily disorder like scarlet fever or appendicitis, but in which the bodily disorder is partly or wholly related to the emotional life of the individual. It is generally accepted that life is difficult and that these difficulties can manifest themselves sometimes in a distortion of the way the mind works, and at other times in a distortion of the way the body works.

As soon as an attempt is made to look into the various ways in which psycho-somatic disorder can arise, it is found that the subject is a vast one, and a statement of psycho-somatic disorder cannot be covered except in a large book written by a team of writers. Moreover, psycho-somatic disorder merges into the universal problem of the healthy interaction between the psyche and the soma; that is to say, between the personality of an individual and the body in which the person lives.

If in order to begin to think about the subject we force ourselves to make a sort of classification, we can say that there are three main ways in which the body is affected by the mind, but before enumerating these I would like to point out that when I use the word "mind" I am not referring to activities of the split-off intellectual processes. I am referring to all that there is of the person, except for the body.

1. Phases of Excitement

The most obvious way in which the body becomes affected has to do with phases of excitement. From time to time the person becomes excited: that is to say, in some way or other instincts are aroused. It does not matter what is the nature of the instinct; once the instincts have been aroused either through the rhythm that comes from within

1. From the journal *Physiotherapy* (June 1969).

or in reaction to stimuli from outside (whether real or imagined), then the body has started along a path which in terms of pure physiology ought to lead to a climax: hunger leading to a meal; a certain type of sensation that leads naturally to an excretory activity; or sexual excitement that can end in genital orgasm; or an accumulation of aggressive impulses that can lead to a fight. Naturally some of these physiological awakenings are more easily brought to a state of satisfaction than others, but the principle is the same: that once excitement has started, then the person whom we are thinking about has to manage either to bring it to a climax (go and eat an apple) or else to live through a phase in which the body has to absorb the changes that belong to excitement without there being any climax. Sleep is one of the ways in which the slate can be washed clean again, or indeed a climax may be reached in association with a dream.

In the early stages of an excitement—that is to say, a change in the physiology of the body that has associated with it some kind of exciting idea—it is comparatively easy for the individual to manage life until the excitement and its effects have died down. It will be readily understood, however, that the further the excitement has proceeded, the more difficult it is for the individual to accommodate the phase of failed climax. Life is quite a lot concerned with the management of these failed climaxes, and they can give rise to such inconvenience that people will organise themselves as far as possible to be distracted so that over long periods of time excitements do not arise. This can be very convenient, but of course an excess of this can be boring. Everyone could write a book called "The Technique for Living," which would be a description of the ways he or she has learned to adapt in order to avoid the beginnings of excitements, and alternatively to arrange for excitements to reach a climax.

Perhaps this is one of the difficulties that life presents which cannot be taught, although people do get help from knowing that the problem is an inherent one.

2. The Effects of Mood

In a different way the body becomes involved in association with mood. In depression the person who is depressed is managing the conflicts that arise in what might be called the "soul" by an over-all control. This comes down automatically like a cloud. The organisation of inner reality which gives the feeling of depression happens unconsciously; that is to say, apart from anything that could be called deliberate. In the same way the cloud lifts when things are ready for the cloud to lift. This over-all control can affect the body, and in some kinds of depression the whole physiology of the body is at a low ebb. The tissues are less alive and a little nearer to being dead.

Here is a group of psycho-somatic disorders, then, which do not respond much to things that we can do to the body. The main thing is that the person shall be helped through the depression mood. During the depression the conflict between what might be called "good" and "evil" that is going on within can be dramatised in bodily terms so that there is a great deal of complaint of pain and discomfort during the depression, and if any actual physical illness exists then this can be exploited.

Here is obviously a difficulty for doctors because it is in the case of these patients that the doctor is either sidetracked from seeing actual disease that exists, or else he too easily plunges into physical treatments and operative procedures when the trouble is really in the patient's psyche, not in the soma.

It is to be noted that a depressed condition tends to have associated with it poor muscle tone, or a compensating tenseness and rigidity. Similarly, postural faults go with the patient's hopelessness about the state of affairs in the personal inner reality. In giving treatment the physiotherapist is working all the time against the handicap of the patient's inner deadness.

3. Disturbance of Personality

In the third group in this rather crude classification there is a disturbance of a more primitive kind in the personality, and it is not possible to describe what is meant by this without making some kind of a statement about the way that people develop from the beginnings of their lives so that they eventually become healthy psycho-somatic persons. The rest of this article will be an attempt to make a statement of this kind.

Statement of the Phases of Early Development

It is important for the physiotherapist to have understanding in this area because it is here that physiotherapy comes into its own. In other words, it is here, in the treatment of persons who are ill in this third

way, that physiotherapy joins up with the entirely natural management that most mothers are able to afford in the care of each baby. I
say each baby because I am referring to matters that belong to the
very beginnings of life; just as each baby is an only child at the beginning, so it is true that in physiotherapy it is necessary during the treatment to give the patient full attention. I mention this to illustrate the
close connection that there is between the physiotherapy of men and
women of any age and the early care that a mother is able to give her
baby. In fact the training for a physiotherapist should include opportunity for close observation of uninformed natural baby-care.

Formation of the Personality

Once attention has been drawn to the fact, it is not difficult for anyone to see that what a person is like at any one moment cannot be
properly assessed without reference to the whole development from
the beginning. It is not certain at what age we have to think of the
individual as starting to be a human being, but certainly there is no
harm done in thinking that significant things have already started up
by the time of the baby's birth. We tend to think of the beginning as
a summation of beginnings, and so get round the difficulty of dates,
because what happens in the first days and weeks of life may of
course be corrected, but if the pattern of an abnormality is set, who
can say at what moment it became set?

In the description that follows tracing the development of the human personality, a great deal has had to be left out, but features essential for the physiotherapist have been retained. The new human
being bringing into the world inherited potential immediately becomes affected by the type of care that happens to be provided. In the
vast majority of cases the mother is able to start up in a satisfactory
way because she is orientated just to this one thing, the care of the
baby that she has been carrying for nine months. Soon she will become distracted, will begin to find again that other things in the world
have importance beside the care of her baby; and she may of course
be ill or in some way prevented from giving herself over to the continued care of her baby. In the vast majority of cases the new baby is
given satisfactory physiotherapy at the beginning in the shape of a
combination of physical and psychological care which makes it unnecessary for us to distinguish between psyche and soma.

It will be a useful over-simplification to say that for a baby that has been started off in this way and whose baby care has not been significantly disrupted, the physiotherapist is not likely to be needed later in that individual's life (omitting deliberately reference to the place of physiotherapy in the treatment of physically determined diseases). Contrariwise, the physiotherapist will indeed be needed where the child has experienced a traumatic disruption of baby-care techniques. (At the extreme where a child has not received natural physiotherapy at the beginning, it is not likely that the physiotherapist can in later life make up for such a gross deficiency of management, but often an attempt will be made.)

It is necessary to take as a basic principle the inherited tendency of each new individual towards growth and development. Under good enough environmental conditions the individual carries a tendency, amongst other things, towards integration of the personality. Out of a relatively unintegrated state each boy or girl baby tends eventually to become a unit, and an autonomous unit. At first the mother lends her unity to the child, and under her aegis the child is a whole person, and very gradually comes to be and to remain a unit when separate and apart from her. From this it can be readily understood that in the early stages there is very great dependence, near absolute at first, and the most difficult thing in child care is the mother's graduated failure of adaptation that is designed to meet the individual child's growing need to strive for a personal way of life.

These things cannot be learned nor can they be done by machinery. They depend entirely on human care and understanding, and a collection of things that can be gathered together and described by the word "love." It can be said of psychotherapy and of physiotherapy, which is part of psychotherapy, that the therapist is giving professionally and at a late date precisely that which is normally given out of love at at earlier date.

There is one aspect of integration and of the general process of growth and development which particularly concerns the physiotherapist. This has to do with the relationship of the person in the child to the body of the child. It is not easy to find the right words to describe this process. It is not clear what to call that part of the personality which in health becomes closely bound up with the body and its functions, but which needs to be considered separately. One can use the word "psyche," but this may suggest to the reader something that is connected with the spirit and even with spiritualism; and certainly one does not mean the mind, which can be taken to refer to the intellect and with being clever or dull, and which when split off provides the area in which thinking, and thinking things out, has a kind of life of its own.

In the use of the term "psycho-somatic illness" these difficulties do not arise, because somehow or other we know that we are talking about the inter-relationship between the functioning of the body and that of the personality (not the intellect).

One wants to be able to say that the psyche and the soma (that is to say, the person and the body that together are that person) do not start off as a unit. They form a unit *if all goes well in the development of that individual;* but this is an achievement. We can by no means take for granted that in every case the baby's psyche and soma will come to work as a unit with the child living in the body and the body functioning according to the child's enjoyment of his or her body. It is a part of integration that the child and his or her body can be what we mean when we talk about that child. When we say, "Billy has a nice face," we do not mean that there is a face there that is nice and forget that there is a person who owns that face. Or when we say, "Susan, come here!" we do not forget that Susan has to use her body either to do what we say or to go in the opposite direction. We take it all for granted except when the partnership goes wrong.

Although a tendency towards the development to which I am referring is inherited by every boy and girl, nevertheless the development cannot take place unless the person who is looking after the child is able to manage the baby and the baby's body as if the two form a unit. There are some mothers, or people who care for children, who make good contact with the baby as a person but who seem to be unable to know what the baby's body is feeling like or needing; and similarly there are others who are naturally good at physical care but who seem to be ignorant of the fact that there is a human being becoming lodged in the body that they are bathing and cleaning up. When those who care for a baby or small child have this kind of a difficulty of their own, then the child they care for cannot become integrated into a unit.

In that case the basis for a psycho-somatic split is laid down. The inherited forces tending towards unity strive to produce unity, but success is only relative and the child is left with a tendency to lose the ability simply to live as a psycho-somatic unit. This is a reason why the physiotherapy student can learn so much from watching ordinary infant care, and of course there are also the physiotherapist's memories, mostly beyond recall but still influential, of having been a baby being cared for.

One can constantly ask, where does the physiotherapist come in in correcting these faulty managements? Probably it is the *psycho*therapist who is most needed, or the specialised teacher, when in the early history of the child the mother or mother-substitute was better at making a relationship to the body than to the person of the baby. It could be expected that the *physio*therapist comes in where in the early history there was good contact on the basis of a communication as between people but a low degree of recognition of bodily needs. To repeat, the physiotherapist makes a professional job out of the same thing which was called loving care in early management.

But what if the physiotherapist should forget that there is a person being ministered to, and that the care of the body is only half of the task?

A physiotherapist may be surprised to find how important the human relationship becomes when what has been learned of techniques is being put into practice. As in all therapy, the therapist gets some of the temporary and special relationship, dependence, love, suspicion, even hate, that the psycho-analyst calls "transference." The psycho-analyst actually uses this "transference" for the main part of his work, but the same can be found, and it needs to be accepted as a natural development, when it is the body that is being manipulated or eased. Always what you do is important because you who do it are human and not machines. It is well to remember this as a basic principle, something to lay alongside all the specialist techniques that are learned by the physiotherapy student.

When we talk of small children we expect the parents to be able to tell us a whole lot of things that their child especially enjoys, perhaps the bath, or snuggling down in bed, or being lifted up by the arms, or a game of swimming in the air. All these things and the physical contacts that go with them belong to the life of parents and infants, and the physiotherapist should not be surprised to find that a great deal that is being done professionally in the department is done in terms of human contact and communication that is other than physical. Even being reliably on time, or having the room warm and draught-free, can be a communication, implying: "I know about your basic needs."

An example of an extreme kind of deficiency which the physiotherapist finds herself or himself correcting comes from faulty holding

568 On Other Forms of Treatment

and handling of the simplest possible kind. For instance, when a mother who through identification with her infant (that is to say through knowing what the baby is feeling like) is able to hold the baby in a natural way, the baby does not have to know about being made up of a collection of parts. The baby is a belly joined on to a chest and has loose limbs and particularly a loose head: all these parts are gathered together by the mother who is holding the child, and in her hands they add up to one. In faulty handling the parts add up to more than one. A gross example of mishandling occurs when a mother fails to deal satisfactorily with the head so that suddenly the baby is in two parts, body and head. This produces the very greatest mental pain. If this sort of faulty handling happens regularly in the pattern of the management of a child, then that child is permanently affected and may eventually come to the physiotherapist for pathological rigidity in the neck region. In any case, when the physiotherapist has to deal with spinal troubles *that are not due to physical disease,* these troubles can quite properly be related to a history in the individual case of faulty holding and handling at the critical stage when the psyche and the soma had not yet become welded into a unit.

There is a limit to the use that can be made of this kind of theory. Certainly there is no point in trying to blame someone for something that happened in the past. Nevertheless, it is easier to do one's work if the aetiology of the illness can be to some extent understood, especially when, as in the case of physiotherapy, the work that is being done professionally is so often a deliberate attempt to do what is usually done quite naturally and unselfconsciously by those who look after their own children in a way that enables the inherited growth tendency to become realised.

In this brief account I have not tried to be comprehensive either in the presentation of a theory of individual development or in the construction of a theory of physiotherapy. What I have tried to do in tackling this enormous subject is to give some deliberately over-simplified lines of thought which the physiotherapist can use in construction of a personal attitude to this important kind of professional work.

Postscript: D.W.W. on D.W.W.

January 1967

In January 1967, four years before his death, Winnicott was asked to address the 1952 Club (a society of senior British analysts who meet informally for discussion of ideas) on the subject of the relationship of his theory to other formulations of early development—an exercise which he preferred to call "D.W.W. on D.W.W." This gave him the opportunity to review chronologically the development of his ideas and to speak about those whose work he felt had influenced him at various stages. It seems fitting that this last collection of papers addressed to those who have a particular investment in psycho-analysis should end with a transcript of this talk.

Winnicott began the proceedings of the evening by passing round an extract of his statement, with spaces left to be filled in as the audience thought appropriate. It is reproduced here without alteration.

The actual talk survived only in the form of a rather poor recording, and this, together with the extreme informality of the language, made it difficult to transcribe and edit. It was a marathon effort lasting for an hour and a half, and the main part of it is given here, including all that Winnicott said directly about his own history and about the development of his ideas.

EDITORS

D.W.W. ON D.W.W.
1952 Club
January 1967

The Method of Investigation. *P-A*	Freud
Protest against reference to	Alice Balint
universal regression from Id	Ribble
satisfaction-frustration in	Suttie
Oedipal triangle	Lowenfeld

569

Positive—examination of *actual*
infant-parent relationship

Diagnosis	Theory of psycho-neurosis	
	Freud	Freud
	Klein for depression and paranoia	Klein
	Schizophrenia and	
	schizoid phases	

1940   Delinquency

$\overline{\quad}$

Hope—   AST[1]   Stealing
                  Aggression

$\overline{\quad}$

till secondary gains

Delinquency   Object relating
                Controls

Classification of Environment (postponed)
   became facilitating environment   Greenacre

P.M.P.[2]
Adaptation, de-adaptation

Dependence
   Individual maturational processes   Bowlby
   Heredity
   Conflict-free sphere in Ego   Hartmann
                                          A
Primitive Emotional Development   B
                                          C

Study of Individual without loss
   of interest in environment

Early is not Deep
   add Delusional Transference   Little

Real ME   FEELINGS   Fairbairn

                movement
Aggression   object in the way
                aggression
              = NOT-ME found by aggression   Erikson
                (becoming complex)   Laing

Object Seeking   Transitional phenomena
            Essential Paradox

I AM   A paranoid position

Alone, in the presence of
    second paradox

Environment as experienced
    added up as memories
    integrated into belief in environment
  = self control

---

add root of paranoia
    in I AM + introjected environment

---

mania: return of repressed
    i.e.   deprivation of environmental controls
            identification with environment
    price: loss of identity
                    creative spontaneity
(Practical applications)

Meanwhile: exploiting Klein contribution
compare dissociation ("splitting") with repression

Hence I AM stage
    integration to unit
        capacity for concern
                    depressive mood   Klein
        "value of depression"

In terms of management: the teaching of
    skills—vis à vis reparation

In Social Work
    The holding technique
        feed-back to P-A

Psyche-soma—relative to intellect
    Intellect exploited
    Psycho-somatic disorder:
        a call back to the body ego from
        flight to the intellectual

    Psycho-somatic patient splits medical care

Two categories of people
        A.   Carry around "having been mad"
        B.   Not so
Mad means breakdown of ego-defences (as existed at
    the time, including mother's ego-support) with clinical
    appearance of archaic or unthinkable anxiety:

> falling forever
> de-integration   Fordham
> disorientation
> depersonalisation etc.

Panic   as a defence against unthinkable anxiety

Winnicott axiom
A. Fear of madness, madness that was
B. Drive to remember by experiencing

                         Aetiology
Surprise

Psychosis	Privation
AST	Deprivation
Psycho-neurosis	Internal strains and stresses in "not too bad" environment

Concept of good-enough mother   Hartmann

Mother's adaptation   P.M.P.
        based on identification
        not mechanical
        not primarily via contraptions   cf. in autism

Contribution to concept of sublimation   Freud
        Three areas for living
        A. Psychic personal reality (inside)
        B. Relationships to objects
                Behaviour in the actual world
        C. Cultural
                Located in potential space between
                child playing alone and "mother"
                whose presence is necessary

Implications for Ego theory
    Ego area (not conflict-free sphere)
        based on actual living experiences that may or
        may not have reality in a child's life

    Theory of actuality
    as a projection

But dependence, especially at stage of subjective object
        Example: survival of actual after aggressive out-
                        burst leads to (or reinforces) the
                        capacity for fantasy, hate instead
                        of annihilation

Add: Excitement (non-orgiastic) at the junction of
the subjective and what is objectively
perceived—between continuity and
contiguity

Additional Notes
Application of these ideas to
    Practice of midwifery
    Theory of separation
    Talking to parents and those with care of children
    Social work theory
    Psychotherapy, exploitation of first interview
    Concept of health
          richness of potential
          adulthood

                sex
        maturity

           wisdom

                                      Anna Freud
    Regression   Kris
    Adolescent doldrums
    Family functioning
    Democracy as a development of
    the functioning family

---

1. Antisocial tendency.—EDS.
2. Primary maternal preoccupation.—EDS.

I've realised more and more as time went on what a tremendous lot I've lost from not properly correlating my work with the work of others. It's not only annoying to other people but it's also rude and it has meant that what I've said has been isolated and people have to do a lot of work to get at it. It happens to be my temperament, and it's a big fault.

Let me interrupt myself for a moment, to say that I made some notes. These notes are a little bit along the lines of what I'm going to say. They're not even properly corrected, let alone having vital significance for hanging on walls; but I thought that if you had a pencil you might feel like writing down Hartmann and Hoffer, you know, in the corner at the edge. At the right-hand edge I left room for you to write all sorts of names in so that you can help me, because I'm now getting to the stage where I really would like to be more correlated.

The other side of the thing is that, with me just as with other people, the development of thought has been along the line of something that has to do with growth, and if I happen to be like somebody else, it just turns up because we're all dealing with the same material. In fact, the series of papers which have meant anything to me have been a continuation of something that happened in my long ten-year analysis with Mr Strachey in which I had a series of dreams. I don't remember any of them, but the point is that I knew that other people had written on this same subject. I also knew that these dreams were different from the others. They were not for analysis; they were consolidations of work done. And I always said that if I'd started at the beginning I'd have written down these dreams so as to collect them one day, but I never did of course. If you started doing this, you'd never dream them. So then after the end of analysis, these things take the form of papers we feel we must write and the amazing thing is that people can be found to listen. I'm really tracing a sort of compulsion; and if only I could do it well it would be a wonderful opportunity.

At the beginning I do know that—like everybody, I suppose, in this room—as soon as I found Freud and the method that he gave us for investigating and for treatment, I was in line with it. This was just like when I was at school and was reading Darwin and suddenly I knew that Darwin was my cup of tea. I felt this tremendously, and I suppose that if there's anything I do that *isn't* Freudian, this is what I want to know. I don't mind if it isn't, but I just feel that Freud gave us this method which we can use, and it doesn't matter what it leads us to. The point is, it *does* lead us to things; it's an objective way of looking at things and it's for people who can go to something without preconceived notions, which, in a sense, is science.

At the beginning there was myself learning to do analysis as a paediatrician having had a tremendous experience of listening to people talking about babies and children of all ages and having had great difficulty in seeing a baby as human at all. It was only through analysis that I became gradually able to see a baby as a human being. This was really the chief result of my first five years of analysis, so that I've been extremely sympathetic with any paediatricians or anybody who can't see babies as human, because I absolutely couldn't, however I used to try. So this thing happened and then I became very interested in it all.

When I came to try and learn what there was to be learned about psycho-analysis, I found that in those days we were being taught about everything in terms of the 2-, 3-, and 4-year-old Oedipus complex and regression from it. It was very distressing to me as someone who had been looking at babies—at mothers and babies—for a long time (already ten to fifteen years) to find that this was so, because I knew that I'd watched a lot of babies start off ill and a lot of them become ill early. For instance, I've had a lot of experience like the one I had this week of two very intelligent and normal parents who brought to me the problem of their little baby of 22 months. This baby, at the age of 16 months, had developed a very well organised obsessional neurosis. The parents said, "Well, what do we do?" and I was able to take the psycho-analytic theory and say to them, "Do this." And they did it and the child dropped the obsessional organisation and went forward. It was an absolutely direct application. It seems to me that to have said this now is just simply ordinary experience, but saying it in 1935 in this country would have met with the objection "But it can't happen." There wasn't an audience for that, because of the fact that to have an obsessional neurosis one would have had a regression from difficulties at the Oedipal stage at 3. I know that I overdo this point, but it was something that gave me a line. I thought to myself, I'm going to show that infants are ill very early, and if the theory doesn't fit it, it's just got to adjust itself. So that was that.

Now, there were people talking about these things before I came on the scene. I'm abysmally ignorant of what Miss Freud was doing until she came to this country. After then I'm able to catch up because she herself grew and I watched her growing through the experiences in the War Nurseries and she changed, I think, tremendously. She found in a practical job which people were doing and which she was supervising that things were happening which really influenced her, and it was a great pleasure to watch her. I think that she made a terrific contribution, but I didn't know at the time the work that she was doing before this. I also know that Alice Balint was interested in the things that I'm talking about. There were other people who weren't analysts who were talking about these things: there was Suttie, and Margaret Lowenfeld who had a tremendous experience of teaching from the very early twenties about mothers and babies; and Merrill Middlemore too.

Now, as regards the psycho-neuroses, I felt that Freud's theory and his developing scheme for things, as far as I could gradually come to learn them, covered the subject; and as far as I know I made no contribution at all in that area. As you know, I came very much in 1930—

1940 into the learning area of Mrs Klein, and she took the trouble to try to help me with cases and tell me about her own work. I took over from her, without always understanding the patterning, a very great deal which I think was original from her point of view. It really comes down to the localisation of fantasy by the patient or the child in the inside. Mrs Klein didn't like that way of putting it: I talked to her about it and she said that wasn't right. But from my point of view, people knew about inner psychic reality through Freud and they knew about fantasy and dream, but it was she who pointed out the importance of the localisations of all that goes on between eating and defaecation and that it had to do with the inside of the body. And I felt that she taught me all this, without which I couldn't do psychoanalysis of children at all, and I couldn't have stopped that child from becoming seriously neuroticised by telling the mother what to do.

Now where did I begin to wake up a bit? I got completely lost in the long controversy that went on during the war and ruined all our scientific meetings, when people were fighting for the rights of Mrs Klein. It had to be done, but it left me completely cold; I didn't know anything about it and I kept out of the way entirely. I find it difficult, even now, to understand. But what happened to me was that I began to be interested in the environment, and this has led to something in me. Now who else was doing this? I don't think I know at the moment. The point is that I was at that time having analysis with Mrs Riviere who was a great friend of Mrs Klein's, and I said that I was writing a paper on the classification of the environment, and she just wouldn't have it. This was a pity really because I'd got a tremendous amount from my five years with Mrs Riviere, but I had to wait a long time before I could recover from her reaction.

I'd just been through a ten-year period in which I did practically nothing but child analysis, but it was wasted really because the fact is that Miss Freud didn't want it because she said that if I gave a case, even if it was a straightforward clinical case, I would give it with a Kleinian slant; and Mrs Klein didn't want it because I wasn't a Kleinian. So I just had to drop the immediate application to teaching and for a little while do work of other kinds.

There was a war on, and there were hostels for difficult children, and working there in Oxfordshire I at last came into touch with maladjusted children whom I'd always avoided having in my clinic because they disrupt any clinic. If you've got three maladjusted children you're preparing reports for the courts, and all the interesting cases you can do something for immediately are wiped out. You're just doing this useless thing, and I'd always sent on my antisocial children to other clinics; and I'm very glad I did in all of the twenty years from 1923 onwards because I was able to have a very large number of children that I could do something for in a very short time. I said to Mrs Riviere one day, "There's only just a line like that between me and the theory of delinquency, and one day that's going to be something and then I'm going to be separate. And I feel it coming up, you know." Only I couldn't do it while I was in analysis with her because—I don't say Mrs Klein minded it, but—the psycho-analysts were the only people for about ten or fifteen years who knew there was anything *but* environment. Everybody was screaming out that everything was due to somebody's father being drunk. So the thing was, how to get back to the environment without losing all that was gained by studying the inner factors.

I think it was a very important contribution from my point of view when suddenly in a lecture I found myself saying that the antisocial act of the delinquent belongs to the moment of hope. So then I had to invent the term "antisocial tendency" to join it up with your child who steals a penny out of somebody's purse or goes and steals some buns from the larder which he has a perfect right to. I wanted to join that up with the tendencies that can lead to delinquency. In delinquency, which doesn't mean anything definite, the secondary gains have become more important than the original cause, which is lost. But my clinical material brought me to the fact that the thing behind the antisocial tendency in any family, normal or not, is deprivation; and the result of deprivation is the doldrums, or hopelessness, or depression of some kind, or any other major defence. But as hope begins to turn up then the child reaches out, trying to reach back over the deprivation area to the lost object. This is an important thing, and life was different for me after this because I now knew what to do with my friends who were bringing their children to me because they had an antisocial tendency in a perfectly good home. I found that before the secondary gains turn up this was something not difficult to treat but easy—though not in every case. I think that was a contribution. I don't know anybody who was actually doing this then, and if there was I'd like to know.

Fortunately I've always had to give lectures—like everybody here, I think—but I've found the most valuable thing has been having to lecture to people who aren't analysts. Susan Isaacs in 1936 gave me the job of giving ten lectures a year at the Institute of Education, which I did for about fifteen years, and that was very important to me. I was supposed to be lecturing on rheumatic fever at the beginning, and the early diagnosis of pain so that people didn't get heart disease; but fortunately before long rheumatic fever died out. Anyhow it was found that half the people sent as rheumatic were depressed and half the people sent as choreic weren't choreic at all—they were cases of common anxious fidgetiness; so we got down to looking at all that. But having to lecture to social workers and teachers and parents and all sorts of people is tremendously important. Somebody, perhaps a parent or a social worker, said, "Look here, I understand this about reaching back over the gap for the object, but you haven't described why another kind of antisocial tendency is destructive." And it took me three or four years to come round to the very simple thing, which is of course that there are two kinds of deprivation. One is in terms of loss of object and the other is in terms of loss of frames, loss of controls. In a sense you could say loss of mother and loss of father—the paternal father, not the standing-in-for-mother father. The thing is the frame, the strength—the deprivation in terms of that. Then a very complicated thing happens when the child becomes all right and begins to feel confidence in a man or a structure or an institution. He begins to break things up to make quite sure that the framework can hold. This showed me that the antisocial tendency has two aspects to it.

The other thing arising out of this is that when a child is deprived of an environmental control what he does is to become a controlling system identified with the parental situation or with the environment and completely loses his identity. This is the reason why when the controls begin to be re-imposed and these children begin to get confidence and to hand over the controls to someone else, and to establish themselves again, the first thing they have to do is to prove that the controls will be sufficient. When this works, the children will be very aggressive. You could say that they have maniacal attacks sometimes—but the point is that they are beginning to exist. You get an idea here of the extreme importance of the situation for seeing the difference between fact and fantasy, because these children come to know that they have destroyed the world ever so many times just like a baby does with the parents, normally, and yet the world is still there. So they begin to see that there's a fantasy of destruction which is different from reality, and this is the lesson they have got to learn because they didn't learn it when they were babies.

It's quite possible for me to have got this original idea of mine about the antisocial tendency and hope, which has been extremely important to me in my clinical practice, from somewhere. I never know what I've got out of glancing at Ferenczi, for instance, or glancing at a footnote to Freud.

Now we get to the facilitating environment and the maturational process. There's something from Greenacre here that I've culled without acknowledgement, particularly in developing the theories around the maturational processes, heredity and the tendencies that go on to make a human being; and the interaction of this with the environment. Here we have to bring in Hartmann's "conflict-free sphere" which really, I think I'm right in saying (he didn't mind when I said it to him), has to do with the inherited tendencies. Then I found I had to formulate a sort of theoretical basis of environmental provision starting at the beginning with 100 percent adaptation and quickly lessening according to the ability of the child to make use of failure of adaptation. This has been said in other terms. Mrs Riviere has stressed the mother's failures as being as important for object-relating as the successes, and there is other work in which you can trace these ideas. But I'm not sold on just taking over the concept of "symbiosis" because this word for me is too easy. It's as if, as in biology, it just happens that two things are living together. I believe it leaves out the extremely variable thing which is the ability of the mother to identify with the infant, which I think is the living thing in this which I've called "primary maternal preoccupation." Her ability varies with different children not with her temperament but with her experiences, and with the way that she is at the time, and this seems to me to be a more fruitful line of enquiry.

This brings me to dependence and adaptation theories. It's interesting to me that Mrs Klein's digging further and further back into the conflicts and processes in the individual infant I found more and more difficult. Then one evening Fairbairn came down to talk to us, and this was the sort of evening that goes right beyond my comprehension, and yet it undoubtedly had tremendous importance. The question was whether the first introjection is of a good or a bad object—the sort of thing I'm no good at. At that time I couldn't see anything in Fairbairn. I saw later that he'd got an extremely important thing to say which had to do with going beyond instinctual satisfactions and frustrations to the idea of object-seeking. He and Mrs Klein had several things in common. I couldn't see that for years and years. But I didn't get involved in Mrs Klein's theories which are based on the concept of the death instinct and of the hereditary factors that seemed to me to be stressed in her Envy paper. This didn't matter, because by that time she'd contributed such a tremendous amount. That's something that the future has to talk about, not me. But you can see how by this time I was thoroughly sunk in the word "dependence" and couldn't talk about the infant without taking into account dependence and adaptation; and without seeing that the mother's ability to de-adapt at the pace that her particular infant at the moment could make use of was an extremely subtle thing which belongs to life, and that health and ill-health have sometimes to be thought of in these terms. Therefore I could never quite get into proper communication with Melanie Klein again, but it didn't matter because she and I agreed to differ. She had a terrific brain, and she said, quite rightly, "I've always acknowledged the importance of the environment in all my writing but I'm talking about the individual." Well, that was fair enough. I was trying to say something she didn't like and I don't know yet whether she's right or not; but it had to do with the fact that at the beginning it seems impossible to talk about the individual without talking about the mother, because to my mind, the mother or the person in that place is a subjective object—in other words has not been objectively perceived—and therefore how the mother behaves is really part of the infant. And I find it's almost like trying to count the number of fairies on the end of a pin to see how far you can go back talking about what's happening in an infant leaving out the fact that the environment is, at the beginning, part of the infant. I think that the difficulty is that there's a paradox, and it's the same paradox that turns up in transitional phenomena, which I tried to work out to deal with it. The paradox is that the environment is part of the infant and at the same time it isn't. The infant has to accept this eventually in order to become a grown-up at all. It comes out in the transitional phenomena theory because if we take the simple case where there's a transitional object we know that we won't ask the baby, "Did you create that object or did you find it?" because we know that the two things are true and that he wouldn't have created it if it hadn't been there, but that he did create it; and this is an extremely difficult concept unless one just says there's a paradox and we've got to accept it. It seems to me to have quite a lot of philosophical importance, only I don't happen to be a philosopher. It has importance to the whole of object-relating where objects can be seen creatively.

Now there was one thing that I needed and I couldn't get at myself, which was the full use of the delusional transference concept. This is one of the most difficult things we have to deal with in analysis, and from my point of view I really took this bit from someone. If Margaret Little hadn't been able to make this clear, I was hung up in a way I think a lot of analysts are hung up. I think you can still hear people unable to take a delusional transference, which is one of the most difficult things we have to do. So that's one little bit of my life where I really did get something from somebody else, almost as if I stole it out of my mother's handbag.

Then an important thing that happened to me was recognising that early is not deep, and this helped me a lot in my attempt to make full use of Klein without getting bogged down. I suddenly realised—in Paris or somewhere—that early isn't deep: that it takes an infant time and development before depth comes in, so that when you're going back to the deepest things you won't get to the beginning. You get to something like 3 or 2 or 1½, and this was very important for me because some mechanisms that have to do with the schizoid groupings seem to belong to early and not to deep, and depression belongs to deep and not to early. And I think this has an effect on our theory of the origin of aggression, because I really believe there's something to be said for talking about aggression (in terms of development in the infant) as being the child's *movement*—that is, muscle erotism—and something happens to be in the way. It seems to me that this is the beginning of aggression. If you're going to talk about hate, that's a long way further on, and a maniacal episode is also a long way from somebody just happening to kick something because it was in the way when he liked kicking. So I got a glimpse of how I might understand a bit better about the origins of aggression, looking at these two different ways of getting at the beginning of it in the individual.

You can see that there is, incidentally, a corollary to this. I was getting away from the necessity of a verbal interpretation in its fullest form. I've been through the long process of interpreting everything I could possibly see that could be interpreted, you know, feeling awful if I couldn't find anything, and pouncing on something because I found I could put it into words. I've been through all that and realised that in certain cases it was no good at all, along with other people who I know had done the same things. Balint had written on this and others have written since, and many things have been said in the last forty years on the subject of silent hours and of long periods of dependence. Since realising this I've had to deal with a lot of silent phases in analysis that lasted a long time, and it's very difficult to know when it's wasted time and when it's extremely productive, but nevertheless all this is now something I love to study. Today, this afternoon, a patient brought me a dream—a patient who's getting near the end of analysis—and suddenly I saw ahead to a solution of where he was getting to, so I let him have my idea of where he was, and he was so dissatisfied that the dream he'd brought with his own meanings to it had been treated in this way. He was absolutely angry with me and absolutely hopeless and he said, "When will you ever learn?" If I was right, I'd taken away his opportunity to be creative, to bring it next time and the time after; and if I was wrong I'd interrupted his reaching an important bit of understanding through this dream. It was as much as he could take at the time. We got through it in the end because I've done it before. He said, "As a matter of fact I've had a very satisfactory day today, but there's only one thing marring it. This evening I shall be worrying about you because you'll be thinking what a rotten analyst you were." At any rate, there's so much that goes on in analysis if it isn't just a straightforward psycho-neurotic case.

I now became aware that Fairbairn had made a tremendous contribution, even if we only take two things. One is object-seeking, which comes into the area of transitional phenomena and so on, and the other is this thing of feeling real instead of feeling unreal. Our patients, more and more, turn out to be needing to feel real, and if they don't then understanding is of extremely secondary importance. The awkward thing is if they're going to be analysts: they want a bit of understanding then. But the vast majority of my patients haven't been analysts, and I've had to be contented if they went away feeling more real than they came. No doubt a lot of people have been on to this— Erikson, and I expect many more.

I can't cover all that I want to. I will just say that I don't know whether you'd like to discuss any of this or would like to help me in a letter to try and make amends and join up with the various people all over the world who are doing work which either I've stolen or else I'm just ignoring. I don't promise to follow it all up because I know I'm just going to go on having an idea which belongs to where I am at the moment, and I can't help it.

Acknowledgments

For permission to reproduce material already in print, we acknowledge with thanks the following:

For articles from journals: *British Journal of Medical Psychology; British Journal of Psychology; British Medical Journal; British Medical Students' Journal; Child Care News; International Journal of Child Psychotherapy; International Journal of Psycho-Analysis; The Lancet; Nature; New Society.*

For articles from books: Basic Books, Churchill-Livingstone; Free Association Books; The Hogarth Press; Methuen and Co.; The Pergamon Press; Tavistock Publications.

Special thanks are due to the Squiggle Foundation for help with the transcription of old tapes. We also wish to thank Mr. B. E. Eaden of the Cambridge University Library for his unstinting assistance and courtesy.

EDITORS

Index

abandonment: by analyst, 33; by mother, 47

Abraham, K., 396, 413, 416

absence: of mother, 58, 357ff

abstract painting, drawing, 143–144, 167, 274, 343

acting out: and analyst's mistakes, 99; of GP's patients, 442; of masturbation fantasy, 62; of memory of being put down, 33

actress, 49

adaptation: de-adaptation and, 146, 445, 565, 580; diminishing, 101; and externalisation of object, 254; of analyst to patient, 99, 132, 163, 209, 448; of mother to infant, 44, 97, 101, 145–146, 156, 179, 254, 434, 445, 448, 570, 572, 580; of patient to analyst, 209

adolescence, 61–63, 71–72, 325–326, 330–332, 435–436; acne in, 282–283; destructiveness in, 239; doldrums in, 573; homosexual identifications in, 62, 369–372; masturbation in, 37, 61–62; organisation of defences in, 120; phase of indeterminate sex in, 62, 371; re-enactment in, 285; reactive pacifism of, 233; sexual activity in, 332, 333, 337

adolescent: relationship to mother, 334–340

adoption, 280–281, 424

affection, 55, 149, 150, 203

aggression, 30, 60, 226, 287, 570, 578; fusion of, with erotic components, 101, 239, 453–454; inherited, 447, 451; lack of, 235–237; object-relating and, 101; and primitive love impulse, 315–316; psycho-analytic study of, 458–459; repression of, 31; roots of, 225–226, 245–246; theory of, 581

alcohol, use of: to control disintegrative anxieties, 187–188; to release spontaneity, 466

aliveness: destructiveness and, 239

alone in the presence of, 571

ambivalence: achievement of, 61, 134, 145, 147; in mother, 146, 250; neurotic, 535; psycho-neurosis and, 69–70; splitting and, in Fairbairn, 418–419

American Psychoanalytic Society, 396

anal level, 46–47

analysis, 29, 91–92, 96–99; collusion in, 91–92, 97, 106, 220; deep regression in, 46; dependence in, 452; destruction and constructive activity in, 249; environmental failure in, 32; environmental influence as traumatic idea in, 175; failure of, 220; first interview in, 319–320; frustration in, 50; futility in, 91–92, 170; holding environment and, 32; interminability in, 170, 172, 220, 227, 450–452; lack of sense of achievement in, 249; mistaken treatment of split-off part in, 174; mistakes in, 81–83; need for theoretical knowledge in, 169; non-use in, 234; of child with depressed mother, 248; of dreams, 202; of psychotic patients, and body fantasy, 533; of superego compared with paranoid anxieties, 470; physical contact in, 32, 257–258; play in, 28–29, 159; re-experiencing of intolerable anxiety in, 74–75, 125–126, 128; reassurance in, 320; silence in, 81–86, 210, 581–582; slowness of, 169; use of toys and pencil and paper in, 28–29; vs. self-analysis, 219, 224; withdrawal and regression in, 149–150. *See also* analyst; psychoanalysis; psychotherapy; therapist

analyst: abandonment by, 33; acceptance of presents by, 150–151; adaptation of, 132, 163, 209, 448; as qualitative factor in environment, 464; attitudes of, 208; avoidance of borderline cases and, 129; capacity for cathexis in, 100; confidence in, 32; cough of, and patient's irritation, 49; delusional transference and, 83, 133,